Ontology Learning and Knowledge Discovery Using the Web:

Challenges and Recent Advances

Wilson Wong
The University of Western Australia, Australia

Wei Liu
The University of Western Australia, Australia

Mohammed Bennamoun
The University of Western Australia, Australia

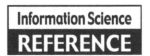

Senior Editorial Director:	Kristin Klinger
Director of Book Publications:	Julia Mosemann
Editorial Director:	Lindsay Johnston
Acquisitions Editor:	Erika Carter
Development Editor:	Joel Gamon
Production Editor:	Sean Woznicki
Typesetters:	Jennifer Romanchak and Mike Brehm
Print Coordinator:	Jamie Snavely
Cover Design:	Nick Newcomer

Published in the United States of America by
Information Science Reference (an imprint of IGI Global)
701 E. Chocolate Avenue
Hershey PA 17033
Tel: 717-533-8845
Fax: 717-533-8661
E-mail: cust@igi-global.com
Web site: http://www.igi-global.com/reference

Library of Congress Cataloging-in-Publication Data

Ontology learning and knowledge discovery using the Web: challenges and recent advances / Wilson Wong, Wei Liu and Mohammed Bennamoun, editors.
    p. cm.
  Includes bibliographical references and index.
  ISBN 978-1-60960-625-1 (hardcover) -- ISBN 978-1-60960-626-8 (ebook) 1. Ontologies (Information retrieval) 2. Data mining. I. Wong, Wilson, 1981- II. Liu, Wei, 1972 July 14- III. Bennamoun, M. (Mohammed)
  TK5105.88815.O587 2011
  006.3'12--dc22
                    2010043008

British Cataloguing in Publication Data
A Cataloguing in Publication record for this book is available from the British Library.

All work contributed to this book is new, previously-unpublished material. The views expressed in this book are those of the authors, but not necessarily of the publisher.

Editorial Advisory Board

Table of Contents

Section 1
Techniques for Ontology Learning and Knowledge Discovery

Section 2
Applications of Ontologies and Knowledge Bases

Section 3
Emerging Trends in Ontology Learning and Knowledge Discovery

Detailed Table of Contents

Section 1
Techniques for Ontology Learning and Knowledge Discovery

Section 1 starts off with Chapter 1 presenting a condensed view of the current work in ontology learning, with a particular focus on a variety of emerging knowledge sources, most of which are Web-based, for discovering domain concepts and labelling the relations between them. As a proof of concept, the authors put forward a generic framework for learning lightweight ontologies using unstructured data sources on the Web such as FreeBase, Flickr, Twitter, and Technorati. Three use cases in tourism, waste management, and climate change, respectively, are presented to demonstrate the applicability of the presented framework to real-world problems as well as for discussing possible pitfalls in ontology learning.

This chapter complements the review in Chapter 1 by focusing on natural language processing techniques for ontology learning, with a particular emphasis on deep semantic analysis methods. The authors discuss both shallow as well as deep techniques for natural language processing, and describe their applicability to each step of learning ontologies from text documents, especially those from the

Web. In particular, the authors discuss the use of lexico-syntactic patterns based on dependency grammars coupled with Web resources for learning ontologies, and explain why this move can be considered as a step towards deeper semantic analysis in ontology learning.

Marian-Andrei Rizoiu, University Lumière Lyon 2, France
Julien Velcin, University Lumière Lyon 2, France

This chapter initiates the transition from the lexical layer in Chapter 2 to the concept layer of ontologies by looking at the application of topic extraction techniques for ontology learning. The authors provide a thorough review of clustering and term extraction techniques, and describe how these techniques are assembled together into an unsupervised learning system for extracting meaningful topics. The chapter also includes some results from an initial experiment with system using the Reuters-21578 corpus. While the extracted topics are not full concepts as yet, they nevertheless provide an excellent starting point for constructing concepts in ontology learning.

Louis Massey, Royal Military College of Canada, Canada
Wilson Wong, The University of Western Australia, Australia

This chapter presents a revolutionary approach for identifying topics from text that is fundamentally different from the existing techniques reviewed in Chapter 3. The authors discuss how the approach, which is inspired by human cognition, allows 'meaning' to emerge naturally from the activation and decay of unstructured text information retrieved from the Web. Using the unstructured texts in Web pages as a source of knowledge alleviates the laborious handcrafting of formal knowledge bases and ontologies which are required by many existing techniques. The authors discuss the results from some initial experiments comparing the use of WordNet versus Web pages from Yahoo! search on the Reuters-21578 corpus to illustrate the power of this new approach.

Ziqi Zhang, University of Sheffield, UK
Fabio Ciravegna, University of Sheffield, UK

This chapter offers an alternative, classification-based view of concept discovery using named-entity recognition techniques as opposed to the notion of topics in Chapter 3 and 4. The authors provide a thorough review of named-entity recognition techniques with an emphasis on those using the Web for background knowledge. The authors then propose a novel method that automatically creates domain-specific background knowledge by exploring Wikipedia for classifying terms into predefined ontological classes. The authors also demonstrate the potential use of this method for ontology population.

This chapter extends the discussion on discovering concepts from the perspective of topics and named entities in Chapter 3, 4, and 5 to ascertaining the taxonomic, also known as hierarchical, relations between concepts. The authors describe several approaches for placing new concepts in existing hierarchies, creating new hierarchies by means of crowdsourcing, and visualising hierarchies, all of which are essential to the semi-automatic creation and maintenance of concept hierarchies. The authors also discuss how unstructured text provided by Web search engines, existing structured resources such as Medical Subject Headings (MeSH) and WordNet, and collaborative editing come together as important resources for the above three tasks.

Chapter 7

This chapter extends the discussion in Chapter 6 on taxonomic relations to include relations of type "related" between concepts. The authors present a novel approach based on probabilistic topic models using Latent Dirichlet Allocation to automatically learn both the "broader" as well as the "related" type of relations from unstructured text corpus. The authors generated around 7,000 ontological statements expressed in terms of the two types of relations from abstracts of publications in the Semantic Web research area.

Section 2
Applications of Ontologies and Knowledge Bases

This chapter begins Section 2 by looking at a popular application of ontologies since the post-genomic era, which is the assignment of functions to uncharacterized proteins. Since proteins mostly interact with other bio-molecular units to execute their functions, the functions of unknown proteins may be discovered by studying their associations with proteins having known functions. This chapter compares neighbourhood-based and global techniques for the automated prediction of protein functions based on the analysis of the patterns of functional associations in interaction networks such as the Gene Ontology (GO). The authors briefly discuss how the taxonomic structure in GO, or in other words, the interrelations between function terms, is used to compute semantic similarity to enhance predictions using these techniques.

Chapter 9

Marco A. Alvarez, Utah State University, USA
Xiaojun Qi, Utah State University, USA
Changhui Yan, North Dakota State University, USA

This chapter proceeds with the discussion raised in Chapter 8 on the use of the Gene Ontology (GO) to compute semantic similarity. The authors first provide a brief review of the current advances and challenges in the development of techniques for calculating semantic similarity between GO terms. The authors then introduce a new technique that exploits the different properties of GO to calculate semantic similarities between pairs of GO terms. In this chapter, the authors combine information about the shortest path between terms, the nearest common ancestor for a pair of terms, and the extent of overlap in the definitions of terms for computing similarity.

Chapter 10

Toby Burrows, The University of Western Australia, Australia

This chapter shifts the discussion from the biomedical domain in Chapter 8 and 9 to the use of ontologies in projects and services for the humanities. The author reviews several examples including the EU VICODI project which uses ontologies to aid the searching a European history portal, the CIDOC conceptual model that can be found in a range of museum documentation projects such as CLAROS, which combines large database records for Greek and Roman art objects, and other smaller scale applications of more specific ontologies. The author explains that the slow progress in applying ontology learning techniques in the humanities can be attributed to the complexity of the linguistic and conceptual environment of the domain. The author discusses four recent projects on the learning of ontologies from major collections of classical literature, 18th-century French writings, 13th-century Latin documents and 18th-century accounts of trials.

Chapter 11

Aba-Sah Dadzie, University of Sheffield, UK
Victoria Uren, University of Sheffield, UK
Fabio Ciravegna, University of Sheffield, UK

This chapter concludes Section 2 by focusing on the application of ontologies to improve knowledge management in organisations. The authors present a knowledge framework that integrates a number of tools to provide alternative perspectives on data to suit different users and tasks across multiple communities of practice. This framework uses domain ontologies to guide users in data exploration and analysis and support the contextualisation and codifying of information into knowledge. The authors evaluate the framework with end users in the aerospace engineering domain, using a simulation of an information retrieval case. The participants found that the ontology-guided hypothesis exploration and investigation aided the contextualisation of information, leading to an increase in the confidence with which they came to conclusions about the simulated issues.

Section 3
Emerging Trends in Ontology Learning and Knowledge Discovery

Chapter 12

Konstantinos Kotis, University of the Aegean, Greece
Andreas Papasalouros, University of the Aegean, Greece

Section 3 starts off with Chapter 12 that focuses on an emerging data source for learning ontologies. This chapter begins with a discussion on the requirements for the automated learning of ontologies from social data on the Web such as blogs, wikis, and folksonomies. The authors then present two techniques for automatically learning ontologies of social concepts and relations from query logs, and Web 2.0 question/answer applications such as Yahoo! Answer. The authors evaluate the ontology learning technique from query logs using Yahoo! and Google query datasets. The authors also discuss the importance of modelling trust for specifying the degree of confidence that agents, both software and human, may have on the conceptualisations derived from social content.

Chapter 13

Bin Lu, City University of Hong Kong, Hong Kong
Benjamin K. Tsou, City University of Hong Kong & Hong Kong Institute of Education, Hong Kong
Tao Jiang, ChiLin Star Corporation, China
Jingbo Zhu, Northeastern University, China
Oi Yee Kwong, City University of Hong Kong, Hong Kong

This chapter turns the focus from social data in Chapter 12 to another emerging type of data for ontology learning and knowledge discovery. This chapter discusses the potentials and challenges of using linguistically diverse Web data to address the problem of mining the same knowledge across different languages. The authors focus on the mining of parallel sentences and parallel technical terms from comparable Chinese-English patent texts which contain both equivalent sentences as well as much noise. The authors touch on the potential use of the extracted parallel sentences and technical terms for further acquisition of terms and relations, translation of monolingual ontologies, as well as other cross-lingual information access applications.

Chapter 14

Hans Hjelm, alaTest.com, Sweden
Martin Volk, University of Zurich, Switzerland

This chapter generalises the discussion in Chapter 13, and brings the book to an end by reflecting on the fact that a formal ontology does not contain lexical knowledge and hence, by nature is language independent. This chapter focuses on ways to automatically build ontologies by exploiting cross-language information from parallel corpora. In particular, the authors present a framework that provides a setting in which cross-language data can be integrated and quantified for cross-language ontology learning. The authors employ resources such as the JRC-ACQUIS Multilingual Parallel Corpus and the Eurovoc multilingual thesaurus for their experiments. The authors conclude that the combining of information from different languages can indeed improve the results of ontology learning.

Foreword

"To live effectively is to live with adequate information." Norbert Weiner, *The Human Use of Human Beings (1954).*

In half a generation, we have moved from a world in which it was hard to discover information about any given subject into one where we feel surrounded, almost imprisoned, by more than we could possibly hope to digest. But, paradoxically, it is harder than ever to keep ourselves informed. How can anyone read and process the Web, which is updated and augmented every second?

Herein lies the key: whereas in the old world virtually all information was recorded on paper, now everything is electronic. Recent decades have seen computational linguists join forces with information professionals and computer scientists to develop productive ways of digesting vast quantities of electronic text, whether automatically or under human oversight. New paradigms of language processing have sprung from the ready availability of corpora whose size was unimaginable 20 years ago, giving birth to fields such as text mining and information extraction.

The information is readily available, and we have ways of analyzing it linguistically. But to find out what it means we need *knowledge*. Today's bottleneck is in handcrafting structured knowledge sources—dictionaries, taxonomies, knowledge bases, and annotated corpora. Tomorrow's machines will unravel knowledge from information automatically. And to do so, they will employ one of philosophy's most fundamental concepts: *ontology*.

Ontology is the study of the nature of being. It concerns what entities exist and how they can be referred to, grouped together, and categorized according to their similarities and differences. The ontologies used in information science are formal representations of concepts and their relationships with one another. An ontology provides a shared vocabulary that can be used to model a domain and talk about it. The need to relate different pieces of information boils down, in essence, to the deep problem of learning and relating different ontologies. Ontologies have moved from an obscure corner of metaphysics to occupy center stage in the world of information processing.

The time is ripe for this book. Techniques of ontology learning and knowledge discovery are beginning to converge. Prototypes are becoming stronger. Industry practitioners are beginning to realize the need for ontology learning. Wilson, Wei, and Mohammed bring together recent work in the construction and application of ontologies and knowledge bases. They introduce a wide range of techniques that utilize unstructured and semi-structured Web data for learning and discovery.

Section I covers existing and emerging techniques for extracting terms, concepts, and relations to construct ontologies and knowledge bases. It provides a background in natural language processing that moves up from the lexical to the concept layer. Knowledge sources include the Web, Wikipedia, and crowd-sourced repositories. One chapter introduces a new topic extraction technique for concept discovery; another promotes the use of existing deep semantic analysis methods in ontology learning. Section II examines how ontologies and knowledge bases are being applied across different domains: biomedicine, genetics, enterprise knowledge management, and the humanities. Section III focuses on emerging trends: learning ontologies from social network data and improving knowledge discovery using linguistically diverse Web data.

The interdisciplinary nature of ontology learning and knowledge discovery is reflected in this book. It will appeal to advanced undergraduates, postgraduate students, academic researchers and practitioners. I hope that it will lead to a world in which we can all live more effectively, a world in which the ready availability of information is balanced by our enhanced ability to process it.

Ian H. Witten
September 2010

Ian Witten *is Professor of Computer Science at the University of Waikato in New Zealand where he directs the New Zealand Digital Library research project. His research interests include language learning, information retrieval, and machine learning. He has published widely, including several books, such as Managing Gigabytes (1999), Data Mining (2005), Web Dragons (2007), and How to Build a Digital Library (2003). He is a Fellow of the ACM and of the Royal Society of New Zealand. He received the 2004 IFIP Namur Award, a biennial honour accorded for "outstanding contribution with international impact to the awareness of social implications of information and communication technology" and (with the rest of the Weka team) the 2005 SIGKDD Service Award for "an outstanding contribution to the data mining field." In 2006, he received the Royal Society of New Zealand Hector Medal for "an outstanding contribution to the advancement of the mathematical and information sciences," and in 2010, was officially inaugurated as a "World Class New Zealander" in Research, Science, and Technology.*

Preface

It has become sort of a cliché nowadays to mention how rapidly textual information is growing and how the World Wide Web has assisted in this growth. This, however, does not shadow the fact that such explosive growth will only intensify for years to come, and more new challenges and opportunities will arise. Advances in fundamental areas such as information retrieval, machine learning, data mining, natural language processing, and knowledge representation and reasoning have provided us with some relief by uncovering and representing facts and patterns in text to ease the management, retrieval, and interpretation process. *Information retrieval*, for instance, provides various algorithms to analyse associations between components of a text using vectors, matrices, and probabilistic theorems. *Machine learning* and *data mining*, on the other hand, offer the ability to learn rules and patterns out of massive datasets in a supervised or unsupervised manner based on extensive statistical analysis. *Natural language processing* provides the tools for analysing natural language text on various language levels (e.g. morphology, syntax, semantics) to uncover manifestations of concepts and relations through linguistic cues. *Knowledge representation and reasoning* enable the extracted knowledge to be formally specified and represented such that new knowledge can be deduced.

The realization that a more systematic way of consolidating the discovered facts and patterns into an organised, higher level construct to enhance everyday applications (e.g. Web search) and enable intelligent systems (e.g. Semantic Web) eventually gave rise to ontology learning and knowledge discovery. *Ontologies* are effectively formal and explicit specifications, in the form of concepts and relations, of shared conceptualisations, while *knowledge bases* can be obtained by populating the ontologies with instances. Occasionally, ontologies contain axioms for validation and constraint definition. As an analogy, consider an ontology as a cupcake mould and knowledge bases as the actual cupcakes of assorted colours, tastes, and so on. *Ontology learning* from text is then essentially the process of deriving the high-level concepts and relations from textual information. Considering this perspective, *knowledge discovery* can refer to two things, the first denotation being the uncovering of relevant instances from data to populate the ontologies (also known as *ontology population*), and the second, more general sense being the searching of data for useful patterns. In this book, knowledge discovery can mean either one of the two.

Being a young and exciting field, ontology learning has witnessed a relatively fast progress due to its adoption of established techniques from the related areas discussed above. Aside from the inherent challenges of processing natural language, one of the remaining obstacles preventing the large-scale deployment of ontology learning systems is the bottleneck in handcrafting structured knowledge sources (e.g. dictionaries, taxonomies, knowledge bases) and training data (e.g. annotated text corpora). It is gradually becoming apparent that in order to minimize human efforts in the learning process, and to improve the scalability and robustness of the system, static and expert crafted resources may no longer be adequate. An increasing amount of research effort is being directed towards harnessing *collective intelligence on the Web* as an attempt to address this major bottleneck. At the same time, as with many fields before ontology learning, the process of maturing has triggered an increased awareness of the difficulties in automatically discovering all components of an ontology, i.e. terms, concepts, relations, and especially axioms. This gives rise to the question of whether the ultimate goal of achieving *full-fledged formal ontologies* automatically can be achieved. While some individuals dwell on the question, many others have moved on with a more pragmatic goal, which is to focus on learning *lightweight ontologies* first, and extend them later if possible. With high hopes and achievable aims, we are now witnessing a growing interest in ontologies across different domains that require interoperability of semantics and a touch of intelligence in their applications.

This book brings together some of the latest work on three popular research directions in ontology learning and knowledge discovery today, namely, (1) the use of Web data to address the knowledge and training data preparation bottleneck, (2) the focus on lightweight ontologies, and (3) the application of ontologies in different domains and across different languages. Section I of the book contains chapters covering the use of a wide range of existing, adapted and emerging techniques for extracting terms, concepts and relations to construct ontologies and knowledge bases. For instance, in addition to traditional clustering techniques reported in Chapter III, a new topic extraction technique is being devised as in Chapter IV to offer alternative ways for discovering concepts. Chapter II, on the other hand, promotes the new application of existing deep semantic analysis methods for ontology learning in general. The use of semi-structured Web data such as Wikipedia for named entity recognition, and the question of how can this be applicable to ontology learning are also investigated in Chapter V. The focus of Chapter I is on the construction of practical, lightweight ontologies for three domains. As for Chapter VI and VII, the authors mainly investigate the use of a combination of data sources, both local and from the Web, to discover hierarchical and non-taxonomic relations. In Section II, the authors look at how ontologies and knowledge bases are currently being applied across different domains. Some of the domains covered by the chapters in this section include biomedical (Chapter VIII and IX), humanities (Chapter X) and enterprise knowledge management (Chapter XI). This book ends with Section III that covers chapters on the use of social data (Chapter XII) and parallel texts (Chapter XIII and XIV), which may or may not be from the Web for learning social ontologies, incorporating trust into ontologies, and improving the process learning ontologies.

This volume is both a valuable standalone as well as a great complement to the existing books on ontology learning that have been published since the turn of the millennium. Some of the previous books focus mainly on techniques and evaluations, while others look at more abstract concerns such as ontology languages, standards, and engineering environments. While the background discussions on the techniques and evaluations are indispensable, the focal point of this book remains on emerging research directions involving the use of Web data for ontology learning, the learning of lightweight as well as cross-language ontologies, and the involvement of ontologies in real-world applications. We are certain that the content of this book will be of interest to a wide ranging audience. From a teaching viewpoint, the book is intended for undergraduate students at the final year level, or postgraduate students who wish to learn about the basic techniques for ontology learning. From a researcher's and practitioner's point of view, this volume will be an excellent addition outlining the most recent progress to complement basic references in ontology learning. A basic familiarity with natural language processing, probability and statistics, and some fundamental Web technologies such as wikis and search engines is beneficial to the understanding of this text.

Wilson Wong
The University of Western Australia, Australia

Wei Liu
The University of Western Australia, Australia

Mohammed Bennamoun
The University of Western Australia, Australia

Acknowledgment

This book would not have been possible without the efforts put in by the Editorial Advisory Board members and all contributing authors. In particular, a special thank you goes to the following individuals for their help in reviewing the submissions received for this book.

Christian Andrich, *Graz University of Technology, Austria*

Gabor Melli, *PredictionWorks Inc, USA*

Hongbo Deng, *University of Illinois at Urbana-Champaign, USA*

Johann Mitloehner, *Vienna University of Economics and Business, Austria*

Josef Moser, *Graz University of Technology, Austria*

Karin Verspoor, *University of Colorado Denver, USA*

Lipika Dey, *Tata Consultancy Services, India*

Martijn Schuemie, *University Medical Center Rotterdam, the Netherlands*

Sunam Kim, *University of Melbourne, Australia*

Yves Lussier, *University of Chicago, USA*

Jianbin Huang, *Xidian University, China*

The editors would also like to thank Mr. Joel Gamon, the Development Editor at IGI Global for his continuous support and advice.

Wilson Wong
The University of Western Australia, Australia

Wei Liu
The University of Western Australia, Australia

Mohammed Bennamoun
The University of Western Australia, Australia

Section 1
Techniques for Ontology Learning and Knowledge Discovery

Chapter 1
Evidence Sources, Methods and Use Cases for Learning Lightweight Domain Ontologies

Albert Weichselbraun
Vienna University of Economics and Business, Austria

Gerhard Wohlgenannt
Vienna University of Economics and Business, Austria

Arno Scharl
MODUL University Vienna, Austria

ABSTRACT

By providing interoperability and shared meaning across actors and domains, lightweight domain ontologies are a cornerstone technology of the Semantic Web. This chapter investigates evidence sources for ontology learning and describes a generic and extensible approach to ontology learning that combines such evidence sources to extract domain concepts, identify relations between the ontology's concepts, and detect relation labels automatically. An implementation illustrates the presented ontology learning and relation labeling framework and serves as the basis for discussing possible pitfalls in ontology learning. Afterwards, three use cases demonstrate the usefulness of the presented framework and its application to real-world problems.

1 INTRODUCTION

Ontologies, which are commonly defined as explicit specifications of shared conceptualizations (Gruber, 1995), provide a reusable domain model which allows for many applications in the areas of knowledge engineering, natural language process-

DOI: 10.4018/978-1-60960-625-1.ch001

ing, e-commerce, intelligent information integration, bio-informatics etc. Not all ontologies share the same amount of formal explicitness (Corcho, 2006), nor do they include all the components that can be expressed in a formal language, such as concept taxonomies and various types of formal axioms. Ontology research therefore distinguishes between lightweight and heavyweight ontologies (Studer et al., 1998). The manual creation of such conceptualizations for non-trivial domains is an expensive and cumbersome task which requires highly specialized human effort (Cimiano, 2006). Furthermore the evolution of domains results in a constant need for refinement of domain ontologies to ensure their usefulness.

Automated approaches to learning ontologies from existing data are intended to improve the productivity of ontology engineers. Buitelaar et al. (2005) organize the tasks in ontology learning into a set of layers. Ontology learning from text requires lexical entries L^C to link single words or phrases to concepts C. Synonym extraction helps to connect similar terms to a concept. Taxonomies H^C provide the ontology's backbone while non-taxonomic relations R supply arbitrary links between the concepts. Finally, axioms are defined or acquired to derive additional facts.

Data sources for ontology learning typically include unstructured, semi-structured and structured data (Cimiano, 2006). Ontology learning from structured data consumes information sources such as database schemas or existing ontologies. This process is also called *lifting* as it lifts or maps parts of existing schemas to new logical definitions. Since most of the available data out there appear in unstructured and semi-structured forms, a major research focus over the last two decades has been the extraction of domain models from natural language text using a variety of methods. Cimiano (2006) presented an extensive overview of ontology learning methods from unstructured data. Many of the methods involve corpus statistics such as association rules mining (Maedche et al., 2002), co-occurrence analysis for term clustering (Wong et al., 2007), latent semantic analysis for detecting synonyms and concepts (Landauer & Dumais, 1997), and kernel methods for classifying semantic relations (Giuliano et al., 2007). Many corpus-based approaches are based on Harris' distributional hypothesis (Harris, 1968), which states that terms or words are similar to the extent that they occur in syntactically similar contexts. Besides corpus statistics, researchers also apply linguistic parsing and linguistic patterns in ontology learning, building on the seminal work of Hearst (Hearst, 1992), patterns support taxonomy extraction (Liu et al., 2005), detection of concepts and labeled relations in combination with the application of Web statistics (Sánchez-Alonso & García, 2006), or Web-scale extraction of unnamed relations (Etzioni et al., 2008).

The integration of Semantic Web resources has become quite popular in ontology learning in the recent years. In the presented modular and extensible framework, we use structured information to apply semantic constraints on learned ontological elements, for example in the task of detecting non-taxonomic relations where the system penalizes suggested relation label candidates conflicting with the constraints defined. Gracia et al. (2006) describe an unsupervised approach that dynamically uses online ontologies for word-sense disambiguation. d'Aquin, Motta, et al. (2008) provide the Scarlet service for discovering relations between two concepts by harvesting the Semantic Web. Similarly, Aleksovski et al. (2006) extract relations between terms in background knowledge. Alani (2006) proposes a method for ontology construction by cutting and pasting ontology modules from online ontologies. Domain text often misses some of the terms important to a particular domain, since those terms and associated concepts are assumed to be common ground shared by the authors and readers of documents. Additional resources, such as collective intelligence in the form of folksonomies (Specia & Motta, 2007), social networking or micro blogging systems, as well as online ontologies are rich sources to augment knowledge expressed in textual resources. Some authors (Mika, 2007; Heymann & Garcia-Molina, 2006; Tang et al., 2009; Schmitz, 2006) build ontologies solely based on information gathered from social sources.

The presented architecture uses data from social sources together with other evidence with the intention to capture the latest terminology of evolving domains (Angeletou et al., 2007) and to integrate background knowledge about the domain from external data sources. The remainder of this chapter is structured as follows. Section 2 introduces the three evidence sources utilized in the presented ontology learning framework. Section 3 presents the major steps and methods applied in the ontology building process for (i) extracting terms, relations and relation labels as well as (ii) applying ontological constraints. Section 4 demonstrates the potential of the ontology learning architecture by means of real-world use cases in three different domains (tourism, waste management, climate change). The chapter closes with an outlook to future work in Section 5.

2 DATA SOURCES

Methods for ontology construction rely on evidences gathered from relevant data sources such as domain documents, online communities and ontology repositories. Generally speaking, one can distinguish between (i) in-corpus evidence sources which mostly rely on unstructured data such as domain relevant text and Web documents (Section 2.1) and (ii) external sources which provide an outside view of the domain by including social (Section 2.2) and structured (Section 2.3) data in the ontology learning process.

2.1 Unstructured Evidence Sources

From unstructured evidence sources (e.g. relevant Web documents), automated ontology learning systems can extract candidate terms by means of information extraction and text mining techniques - e.g., significant phrase detection, *co-occurrence analysis* and *trigger phrases. Significant phrase detection* determines bi- and tri-gram terms in the domain corpus by comparing the number of a term's observed occurrences to the number of expected occurrences under the hypothesis of independent terms using the log likelihood ratio

(Hubmann-Haidvogel et al., 2009). Co-occurrence analysis locates these terms and unigrams in the domain corpus and compares their frequency in sentences and documents containing seed ontology concepts with their general distribution in the corpus. A chi-square test with Yates' correction for continuity (Yates, 1934) suggests a ranked list of terms, which occur significantly more often with seed ontology concepts, for inclusion into the domain ontology. Trigger Phrases (Grefenstette & Hearst, 1992; Joho et al., 2004) yield concept candidates and relations by matching text fragments that indicate a particular relationship (e.g. hyponym, hypernym and synonym) between terms in the domain corpus.

2.2 Social Evidence Sources

Social evidence sources query Web 2.0 applications such as tagging systems, social networking and micro-blogging services to retrieve candidate concepts for the extended ontology based on a set of given seed ontology terms. Delicious[1] and Flickr[2], for example, provide an API to retrieve the number of entities which have been labeled with a specific tag (= tag popularity) and to determine related tags. Technorati[3] does not offer such an API. Therefore, we had to implement a method to compute related tags based on the tags in the top 100 blogs returned for a target tag. The same strategy has been applied to Twitter[4]. Comparing tag popularities by applying similarity measures such as the dice coefficient or pointwise mutual information yields suggestions for relations between tags.

2.3 Structured Evidence Sources

Structured evidence sources include repositories such as DBpedia (Bizer et al., 2009), Freebase[5] and OpenCyc[6], which provide ontological data including concepts, relations and instance data; their integration is the goal of the Linking Open Data[7] initiative. Several search engines such as

Figure 1. A generic ontology learning process

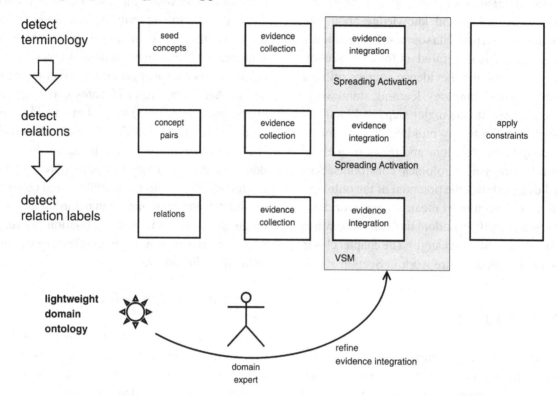

Swoogle[8] specialize in sharing ontologies via standardized formats, others like Sindice[9] concentrate on providing triple-based instance data from RDF and microformats. Many engines offer both conceptual data as well as instances; e.g., Watson (d'Aquin, Sabou, et al., 2008), Falcons[10], and SWSE[11].

3 METHOD

Figure 1 outlines the process of constructing lightweight ontologies. In the initial step, domain experts identify seed terms or a seed ontology. The system then detects relations between these terms, and identifies labels for these relations. These steps are independent of each other and can be performed using different extension frameworks that use the process outlined in Figure 1 to learn concepts, relations and relation labels.

Evidences from unstructured, structured and social sources help identify possible candidates for integration in the domain ontology. Methods such as spreading activation (Crestani, 1997) or the vector space model (Salton et al., 1975) integrate these evidences and provide a ranked list of candidates. Applying domain constraints on the collected data penalizes entries that violate ontological constraints. Domain experts help to refine and optimize the ontology learning process by providing feedback on the suggested concepts, relations, and relation labels (Figure 1). The following section will outline each step of the learning process in more detail and describe our implementation of the proposed ontology building method, which comprises (i) the framework introduced in Liu et al. (2005) for term extraction and relation detection, and (ii) the relation labeling component presented in Weichselbraun et al. (2010), which applies constraints to ensure that

Figure 2. Ontology learning framework using spreading activation for evidence integration (Liu et al., 2005)

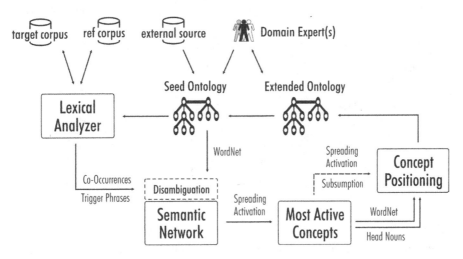

Table 1. Example evidences collected by the ontology learning framework

Seed Term	Evidence	Candidate Term
climate change	wl:coOccurs	carbon dioxide
energy sources	wl:meronym	Oil
energy	wl:hyperonym	renewable energy
climate change	wl:delicious	Gas

its suggestions are consistent with the domain model.

3.1 Term Extraction

Figure 2 presents an implementation of the first two steps in the ontology construction process outlined above which follows Liu et al. (2005).

The ontology extension architecture assembles evidences from unstructured data sources such as Web pages, blogs and media archives. Plugins extract evidences such as co-occurring terms, Hearst patterns and WordNet relations from this data and forward them to the evidence integration component. Social sources such as Delicious, Flickr, Twitter and Technorati could be integrated in this step as well.

The system then collects all evidences as RDF statements in a semantic network as illustrated in Table 1. Reification adds relation meta data such as significance values, number of occurrences and weights to the suggested concepts.

The left site of Figure 3 shows an example entry for the term *climate change*, which co-occurs with *carbon dioxide* with a significance of 12.982 according to a Chi-squared test with Yates correction.

Liu et al. (2005) use spreading activation to transform the data collected in the semantic network into a ranked list of candidate terms for integration in the domain ontology. Per evidence source heuristics translate evidences into spreading activation weights and build a spreading activation network which will be used for the ranking process. The subjects of the statements

Figure 3. Transformation of RDF statements to spreading activation weights

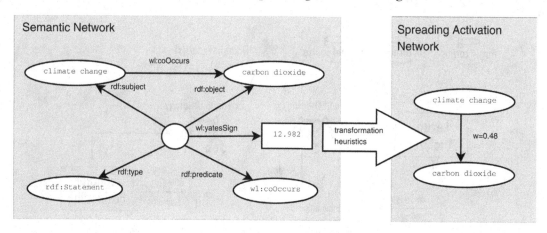

collected in the semantic network are transformed into sources, the objects into sinks and evidence type and annotations into the appropriate weights (Figure 3, for details see Liu et al. (2005)). Activating the source nodes yields activation energy levels for the collected evidences which correspond to their ranking resulting from the evidence integration step.

Angeletou et al. (2007) note that the integration of structured and social evidences introduces new and evolving vocabulary into the domain ontology. External sources also cause the problem of including unrelated terms, or terms that are irrelevant in the context of the ontology. Figure 4 provides such an example. Terms which are connected with bold lines to other concepts have been determined by a social source (Delicious). Most of the included vocabulary such as methane, environment, greenhouse, etc. is intuitive, but the relations *cooling → overclocking* and *ice → machine* clearly introduce terms that are irrelevant in this particular context.

One potential strategy to prevent the inclusion of such concepts is the use of a disambiguation process, which includes additional context terms for ambiguous seed terms. The importance of a proper selection of social and structured evidence sources should not be underestimated. For instance, including Flickr into the extension process

of an ontology which focuses on abstract concepts would probably not be an excellent choice, although the impact of a single source might be reduced by combining multiple social and structured sources.

Another risk of external sources is that they might lead to shifts in the ontology's focus. Therefore, it is extremely important to balance in-corpus sources and external sources and to include safeguards, such as rules which enforce a certain relationship between external and internal concepts, which ensure a proper focus of the extended ontology.

3.2 Relation Detection

The relation detection process (step 2 in Figure 1) takes concept pairs and populates a semantic network with evidences such as relation types suggested by certain patterns (Hearst, 1992; Joho et al., 2004), subsumption analysis (Sanderson & Croft, 1999) and grammatical relationships between the terms. It is even possible to use the semantic network from the concept detection step for this process.

Evidence specific transformation heuristics translate this data into spreading activation weights (Section 3.1). Subsequently, an iterative process activates new concepts and creates a relation to the

Figure 4. Extended ontology based on new terms from Delicious as an example of social evidence sources

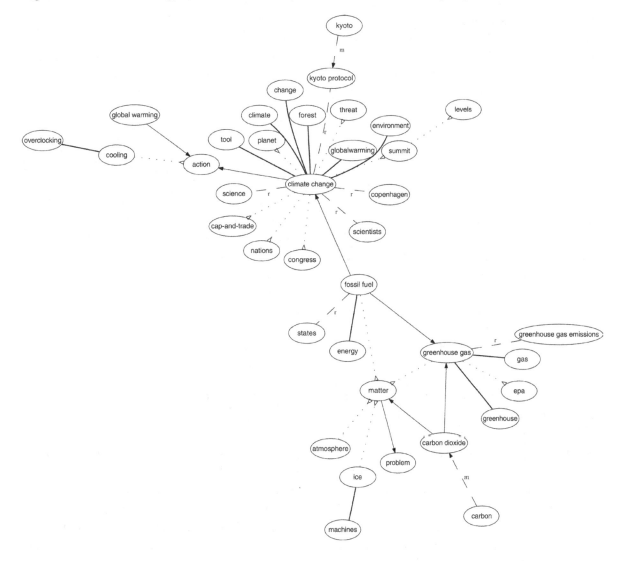

concept with the semantically strongest relation (= the relation with the highest share of the activation energy from the new concept). Depending on the use case, specific preference relations might be limited to seed ontology concepts, or links between new terms might be promoted.

Currently, the relation detection component only detects the *strongest* relation between the candidate term and the other terms in the ontology. Using cut-off levels and additional heuristics will allow the detection of multiple relations and

provide a more fine-grained control over the relation detection process.

3.3 Relation Labeling

Figure 5 presents the relation labeling approach (step 3 in Figure 1) introduced in Weichselbraun et al. (2010) which follows the generic process illustrated in Figure 1.

Based on a set of candidate relations, which are formally described in a relation description ontology, the method starts extracting evidences

Figure 5. Learning relation labels (Weichselbraun et al., 2010)

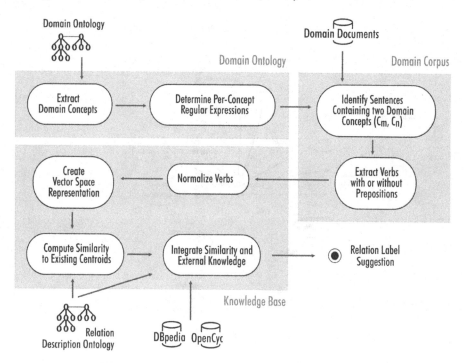

from domain relevant documents which contain the subject and the object participating in the relation. The relation labeling prototype introduced in Weichselbraun et al. (2010) only considers verbs or verbs together with prepositions as evidences. Future versions might consider other part-of-speech tags in the evaluation as well. A vector space model is used to integrate the data – every evidence collected corresponds to a position in the vector space model (Figure 5).

Applying the evidence collection process to known relations defined in the relation description ontology yields vector space representations (centroids) for those known relation labels. The label of newly acquired and therefore unlabeled relations is determined by choosing the label of the semantically closest centroid based on the vector space model with the cosine similarity measure.

3.4 Constraints

In a final step, the proposed process uses constraints to ensure the consistency of the generated ontology, and to refine the ranking of choices based on their conformance with these constraints.

For applying domain and range restrictions (as defined in the relation description ontology) to relation candidates, a concept grounding using an external ontology such as OpenCyc has proven to be beneficial as it allows constraints based on more general concepts such as organization, person, etc. Currently we verify domain, range and property restrictions by enforcing relation label suggestions which fulfill these constraints and penalizing elements violating them. The refined ranking is the base for deciding on the concepts, relations and relation labels to include in the domain ontology.

Figure 6. Tourism ontology (Dickinger et al., 2008)

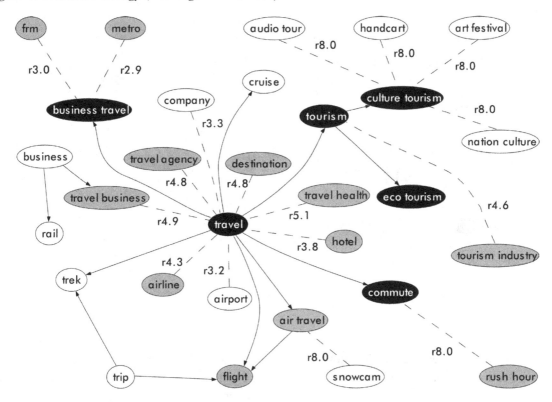

4 USE CASES

This chapter presents three real-world use cases which successfully applied the ontology learning framework introduced in this chapter. The use cases generate ontologies that reflect the knowledge contained in a given corpus. Since knowledge representation experts are not the primary target audience for the resulting structures, the ontologies only contain taxonomic relations indicated by arrows as well as an abstract "related" (r) type to indicate non-taxonomic relationships between terms.

4.1 Tourism Destinations

Dickinger et al. (2008) analyze news media coverage to acquire and structure tourism knowledge using ontology learning. They apply contextual filtering to differentiate between general and tourism-specific news media coverage.

Our ontology learning process extends an ontology of six seed concepts (the black terms in Figure 6) to a lightweight domain ontology which comprises 30 concepts, which were extracted from the input corpus (Figure 6).

Most of the terms and relations included by ontology learning are straightforward to interpret. Nevertheless, there are also a number of unexpected relations such as *culture tourism → handcart, air travel → snowcam* which where added due to a special coverage of certain Web pages (e.g. the CNN and USA Today coverage on "Mormon Hand Track" referring to a cultural tourism attraction). From the ontology engineering point of view, the inclusion of such relations is not necessarily a good thing and might be avoided by (i) using a larger input corpus which reduces the impact of singular events, or (ii) by adding ad-

Figure 7. Solid waste disposal ontology (Pollach et al., 2009)

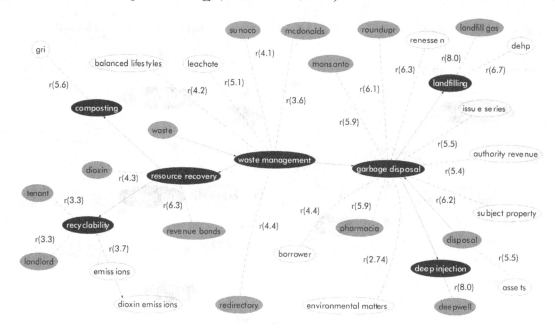

ditional evidence sources such as the ones suggested in Section 2.2 and Section 2.3.

4.2 Communication in Waste Management

Pollach et al. (2009) investigate the Internet coverage of solid waste management on media sites, corporate Web sites and on the Web pages of non-governmental organizations. The authors extend a small seed ontology with the ontology framework introduced by Liu et al. (2005) (Section 3.1) to investigate how well the content of these Web sites corresponds to the perception of domain experts. A detailed analysis of the frequency and sentiment of terms identified reveals that there are significant differences regarding attention and attitude towards the respective topics among the Web coverage of actors such as news media sites, NGOs and companies. Figure 7 visualizes the domain ontology obtained from the ontology extension process.

Black terms indicate the seed ontology, gray terms were added in the first iteration of ontology

extension, white concepts in the second iteration. The method extracted terms such as "landfill gas", "emissions", "dioxin emissions" which are clearly relevant to the domain. Companies addressing environmental issues (McDonalds, Monsanto, Pharmacia, Renessen, Sunoco) got included, as well as environmental programs (Balanced Lifestile, GRI, Redirectory) and chemical substances (DEHP, RoundupR). The usefulness of terms such as "borrower", "issue series" and "assets" is less clear, but were included since they co-occur quite frequently with some of the seed terms. Including external evidence sources into the ontology learning process (Section 2) would reduce the impact of such relations derived from in-corpus evidence sources.

4.3 Media Watch on Climate Change

The Media Watch on Climate Change Hubmann-Haidvogel et al. (2009) builds contextualized information spaces by enriching documents with geospatial, semantic and temporal annotations. Ontology learning (relying on the frameworks

Figure 8. Media Watch on Climate Change (Hubmann-Haidvogel et al., 2009)

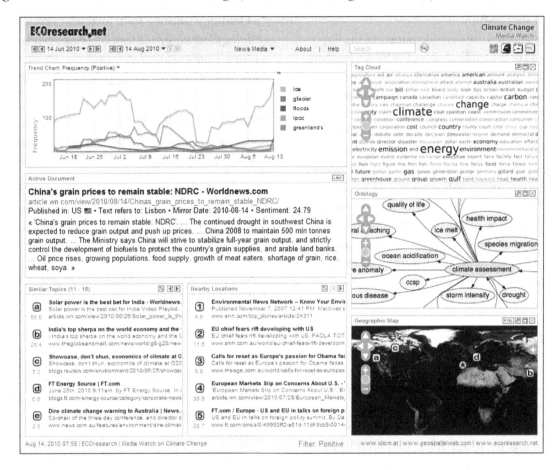

presented in this chapter) is used to create lightweight domain ontologies for structuring the information in the contextualized information space, and to provide means for navigating the repository (Figure 8).

As in the previous use cases, the authors only consider taxonomic relations and a general non-taxonomic *related* type in the ontologies to prevent them of getting too complicated for (non-expert) users to read and understand. Geographic maps, semantic maps and tag clouds complement the ontology view and provide context information on documents and search queries.

5 OUTLOOK AND CONCLUSIONS

This chapter presented a blueprint for a generic ontology extension framework, together with a number of real-world applications. It sheds light on the different aspects of such a framework by (i) suggesting data sources which contain domain knowledge and might act as input for the ontology learning process, (ii) presenting a set of techniques to assemble the necessary components and achieve useful results for different application domains, (iii) stressing the balance necessary between in-corpus evidence and evidence from external sources to ensure a proper focus of the extended ontology, (iv) discussing actual implementations of these techniques and finally, (v) presenting use cases where these techniques have already been applied successfully.

The selected use cases demonstrate the importance and broad applicability of ontology learning. Simple lightweight ontologies help to structure knowledge and to navigate complex information spaces, and indicate how different actors perceive a domain. Future research will focus on the identification and inclusion of new data sources for ontology extension, the improvement of evidence plugins (e.g., by including more sophisticated information extraction and text mining algorithms), the optimization of transformation heuristics, the improvement of the balance between external and in-corpus evidences, and the integration of user feedback into this process.

REFERENCES

Alani, H. (2006). Position paper: Ontology construction from online ontologies. In L. Carr, D. D. Roure, A. Iyengar, C. A. Goble, & M. Dahlin (Eds.), *Proceedings of the 15th International Conference on World Wide Web (WWW 2006)* (pp. 491–495). Edinburgh, Scotland, UK: ACM.

Aleksovski, Z., ten Kate, W., & van Harmelen, F. (2006). Ontology matching using comprehensive ontology as background knowledge. In P. Shvaiko et al. (Eds.), *Proceedings of the International Workshop on Ontology Matching at ISWC 2006* (pp. 13–24). Athens, GA, USA: CEUR.

Angeletou, S., Sabou, M., Specia, L., & Motta, E. (2007). *Bridging the gap between folksonomies and the Semantic Web: An experience report* (vol. 2).

Bizer, C., Lehmann, J., Kobilarov, G., Auer, S., Becker, C., & Cyganiak, R. (2009). DBpedia - a crystallization point for the Web of data. *Journal of Web Semantics: Science. Services and Agents on the World Wide Web, 7*(3), 154–165. doi:10.1016/j.websem.2009.07.002

Buitelaar, P., Cimiano, P., & Magnini, B. (2005). 7). Ontology learning from text: An overview. In *Ontology learning from text: Methods, evaluation and applications/frontiers in artificial intelligence and applications (Vol. 123*, pp. 3–12). Amsterdam, The Netherlands: IOS Press.

Cimiano, P. (2006). *Ontology learning and population from text: Algorithms, evaluation and applications*. Springer.

Corcho, O. (2006). Ontology based document annotation: Trends and open research problems. *IJMSO, 1*(1), 47–57. doi:10.1504/IJMSO.2006.008769

Crestani, F. (1997). Application of spreading activation techniques in information retrieval. *Artificial Intelligence Review, 11*, 453–482. doi:10.1023/A:1006569829653

d'Aquin, M., Motta, E., Sabou, M., Angeletou, S., Gridinoc, L., & Lopez, V. (2008). Toward a new generation of Semantic Web applications. *IEEE Intelligent Systems, 23*(3), 20–28. doi:10.1109/MIS.2008.54

d'Aquin, M., Sabou, M., Motta, E., Angeletou, S., Gridinoc, L., & Lopez, V. (2008). What can be done with the Semantic Web? An overview of Watson-based applications. In A. Gangemi, J. Keizer, V. Presutti, & H. Stoermer (Eds.), *Proceedings of the 5th workshop on Semantic Web applications and perspectives (swap2008)* (Vol. 426). Rome, Italy: CEUR-WS.org.

Dickinger, A., Scharl, A., Stern, H., Weichselbraun, A., & Wöber, K. (2008). Applying optimal stopping for optimizing queries to external Semantic Web resources. In P. O'Connor, H. Wolfram, & G. Ulrike (Eds.), *Information and communication technologies in tourism 2008, Proceedings of the International Conference in Innsbruck, Austria, 2008* (pp. 545–555). Vienna, Austria/New York, NY: Springer.

Etzioni, O., Banko, M., Soderland, S., & Weld, D. S. (2008). Open information extraction from the Web. *Communications of the ACM, 51*(12), 68–74. doi:10.1145/1409360.1409378

Giuliano, C., Lavelli, A., & Romano, L. (2007). Relation extraction and the influence of automatic named-entity recognition. *ACM Transactions on Speech and Language Processing, 5*(1), 1–26. doi:10.1145/1322391.1322393

Gracia, J., Trillo, R., Espinoza, M., & Mena, E. (2006). Querying the Web: A multiontology disambiguation method. In D. Wolber, N. Calder, C. Brooks, & A. Ginige (Eds.), *Proceedings of the 6th International Conference on Web Engineering (ICWE 2006)* (pp. 241–248). Palo Alto, CA, USA: ACM.

Grefenstette, G., & Hearst, M. A. (1992). A method for refining automatically-discovered lexical relations: Combining weak techniques for stronger results. In *AAAI Workshop on statistically-based natural language programming techniques* (pp. 64–72). Menlo Park, CA: AAAI Press.

Gruber, T. R. (1995). Toward principles for the design of ontologies used for knowledge sharing? *International Journal of Human-Computer Studies, 43*(5-6), 907–928. doi:10.1006/ijhc.1995.1081

Harris, Z. (1968). *Mathematical structures of language*. John Wiley & Sons.

Hearst, M. A. (1992). *Automatic acquisition of hyponyms from large text corpora* (pp. 539–545). Nantes, France: Coling.

Heymann, P., & Garcia-Molina, H. (2006, April). *Collaborative creation of communal hierarchical taxonomies in social tagging systems* (Technical Report No. 2006-10). Computer Science Department.

Hubmann-Haidvogel, A., Scharl, A., & Weichselbraun, A. (2009). Multiple coordinated views for searching and navigating Web content repositories. *Information Sciences, 179*(12), 1813–1821. doi:10.1016/j.ins.2009.01.030

Joho, H., Sanderson, M., & Beaulieu, M. (2004). A study of user interaction with a concept-based interactive query expansion support tool. In S. McDonald & J. Tait (Eds.), *Advances in information retrieval, 26th European Conference on IR research (ECIR 2004)* (Vol. 2997, p. 42-56). Sunderland, UK: Springer.

Landauer, T., & Dumais, S. (1997). A solution to Plato's problem: The latent semantic analysis theory of acquisition, induction and representation of knowledge. *Psychological Review, 104*(2), 211–240. doi:10.1037/0033-295X.104.2.211

Liu, W., Weichselbraun, A., Scharl, A., & Chang, E. (2005). Semi-automatic ontology extension using spreading activation. *Journal of Universal Knowledge Management, 1*, 50–58.

Maedche, A., Pekar, V., & Staab, S. (2002). Ontology learning part one-on discovering taxonomic relations from the Web. In Zhong, N., Liu, J., & Yao, Y. (Eds.), *Web intelligence* (pp. 301–322). Springer.

Mika, P. (2007). Ontologies are us: A unified model of social networks and semantics. *Journal of Web Semantics, 5*(1), 5–15. doi:10.1016/j.websem.2006.11.002

Pollach, I., Scharl, A., & Weichselbraun, A. (2009). Web content mining for comparing corporate and third party online reporting: A case study on solid waste management. *Business Strategy and the Environment, 18*(3), 137–148. doi:10.1002/bse.549

Salton, G., Wong, A., & Yang, C. S. (1975). A vector space model for information retrieval. *Communications of the ACM, 18*(11), 613–620. doi:10.1145/361219.361220

Sánchez-Alonso, S., & García, E. (2006). Making use of upper ontologies to foster interoperability between SKOS concept schemes. *Online Information Review, 30*(3), 263–277. doi:10.1108/14684520610675799

Sanderson, M., & Croft, W. B. (1999). Deriving concept hierarchies from text. In *22nd Annual International ACM Sigir Conference on research and development in information retrieval* (pp. 206–213). Berkeley, CA.

Schmitz, P. (2006). *Inducing ontology from flickr tags*. In Collaborative Web tagging workshop at WWW 2006. Edinburgh, Scotland.

Specia, L., & Motta, E. (2007). *Integrating folksonomies with the Semantic Web*. In The Semantic Web: Research and applications, 4th European Semantic Web Conference (eswc-2007) (Vol. 4519, p. 624-639). Berlin, Germany: Springer.

Studer, R. R., Benjamins, R., & Fensel, D. (1998). Knowledge engineering: Principles and methods. *Data & Knowledge Engineering, 25*(1-2), 161–197. doi:10.1016/S0169-023X(97)00056-6

Tang, J., Leung, H. F., Luo, Q., Chen, D., & Gong, J. (2009). Towards ontology learning from folksonomies. In *Ijcai'09: Proceedings of the 21st International Joint Conference on Artifical Intelligence* (pp. 2089–2094). San Francisco, CA, USA: Morgan Kaufmann Publishers Inc.

Weichselbraun, A., Wohlgenannt, G., & Scharl, A. (2010). Refining non-taxonomic relation labels with external structured data to support ontology learning. *Data & Knowledge Engineering, 69*(8), 763–778. doi:10.1016/j.datak.2010.02.010

Wong, W., Liu, W., & Bennamoun, M. (2007). Tree-traversing ant algorithm for term clustering based on featureless similarities. *Data Mining and Knowledge Discovery, 15*(3), 349–381. doi:10.1007/s10618-007-0073-y

Yates, F. (1934). Contingency table involving small numbers and the χ^2 test. *Supplement to the Journal of the Royal Statistical Society, 1*(2), 217–235. doi:10.2307/2983604

ADDITIONAL READING

Fellbaum, C. (1998). Wordnet - an electronic lexical database. *Computational Linguistics, 25*(2), 292–296.

Jurafsky, D., & Martin, J. H. (2000). *Speech and language processing: An introduction to natural language processing, computational linguistics, and speech recognition. Prentice Hall. Powers, S. (2003). Practical RDF*. Sebastopol, CA, USA: O'Reilly & Associates, Inc.

Ruiz-Casado, M., Alfonseca, E., & Castells, P. (2007). Automatising the learning of lexical patterns: An application to the enrichment of wordnet by extracting semantic relationships from wikipedia. *Data & Knowledge Engineering, 61*(3), 484–499. doi:10.1016/j.datak.2006.06.011

Segaran, T. (2007). *Collective intelligence - building smart web 2.0 applications*. O'Reilly.

Shadbolt, N., Berners-Lee, T., & Hall, W. (2006). The Semantic Web revisited. *IEEE Intelligent Systems, 21*(3), 96–101. doi:10.1109/MIS.2006.62

Tao, C., & Embley, D. W. (2009). Automatic hidden-web table interpretation, conceptualization, and semantic annotation. Data & Knowledge Engineering, 68 (7), 683 - 703. (Special Issue: 26th International Conference on Conceptual Modeling (ER 2007))

KEY TERMS AND DEFINITIONS

Co-Occurrence Analysis: Co-occurrence analysis determines whether terms are significantly over-represented in designated spans of text. The calculation of statistical significance compares the distribution of terms in a domain-specific target corpus with their distribution in a generic reference corpus to identify candidate terms of inclusion in the extended ontology.

Evidence: Evidence represents the input data for the ontology learning process. The presented framework relies on evidences from unstructured sources (domain text), social sources (for example APIs of Web 2.0 applications and tagging systems) and structured sources (online Semantic Web data and ontologies).

Evidence Integration: Integration of evidences from heterogeneous sources supports the ontology learning process. Combining in-corpus data with social sources, for example, will include an outside view of the domain into the learned ontology.

Sentiment: Sentiment is the emotional attitude towards abstract or real objects of their environment. Measures of individual or organizational bias that distinguish between positive, negative and neutral media coverage are important indicators for investigating trends and differing perceptions of stakeholder groups.

Spreading Activation: Spreading activation is a graph-based, interative search technique inspired by cognitive models of the human brain. It is typically applied to various types of networks (e.g., associative, semantic or neural networks).

Trigger Phrases: Trigger phrases rely on the heuristic that certain phrases (e.g., "renewable energy, especially solar energy ...") often indicate hyponym, hypernym, and meronym relations. Trigger phrase analysis detects these constructs by using pattern matching via regular expressions combined with part-of-speech tags.

Vector Space Model: Vector space models are a common way to represent documents and queries in information retrieval systems, e.g. for computing similarity between documents, or between a query term and a document collection.

ENDNOTES

1   www.delicious.com
2   www.flickr.com
3   www.technorati.com
4   www.twitter.com
5   www.freebase.com
6   www.opencyc.org
7   esw.w3.org/topic/sweoig/taskforces/communityprojects/linkingopendata
8   swoogle.umbc.edu
9   www.sindice.com
10 iws.seu.edu.cn/services/falcons
11 swse.deri.org

Chapter 2
An Overview of Shallow and Deep Natural Language Processing for Ontology Learning

Amal Zouaq
Simon Fraser University - Athabasca University, Canada

ABSTRACT

This chapter gives an overview over the state-of-the-art in natural language processing for ontology learning. It presents two main NLP techniques for knowledge extraction from text, namely shallow techniques and deep techniques, and explains their usefulness for each step of the ontology learning process. The chapter also advocates the interest of deeper semantic analysis methods for ontology learning. In fact, there have been very few attempts to create ontologies using deep NLP. After a brief introduction to the main semantic analysis approaches, the chapter focuses on lexico-syntactic patterns based on dependency grammars and explains how these patterns can be considered as a step towards deeper semantic analysis. Finally, the chapter addresses the "ontologization" task that is the ability to filter important concepts and relationships among the mass of extracted knowledge.

1. INTRODUCTION

Given the large amount of textual data in almost all the aspects of our everyday lives and the fact that natural language is our primary medium for communicating knowledge, there is no doubt that natural language processing (NLP) technologies are of tremendous importance for analyzing textual resources and extracting their meaning. One of the current research avenues where NLP

DOI: 10.4018/978-1-60960-625-1.ch002

should play a leading role is the Semantic Web. In fact, NLP should be considered as one of the pillars of the Semantic Web (Wilks & Brewster, 2009) for its role in the acquisition of domain ontologies. Despite the vast majority of works dedicated to ontology learning based on NLP (Buitelaar & Cimiano, 2008) (Cimiano & Volker, 2005) (Buitelaar et al., 2005), it is clear that the whole potential of the available techniques and representations has not been fully exploited. More precisely, the works from the computational semantics community (Bos, 2008c) have been largely neglected, to my knowledge, in the ontology learning field until now. Advances from this community are of particular relevance since they address important aspects of text understanding that are not available in more shallow techniques. I believe that these deep aspects are essential for building an accurate domain ontology reflecting the content of its source data. This chapter is a tentative to bring this issue to the attention of the research community. This chapter also provides a quick overview over techniques from the computational semantics community that may be of interest for ontology learning. We will look at some of the shallow NLP techniques as well as deeper methods based on dependency grammars and lexico-syntactic patterns which have already been employed for ontology learning. Many of these deeper methods used for ontology learning have not yet reached the required depth that is advocated in computational semantics. They nevertheless can be considered as early attempts towards this goal.

The chapter is organized as follows. After the introduction, Section 2 provides the definition of ontologies and the ontology learning task. Section 3 discusses the various natural language processing techniques that may be used in an ontology learning process. It also provides a quick overview over the available techniques in the computational linguistic and semantics communities including shallow and deep analysis, both at the syntactic level and the semantic level. Section 4 presents a set of projects for ontology learning with a special emphasis on the dependency grammar formalism and the use of patterns based on this formalism. This section emphasizes the links between the presented projects and the various NLP techniques that were used. Section 5 explains an important stage of the ontology learning process which is the ontologization task. We end this chapter in Section 6 with a discussion on a number of issues that require the attention of the research community.

2. BACKGROUND

There are a number of resources that describe what an ontology is, with the most cited definition being the one presented by (Gruber, 93): "*An ontology is a formal specification of a conceptualization*". Although this definition may seem too broad, we can extract from it two keywords that are essential for our understanding of ontologies: formal and conceptualization.

- **The formal characteristic:** In the domain of computer science and formal logic, a formal system designates a system using a **formal language,** a grammar that indicates the well-expressed formulas according to the language and a set of axioms or inference rules to reason over this language. A formal language is defined using a set of symbols.

- **The conceptual characteristic:** Having its root in philosophy, the notion of concept has been widely used in the Artificial Intelligence community. According to (Guarino, 98), a conceptualization must be defined on an intentional level and an extensional level. The intentional level deals with the *meaning* of what is being defined (the domain of interest), while the extensional level describes the instances of that domain.

As it can be seen, an ontology is grounded in the domain of mathematical logic, reasoning and theorem-proving. In fact, it is the main knowledge structure of the *Semantic Web*, whose aim is to provide a set of machine understandable semantics. These semantics are generally organized in a structure called a domain ontology, which is used to express the conceptualization of that domain.

Formally, a domain ontology is represented by a tuple <C, H, R, A, I>, where:

- C represents the set of classes. E.g.: Animal, Human, etc.
- H represents the set of hierarchical links between the concepts. E.g. is-a (Feline, Animal).
- R, the set of conceptual links. E.g. eat(Herbivores, Plant)
- A, the set of axioms, i.e. the rules that govern this domain and make a reasoner able to infer new information.
- I the set of instances, i.e. the objects of the world which can be categorized into the ontological classes C.

Generally, when we think about developing or learning an ontology, we target the first four components (which are considered as steps in the ontology learning process), i.e. the tuple <C, H, R, A>, while the last one (I) is tackled by what is called "ontology population". Ontology engineering has proposed various methodologies that provide guidelines to users for effectively building ontologies through ontology editors. However, one drawback of these methodologies is the huge amount of time and effort required by humans, the so called knowledge acquisition bottleneck. This situation is even worsened when it comes to ontology evolution or mapping. In front of the rapidly growing amounts of electronic data, providing (semi)automatic knowledge extraction tools is a must. This is the reason why this chapter focuses on (semi) automatic ontology learning.

As a process, ontology learning starts with a source of knowledge, extracts the various elements <C, H, R, A>, and produces an ontology, generally expressed using one of the Semantic Web Languages, such as RDF or OWL. There have been many attempts to define (semi)automatic processes from structured documents, including knowledge bases and xml files for instance (Maedche & Staab, 2001). This is mainly accomplished by creating mappings between the original structures and the ontological structures (concepts, taxonomy, etc.). But the main effort of the research community

is directed towards extracting semantics from unstructured sources, such as plain text or Web documents (which cannot be really considered as structured). The democratization of the access to the Web and hence the huge production of Web documents participate greatly to this need as well as the emergence of the Semantic Web, which calls for semantic models attached to the WWW resources. This chapter does not deal particularly with Web content but rather focuses on how texts (and among them textual Web resources) might be a useful knowledge source for acquiring ontologies. Important aspects such as the necessity of extracting the structure of a Web document to guide the learning process or how we might filter Web content are not addressed here. However, we believe that many of the methods and approaches presented here may benefit to ontology learning from the Web.

Ontology learning from texts involves a number of disciplines ranging from lexical acquisition, text mining, natural language processing, statistics and machine learning. These are generally fully intricate in the ontology learning process and are involved at the various levels of ontological acquisition. This chapter focuses particularly on the natural language processing (NLP) techniques ranging from lexical acquisition to shallow and deep analysis methods (both at the syntactic and semantic levels). However, we will also refer to many other approaches from statistics and machine learning, especially when they come as a complement to the NLP process.

There are many reasons why deep NLP may be of great interest. First, because it is the discipline which deals with the understanding of a message conveyed by a text, hence it is an indispensable tool for ontology learning from text. Second, NLP tools are becoming sufficiently robust to be considered as reliable tools for knowledge and model extraction [Bos, 2008c]. Third, NLP methods that have been used until now, in the ontology learning field, remain generally shallow and do not borrow significant insights from the computational linguistics and semantics communities. To conclude, this chapter is a tentative to show the interest of computational semantics (or at least deeper linguistic processing) for the ontology learning field.

3. NLP APPROCHES

There exists a broad range of NLP approaches that may be used for ontology learning. These include shallow NLP and deep NLP methods. The following sections explore these NLP approaches both at the syntactic and semantic levels.

3.1. Shallow NLP

Shallow NLP has been the main approach used by the ontology learning community, primarily for three reasons: its robustness to noise, its low need of training resources (such as tagged corpora) and its efficiency in terms of calculation, which is important if we deal with large amounts of texts. Using Shallow NLP techniques may be applied at the syntactic level and semantic level.

3.1.1. Shallow Syntactic Processing

Shallow NLP, when coping with the *syntactic aspect*, generally designates methods for generating partial analysis of sentences and include tools such as chunkers (dividing sentences into chunks (Abney, 1991)) and parts-of-speech taggers (assigning a syntactic label such as NP to a chunk). An example of a chunked sentence, taken from (Li & Roth, 2001), is: "[NP He] [VP reckons] [NP the current account deficit] [VP will narrow] [PP to] [NP only $ 1.8 billion] [PP in] [NP September]", where NP indicate Nominal Phrases, VP verbal phrases and PP prepositional phrases. Theses chunks could be used, for instance, to identify interesting terms, especially based on NPs.

Shallow NLP may be used in a number of tasks related to ontology learning:

- **Term Extraction:** The most common approach consists in using primarily shallow NLP techniques to extract terms. Terms constitute the linguistic expression of a concept that may be of interest to the domain (Buitelaar et al., 2005). In fact, the nominal phrases extracted by chunkers may constitute the basic vocabulary of the domain model. However, besides identifying these nominal expressions, it is also needed to compute their weight or importance with respect to the corpus. This is generally tackled using statistical measures from information retrieval such as TF*IDF (Salton & Buckley, 1988), Pointwise Mutual Information (Church & Hanks, 90), and so on. The reader is referred to (Nanas et al., 2003) (Zhang et al., 2008) to gain more insight on metrics used for term weighting.

- **Taxonomy Extraction:** Shallow syntactic parsing has also been successfully used for learning hierarchical links in an ontology (Maedche & Staab, 2001) (Cimiano & Volker, 2005). These links are generally identified with lexico-syntactic patterns such as the patterns defined by (Hearst, 92). These patterns are mainly expressed using regular expressions to be fetched over a text or a chunked text.

- **Relation Extraction:** There are only limited possibilities to extract reliable relations using only shallow syntactic parsing. Based again on regular expressions, it is possible to extract some patterns such NP VP NP. But this is far from being sufficient and this does not cope with language ambiguities such as long-distance relationships. Therefore, shallow parsing shows its limits at this level, not to talk about axiom learning, which might only be extracted with deeper syntactic methods.

3.1.2. Shallow Semantic Processing

Besides syntactic parsing, there are also various methods for shallow semantic parsing (also called semantic tagging) which may be used in an ontology learning/population process (Etzioni et al., 2004) (McDowell & Cafarella, 2008). These methods generally require a set of knowledge resources such as frames, templates, or roles, to identify the structures to be found in the corpus. From this perspective, this approach is radically different from learning an ontology based only on texts. Here learning relies on sources that guide the extraction and this supposes that you *know* what you are looking for, contrary to a "blind" approach where you actually *discover* the important concepts and relations.

In such a process, the resulting ontology uses the knowledge resources terminology (roles, frames, concepts) to discover instances of these resources, which in turn nourish the ontology. These resources may include role taxonomies, lists of named entities and also lexicons and dictionaries (Giuglea & Moschitti, 2006). They also generally require a word sense disambiguation algorithm to pick up the right sense of a given word and assign it the right meaning or concept. Shallow semantic parsing is also useful to identify particular semantic relationships such as synonyms, meronyms, or antonyms using pre-specified patterns, such as Hearst patterns (Hearst, 92), or verb subcategorizations (e.g. VerbNet) hence mixing the syntactic and semantic processing perspectives.

Shallow semantic parsing has been mainly used for "populating" ontologies rather than learning them, because it relies on conceptual structures that guide the extraction. Lexical semantics, involving semantic role labeling (Gildea & Jurafsky, 2002) and word sense disambiguation can also be categorized as shallow semantic approaches (although they may rely on **deep syntactic** processing and syntactic grammars).

3.2. Deep NLP

As outlined earlier, deep semantic analysis of texts may prove more appropriate to extract rich domain ontologies, involving not only concepts but also relationships and axioms. Shallow methods may be of interest for some of the ontology learning steps, but they fell short when confronted with more complex understanding of texts. Computational semantics deals with such aspects, and aims at producing meaning representations while tackling very fine-grained aspects of the language such as anaphora resolution, quantifier scope resolution, etc. For example, anaphora resolution identifies the entities referred by expressions such as pronouns. In general, computational semantics aims at grasping the *entire meaning* of sentences and discourse, rather than focusing on text portions alone.

Computational semantics provides a method for extracting representations from natural language and drawing inferences based on these representations. Such a definition enables a clear and straightforward link to the objective of the Semantic Web in general and of domain ontologies in particular: expressing (textual) Web resources content based on a standard language understandable by machines and endowed with inference capabilities. The first essential component for a deep analysis of texts is a syntactic parser based on syntactic grammars.

3.2.1. Syntactic Grammars

Syntactic parsing is performed using a set of grammar rules that assign parse trees to sentences. This set of rules is known as a syntactic grammar. Traditional syntactic parsing (Jurafsky & Martin, 2009) relies also on a lexicon that describes the vocabulary that may be used in the parsed sentences. For instance, WordNet (Fellbaum, 1998) can be considered as a lexicon. There are also statistical parsers (Klein & Manning, 2003) (Jurafsky & Martin, 2009) which learn their knowledge about

Figure 1. A phrase structure parse (Left) and a dependency parse (Right) (Nivre, 2005)

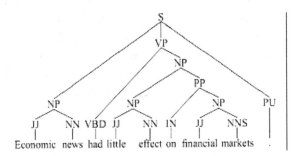 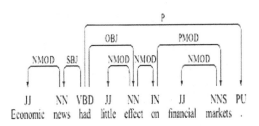

a language using hand-labeled sentences and produce the most likely analyses when parsing sentences. The output representations can take the form of phrase structure tree representations or dependency parses. Phrase structure parses associates a syntactic parse in the form of a tree to a sentence, while dependency parses creates grammatical links between each pair of words in the sentence (see figure 1).

Phrase structure grammars and dependency grammars cannot be considered as opposite approaches but rather as complementary. In fact, many syntactic theories make use of both formalisms. However, despite the fact that these two representations differ from each other only by what is explicitly encoded, as pointed out by (Kübler et al., 2009), "practical experience has shown that it is a non-trivial task to perform an automatic conversion from one type of representation to the other". Dependency parsing seems to regain its central place in the research community (especially with CoNLL shared tasks), with many researchers (Briscoe & Carroll 2006; Zouaq, 2008, Kübler et al., 2009) arguing that dependencies model predicate-argument structures in a more convenient or intuitive form (for further semantic analysis), and that dependency grammar has led to the development of accurate syntactic parsers using machine learning on Treebanks (Kübler et al., 2009). The majority of the approaches for ontology learning are based on the exploitation of the syntactic parses to further extract relevant structures, using patterns and

machine learning. These approaches use syntactic parses for a more fine-grained term extraction (noun compound for instance), relation extraction and axiom learning. Section 4 is dedicated to the presentation of works based on this approach.

3.2.2. Linguistic Grammars and Theories

A long tradition of the linguistic community is the use of grammars that rely mainly on lexical items. By linguistic grammars, we mean grammars which build upon a number of syntactic rules and a lexicon to produce some kind of representations of the sentence or the discourse. These grammars include HPSG grammars (Sag et al., 2003) and CCG grammars (Steedman, 2001), which are among the most used formalisms in the linguistic community.

Linguistic grammars rely basically on two main methods: the unification-based approaches and the lambda-calculus approaches, which may be considered as drawing their roots in formal semantics. Many grammars, such as HPSG, are based on the unification mechanism.

Unification-Based Approaches
The unification based-approaches rely on representations called feature structures that express valid phrase structure rules between syntactic categories (e.g. S→NP VP) and use lexical entries (also described as feature structures) as their content. The phrase structure rules have the form

Figure 2. An example of an HPSG lexical item (Bender et al., 2003)

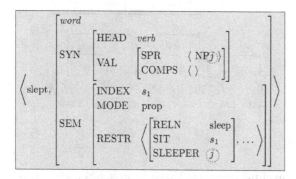

LHS/RHS where LHS is a non lexical category and RHS might be a set of lexical and non lexical categories. These rules guarantee the correct unification of all the semantic features with instances that respect the syntactic features. A lexical item is represented as phoneme coupled with a syntactic and a semantic part. Figure 2 shows a an example of an HPSG lexical item, with a syntactic component (Syn) and a semantic component (Sem), and where the subject of the verb "slept" in the Syn part is the "Sleeper" argument in the Sem part.

Lambda Calculus

Another approach consists in using lambda-calculus as the glue to combine semantic representations, and solve some of the problems of the unification-based approaches (such as coordination processing). In lambda-calculus, all the formulas are regarded as lambda expressions, as well as the combination of variables and lambda expressions.

All the approaches described so far tackle the semantic analysis at the sentence level. The discourse Representation Theory (DRT) (Kamp and Reyle, 1993) was born to address this shortcoming by providing means to parse a discourse. More precisely, DRT enables resolving pronouns to their textual antecedents. The basic unit of the DRT is the Discourse Representation Structure (DRS) which map sentence constituents to objects, properties and predicates and provides discourse

referents (variables) to represent these objects (Figure 3). These referents are then used to resolve a pronominal anaphora. The DRT provides triggering rules associated to particular syntactic configurations as well as transformation methods that output semantic representations.

3.2.3. Summary on Deep NLP

Very few approaches have used these types of grammars for ontology learning or population. To our knowledge, the only exception is the OntoSem project (English & Nirenburg, 2007) which carries out preprocessing, morphological analysis, syntactic analysis, and semantic analysis to build a fact repository. OntoSem relies on a syntactic and semantic lexicon, as well as on an existing ontology and is able to "learn" a concept from the Web based on these resources. Given a specific word, OntoSem builds a corpus of sentences, derived from the Web, containing this word and annotates this corpus using its semantic analyzer. Then the system creates a candidate new concept by collating semantic information from annotated sentences and finds in the existing ontology concept(s) "closest" to the candidate. The objective of the OntoSem project is in fact closer to the goal of shallow semantic processing approaches, which aims at populating an ontology rather than creating its structure. OntoSem, however, uses deep semantic processing techniques to reach this goal.

Given these various NLP-based methods, the main difficulty is to pick up the right method according to the particular task that is envisaged. On way to provide some insights over this kind of decisions is to give an overview on state-of-the art experiences. The following sections present practical examples of systems which are based on dependency grammars and lexico-syntactic patterns and which aim at extracting a whole ontology or a particular ontology component (classes, relations, axioms, etc.).

Figure 3. An example of discourse representation structure

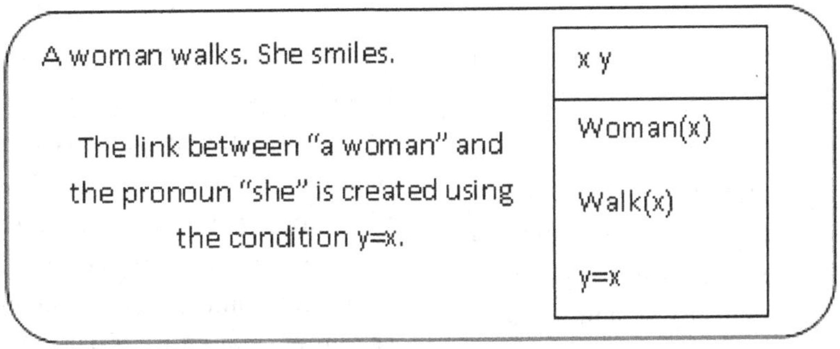

4. Practical Examples of Lexico-Syntactic Patterns

The field of NLP offers now tools and methods mature enough to be considered in the text understanding process, particularly with the availability of robust statistical syntactic analyzers (Bos, 2008a), annotated corpora and semantic lexica such as WordNet (Fellbaum, 1998) or FrameNet (Baker et al., 1998). In this context, using a deep syntactic analysis approach, rather than a shallow one, may bring more insights over the structure and meaning of sentences. Deep syntactic analysis may also be the way to pave the road for deeper *semantic* analysis as well. The following sections show how these deep syntactic analyses have been used in the state-of-the-art to learn ontologies, ontology components and to create semantic analysis.

4.1. Pattern Definition

One of the common ways to exploit a deep syntactic analysis is to find patterns in the syntactic parses. In its broad sense, a pattern is a model, a set of elements that describe a structure of interest. Based on the dependency parses, a lexico-syntactic pattern may be able to define a meaningful structure on which additional computations can be performed depending on the required task. For example, (Snow et al., 2004) define a space of lexico-syntactic patterns as all shortest paths of

four links or less between any two nouns in a dependency tree. In the TEXCOMON project (Zouaq & Nkambou, 2009), each pattern is organized as a tree around a root term, *T*, linked to specific input and output grammatical links. Each node in the pattern represents a variable. An example of such a pattern is: found in Figure 4:

In (Zouaq et al., 2010), patterns are represented by Prolog rules. In both projects (Zouaq & Nkambou, 2009) (Zouaq et al., 2010), these patterns are linked to transformation methods that output some sort of representation (concept maps, logical forms). During the semantic analysis, the basic idea is that these patterns are searched in the parse trees and instantiated with data whenever an occurrence is found. Conceptually, these patterns constitute triggering rules that call transformation methods whenever a meaningful syntactic representation is found.

Other works have proposed pattern models based on dependency grammars. (Stevenson & Greenwood, 2009) give a good overview of the pattern structures that may be used for information extraction, namely: *Subject-Object Model* (Yangarber, 2003), the *Chain Model* that represents the chain from a verb to its descendants (Sudo et al., 2001), the *Linked Chain Model* where a pattern is a pair of chains which share the same root verb but do not share any direct descendants (Greenwood et al., 2005), the *Shortest path Model* which models the shortest route in the dependency tree between any pair of nodes (Bunescu & Mooney, 2005), and

Figure 4.

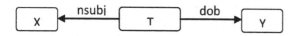

the *Sub-tree Model*, where any sub-tree of a dependency tree can be used as an extraction pattern (Sudo et al., 2003). These patterns are generalized by replacing the lexical items by semantic roles. For example, the sentences "Acme Inc. hired Smith" and "IBM hired Jones last week." will be matched by the generalized pattern: [V/hire](subj[Organisation]+obj[Person]). However, (Stevenson & Greenwood, 2009) do not state how this generalization might be done and this pre-supposes that there are roles (Organization, Person) that are defined, and that a certain form of named entity extraction is performed. This kind of approach is an information extraction one, meaning that one knows what to look for in the texts. This also involves the use of a word sense disambiguation approach to determine the right sense of the words with respect to your terminology.

As already shown, ontology learning from text might not be guided by knowledge structures (named entities, roles, etc.) and may have to perform a meaningful extraction from scratch. Being in one or other situation helps determine the adequate pattern model. However, developing *grammars of meaningful patterns* may prove essential for ontology learning. This intuition is guided by the hypothesis that focusing on meaningful parts of dependency parses may be the most suitable approach for accurate extraction. This hypothesis seems to be confirmed by the experiments in (Stevenson & Greenwood, 2009) (Zouaq & Nkambou, 2009) (Zouaq et al., 2010).

The following sections present two projects in this line of research where I have been deeply involved as well as other projects that have used lexico-syntactic patterns over dependency grammars.

4.2. TEXCOMON

TEXCOMON as illustrated in Figure 5 is a domain-independent ontology learning system that performs a number of steps to produce a domain ontology. First, it analyzes plain text documents and extracts paragraphs, sentences, and keywords. Second, the sentences containing the keywords are selected and parsed using the Stanford parser (Klein & Manning, 2003) (De Marneffe et al., 2006), which outputs a dependency parse. This key sentences' selection helps reduce the search space for important information as well as the time required to parse the corpus.

TEXCOMON relies on a hierarchy of handmade patterns that identify the meaningful grammatical structures which trigger transformation methods. The interest of these patterns is that they enable the extraction of domain terms, taxonomical relationships, conceptual relationships and axioms at the same time, and are completely independent of a domain or a corpus. The process results into the production of multiple Concept Maps, which are in fact, terminological maps that comprise terms related by labeled relationships. These maps may be related by common terms or not. Next, metrics from graph theory such as the *degree of a node* are used to identify the important concepts and relations, which are then exported to a domain ontology. Given this project description, it is clear that the approach of (Zouaq, 2008) (Zouaq & Nkambou, 2009) exploits deep syntactic analysis, but also "deep-shallow" semantic analysis. By this "deep-shallow" analysis, we mean that we do not handle cases such as anaphora resolution and entity co-reference (resolving references to earlier or later entities in the discourse), but we still develop a hierarchy of patterns coupled with transformational methods, thus getting closer to this idea of *grammars of meaningful patterns*. Moreover, there seem to be new initiatives in the computational semantic community (for instance (Bos, 2008b)) that try to build

Figure 5. The TEXCOMON Architecture and an Example of a Concept Map

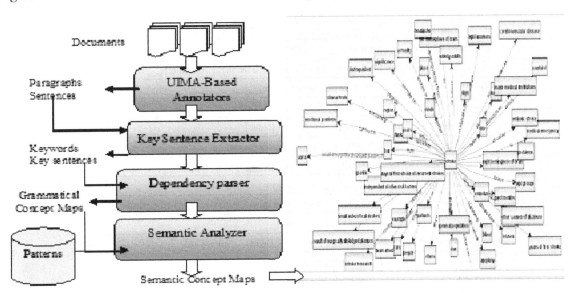

a semantic analysis based on the output of a syntactic parser.

An experiment of TEXCOMON, deeply described in (Zouaq & Nkambou, 2009b), shows that these patterns may be very effective to build a domain ontology by comparison with another ontology learning tool, Text-To-Onto (Maedche & Staab, 2001) (Maedche & Volz, 2001). According to two domain experts, TEXCOMON reaches a mean precision of up to 90% for concept identification on a SCORM corpus dataset while Text-to-Onto obtains 73% on the same dataset. Similarly, relationships precision is also very interesting with up to 84% for hierarchical links and up to 93% for conceptual links.

The purpose of the following project (Zouaq et al., 2010) is to propose a deep semantic analysis using this pattern-based approach.

4.3. The Semantic Analyzer

The aim of the Semantic Analyzer (Zouaq et al., 2010) is to extract logical forms from free texts and to annotate these forms using an upper-level ontology. Semantic analysis is represented as a modular pipeline that involves three steps (Figure.6): 1) Syntactic parsing of texts; 2) Logical analysis using a dependency-based grammar; 3) Semantic annotation based on the upper-level ontology SUMO involving word-sense disambiguation.

This modular process enables the creation of a modular design clearly separating syntactic, logical and semantic annotation or extraction steps. The process is domain-independent and lexicon-independent, and it uses an ontology as a way to formally define semantic roles and make them understandable from one semantic role labelling system to another.

The system also relies on dependency syntactic patterns to extract logical representations. Here, these patterns are exploited as an intermediate step towards an efficient modular semantic analysis based on an existing ontology, SUMO (Pease et al., 2002) and WordNet (Fellbaum, 1998). Each pattern is a Prolog rule that builds a logical representation according to the fired pattern and pattern hierarchy is simply represented by the order of the Prolog rules in the Semantic Analyzer. Table 1 and 2 show the patterns (Core and modifiers

Table 1. Core patterns (Zouaq et al., 2010)

Patterns	Examples
Verb-nsubj-dobj-iobj	{Mary}$_{nsubj}$*gave* {Bill}$_{iobj}$ a {raise}$_{dobj}$
Verb-nsubj-dobj-xcomp	{The peasant}$_{nsubj}$*carries* {the rabbit}$_{dobj}$, {holding}$_{xcomp}$ it by its ears
Verb-nsubj-dobj	{The cat}$_{nsubj}$*eats* {a mouse}$_{dobj}$
Verb-nsubj-xcomp[-dobj]	{Michel}$_{nsubj}$*likes* to {eat}$_{comp}$ {fish}$_{dobj}$
Adjective-nsubj-xcomp	{Benoit}$_{nsubj}$ is *ready* to {leave}$_{xcomp}$
Verb-csubj-dobj	What Amal {said}$_{csubj}$*makes* {sense}$_{dobj}$
Verb-nsubj-expl	{There}$_{expl}$*is* a small {bush}$_{nsubj}$
Adjective-nsubj-cop	{Benoit}$_{nsubj}$ {is}$_{cop}$*happy*
Noun-nsubj-cop	{Michel}$_{nsubj}$ {is}$_{cop}$ a *man*
Verb-nsubj-acomp	{Amal}$_{nsubj}$*looks* {tired}$_{acomp}$
Verb-xcomp-ccomp	Michel *says* that Benoit {likes}$_{ccomp}$ to {swim}$_{xcomp}$
Verb-nsubj	{The cat}$_{nsubj}$*eats*
Verb-dobj	Benoit talked to Michel in order to *secure* {the account}$_{dobj}$
Verb-nsubjpass-prep by	{The man}$_{nsubjpass}$ has been *killed* {by}$_{prep}$ the police
Verb-csubjpass-prep by	That he {lied}$_{csubjpass}$ was *suspected* {by}$_{prep}$ everyone
Verb-nsubjpass	{Bills}$_{nsubjpass}$ were *submitted*

Table 2. Modifier patterns (Zouaq et al., 2010)

Modifiers Patterns (Modifiers)	Examples
Partmod[prep]	There is garden surrounded by houses.
Prep[pcomp]	They heard about Mia missing classes.
Prep (after a noun)	Vincent discovered the man with a telescope.
Prep (after a verb)	Bills were submitted to the man.
Amod	The white cat eats
Tmod	Vincent swam in the pool last night
Advcl	The accident happened as the night was falling.
Ccomp	Michel says that Benoit likes to swim.
Purpcl	Benoit talked to Michel in order to secure the account.
Infmod	The following points are to establish.
Measure	The director is 55 years old.
Num	The director is 55 years old.
Poss	The peasant taps the rabbit's head with his fingers.
Quantmod	About 200 people came to the party.
Advmod	Genetically modified food is dangerous.
Rcmod	Michel loves a cat which Benoit adores.

Figure 6. The Semantic Analyzer Architecture (Zouaq et al., 2010)

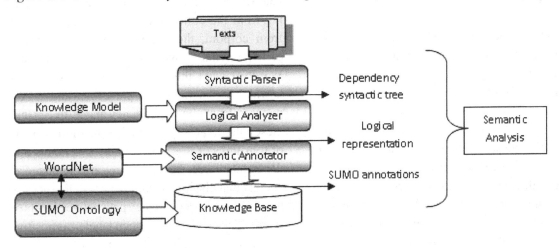

patterns) that are currently implemented as rules in the Prolog Semantic Analyzer. These patterns were discovered using a manual analysis of dependency parses.

Core patterns are used to extract main meaningful syntactic structures in the language while modifiers complete the meaning of core patterns and particular syntactic categories. For example, a preposition after a noun should not be interpreted the same way as a preposition after a verb.

The resulting representation is a predicative flat formula composed of predicates applied to lexical elements, as well as predicates resulting from prepositional relations and predicates indicating if an entity has already been encountered in the discourse. Relationships between predicates are represented through their arguments and referential variables are assigned to the instantiated knowledge model elements. An example of a logical formula created by the semantic analyzer is:

Sentence: *The Guatemala army denied today that guerrillas attacked Santo Tomas Presidential Farm.*

[message(e1, e2), event(e2, attacked, id3, id4), entity(id4, santo-tomas-presidential-farm), resolve(id4), entity(id3, guerrillas), time(e1,

id2), entity(id2, today), event(e1, denied, id1), entity(id1, guatemala-army), resolve(id1)]

We ran experiments to evaluate the performance of the logical analyzer and the semantic annotator in terms of precision and recall. Overall, the logical analyzer reached a very good performance with a precision around 94% and a recall around 80%. The semantic annotator performance depended on the performance of the employed word sense disambiguation algorithm and the corpus. Overall, we were able to obtain a precision/recall of 64.1% (Fine-grained) and 69% (coarse-grained) on Senseval Data (Mihalcea et al., 2004).

As shown in Figure 6, the semantic analyzer (Zouaq et al., 2010) is an example of the shallow semantic approach, since it uses an existing ontology to annotate the representation, and does not lead to a new ontology but it is also a "deep" semantic analysis in the sense that it relies on a grammar of dependency-based patterns. This simply shows what can be done by combining various methods. Moreover, one can imagine how an ontology learning system might benefit from very detailed predicative formulas as the one presented above especially for the extraction of axioms.

4.4. Other Works

Many other works have relied on lexico-syntactic patterns for relation extraction, taxonomy extraction or concept learning. In general, there have been many efforts to build relationship classifiers, which uses machine learning to try to identify a particular type of relationship. Among these works, we can cite the seminal work of (Hearst, 92) on hyponyms as well as successor works such as (Snow et al., 2004), (Girju et al., 2006) for part-of relationships, or (Lin et al., 2003) for synonyms. In general, these classifiers use lexico-syntactic patterns and build models based on seed patterns.

One of the most recent projects, Kleo (Kim et al., 2009), uses a semantic interpreter (built on dependency grammars) that handles a number of linguistic forms such as auxiliary verbs, noun compound, causal verbs, and definitional phrases through rules that create, for instance, causal relationships for causal verbs, or taxonomical links for definitional phrases. Kleo's lexico-syntactic patterns lead to the creation of triples. Kleo builds on the results of Mobius (Barker et al., 2007), which uses the same kind of approach to extract triples from texts. Another interesting example for the extraction of relationships from texts is Espresso (Pantel & Pennacchiotti, 2008). Espresso uses a minimally supervised bootstrapping approach that starts with a set of seed instances for a particular relation (patterns) and learns surface broad-coverage patterns from the Web. These patterns are then ranked based on a metric called "reliability of a pattern" and the algorithm conserves the top k patterns as meaningful structures. These structures are then used to collect reliable instances of the patterns, thus leading to the creation of reliable relationships.

One of the most studied relationships has been the taxonomical link (hypernym-hyponym). This interest might be due to the fact that these links are essential for further reasoning over the obtained structure. An interesting work (Snow et al., 2004) builds a hypernym classifier based on features extracted from dependency trees. Starting from the collection of noun pairs extracted from corpora, the system identifies examples of hypernyms between these noun pairs using WordNet. Next, the system collects the sentences in which both nouns occur, parse them and extract patterns from the dependency parse tree. Here these patterns are represented by the shortest paths of four links or less between any two nouns in a dependency tree. These features are organized as vectors that display the number of occurrences of a given shortest dependency path between pairs of words. These features are then labeled as positive or negative examples of the hypernymy relationships and are used to train the classifier. Another work (Cimiano et al., 2005) relies on a blended approach for learning taxonomies based mainly on lexico-syntactic patterns, the Web and Word-Net. The lexico-syntactic patterns, derived from (Hearst, 1992), are based on regular expressions over part-of-speech tags. Any known hierarchical relationship between each two terms is ranked according to its frequency in the corpus (based on the frequency of the instantiated patterns between these two terms). To deal with the data scarcity problem, (Cimiano et al., 2005) uses the Web to gain more evidence on the hypernymy link. For each pair of terms, the lexico-syntactic patterns are instantiated and sent as queries to Google. The number of hits returned by Google constitutes an evidence of the existence of the hypernymy link. The internal structure of noun phrases (also called string inclusion) may also help to identify taxonomic relations (Velardi et al., 2007). (Cimiano et al., 2005) use supervised machine-learning techniques to derive an optimal combination of the different features.

Finally, regarding concept (or semantic class) learning, many works try to induce semantic classes based on the notion of syntactic context similarity. (Lin & Pantel, 2001) proposed a clustering algorithm, UNICON, which creates lists of similar or related words while taking into account their various senses. UNICON relies on a collocation database where each word is linked to a feature vector composed of the dependency relationships that involve the word as well as their frequency of occurrence. These features are then used to compute the similarity between the words, based on the distributional hypothesis: the more syntactic contexts two words share, the more similar they are. In (Pantel & Lin, 2002), the same approach is reused by the *Clustering by Committee* algorithm. However, it is enhanced by relying on the notion of committees, i.e. sets of representative words for each class. Using these representative elements, (Pantel & Lin, 2002) are able to computer cluster centroids, which describe the members of a possible class in an unambiguous way.

In general, the extraction of semantic classes using this kind of approach goes in pair with the extraction of taxonomical links. For example, (Pantel & Ravichandran, 2004) algorithm is based on co-occurrence statistics of semantic classes discovered by algorithms like *Clustering by Committee* to label their concepts. Once a class and its instances are discovered, it is then possible to create a hyponym relationship between the class and its instances.

5. ONTOLOGIZING THE KNOWLEDGE

As we have seen, there are many approaches that rely on dependency grammars and lexico-syntactic patterns to extract relevant knowledge from texts. Some of these approaches may be purely NLP-based, but in general they rely on a mix of NLP and statistical/machine learning methods. Patterns may be organized as flat lists of structures such as what have been proposed by the majority of the works but also as hierarchies (Zouaq & Nkambou, 2009) or even grammars (Zouaq et al., 2010). The interest of these two structures is to avoid redundancy or inadequate understanding of some syntactic structures, but

also to come up with formal representations of the language (here English). From the NLP side, the employed methods may be shallow methods, such as matching regular expressions over parts-of-speech (Cimiano et al., 2005) or deep syntactic methods that rely on a syntactic parser. Approaches may also be divided between those where patterns are completely hand-built (Zouaq et al., 2010) (Kim et al., 2009), and those which discover automatically these patterns (Pantel & Pennacchiotti, 2008) and evaluate their efficiency. This automatic discovery of patterns should generally be filtered in order to keep only the most accurate ones. Using the Web at this stage to discover new patterns and ascertain the correctness of the discovered ones is a very interesting approach. It provides statistical evidence regarding the correctness of a pattern that corpora are unable to provide due to their size (which cannot compete with the Web).

As we have seen, the previous sections have dealt with the issue of semantic analysis and knowledge extraction from text. Many representation structures may result from semantic analysis, including concept maps, logical forms and discourse representation structures. These representations generally stay at the lexical level, meaning that their basic elements are lexical items, or they might be indexed by semantic roles, in case an ontology/dictionary/lexicon is given to annotate the representations. Therefore, there is a need of discovering structures, hierarchies and clusters in the extracted representations for an effective learning of the ontology (Section 4.4. has already offered a glimpse over this issue).

5.1. The "Ontologization" Task

The difficulty lies here in the ability to build a bridge between the language level and the abstract/conceptual level. This is referred to as the *ontologization* of the extracted knowledge. In fact, there are many reasons for considering this step as the most important one for ontology learning. First, the ability to extract "concepts" from factual data and linking them through conceptual relationships is vital for the production of ontological classes and properties with domain and ranges. Second, most of the automatic approaches for semantic analysis and knowledge extraction generate a lot of noisy data, due to improper syntactic or semantic analysis, or due to a noisy corpus (language issues for e.g.), etc. This ontologization may then be considered as a filtering step.

There have been a raise of interest regarding this issue with many researchers e.g. (Barker et al., 2007) (Pantel & Pennacchiotti, 2008) (Zouaq & Nkambou, 2009) trying to come up with methods and metrics to solve the problem. Basically, these methods may be divided into methods built on statistics and machine learning and methods based on metrics.

5.2. Ontologization through Statistics and Machine Learning

In general, this notion of ontologization may cover two different situations, namely, the ability to find structures/classes in the representations, or the ability to relate the representations to available ontologies. For example, Espresso (Pantel & Pennacchiotti, 2008) focuses on the ontologization of extracted relations. For any relation (x; r; y) between terms x and y, the ontologization task is to identify the WordNet senses of x and y where r holds. From a set of reliable patterns, the algorithm uses a clustering method for ontologizing the extracted relations. (Pantel & Pennacchiotti, 2008) give the following example: Given two instances of the "part-of" relationship: (second section, PART-OF, Los Angeles-area news) and (*Sandag study, PART-OF, report*), the algorithm categorizes them into a common semantic cluster [*writing#2, PART-OF, message#2*]. This categorization uses a metric based on WordNet taxonomy (*writing#2 is a hypernym of both section and study, and message#2 is a hypernym of news and report*) and frequency scores that enable to select the best cluster for each instance. Kleo (Kim et al., 2009)

also relies on an established knowledge base, the Component Library and WordNet, to ontologize the knowledge.

There are also highly supervised machine learning approaches for the task of ontologizing relationships. These approaches suffer from their dependence upon hand-labeled examples, but they may lead to very accurate results. For example, (Gurju et al., 2006) proposes a machine-learning algorithm that learns selectional restrictions from a set of examples. These restrictions are then used to filter the correct patterns. In general, all the clustering algorithms may be considered in this step.

5.3. Ontologization through Metrics

The ontologization through metrics might come as a complement to the previous one (based on machine-learning) or it might be used alone. Many metrics are based on the notion of semantic distance and many algorithms calculate this distance. For example, Espresso (Pantel & Pennacchiotti, 2008) uses also the anchor approach for identifying the ontologized relations. The anchor approach is based on the distributional similarity principle, which states that words which occur in same contexts will tend to have similar meanings. Given an instance (x;r;y), the algorithm fixes first the term y (the anchor) and finds all the set T of other terms that are related by r with y. Based on a similarity metric that makes use of the WordNet taxonomy, the algorithm disambiguates x using the T set. (Basili et al., 2000) also uses a metric called conceptual density to infer the semantic classes of terms involved in a verbal relationship. Again, these semantic classes represent generalizations of the verb arguments using WordNet taxonomy, and they produce a set of possible patterns for each verb. There are also efforts to find concepts using metrics from graph theory. For example, (Zouaq et al., 2009) identify the out-degree of a lexical item (the number of edge whose source is the item) as an important feature and propose to select all the concepts whose out-degree is superior to a given threshold.

6. OPEN ISSUES AND FUTURE RESEARCH DIRECTIONS

Despite the large number of research works devoted to the ontology learning task, there are still many issues that are not well-covered. Among these issues are the problem of knowledge integration and the lack of deep semantic analysis approaches.

As outlined by (Kim et al., 2009) and (Barker et al., 2007), many extracted structures are just relational triples (Banko et al., 2007) that are more lexically-based than conceptual. The notion of ontologizing the knowledge is a step towards this goal but it requires a more thorough approach.

To my knowledge, there are very few, if any, works that use one of the techniques and grammars mentioned in section 3.2.2 to understand the meaning of texts. While there has been a significant move towards deep syntactic analysis during these last years, the same conclusion does not hold regarding shallow versus deep semantic analysis. However, these approaches are the only way to build really interesting ontologies reflecting the content of texts and to integrate information from multiple sources into a single coherent unit. An interest in these questions can be observed in (Barker et al., 2007), where the envisaged future work lists many of the required semantic analysis steps. In Kleo (Kim et al., 2009), the idea of knowledge integration is evoked and relies on graph-matching techniques and on an existing knowledge base to link the new extracted knowledge to the already available one. However, I believe that relying on an existing huge knowledge base is a wrong assumption, simply because such initiatives have been taken since the beginning of artificial intelligence (Cyc, etc.) and have not proven their interest due to the huge amount of required time and efforts, and due to scalability issues. Despite

this aspect, a very interesting proposition of their work is to use abduction to add new propositions and to recover some linkage between the output logical forms, thus contributing to knowledge integration.

Another concern is related to the accuracy of the syntactic parses, especially when parsers are confronted with the diversity of Web texts. Despite major advances in the field, one cannot count on entirely correct parses. Semantic analysis systems should then incorporate mechanisms for filtering and checking the accuracy of the syntactic aspects (Banko et al., 2007) and the semantic aspects. One way to do this is to rely on redundancy across multiple texts (Wilks, 2008), and the Web, which might provide a statistical evidence of the interest of a given pattern, or extracted data. Other research works advocate the necessity of reasoning over inconsistent ontologies or repairing the inconsistency of learned ontologies (Haase & Volker, 2008) (Qi et al., 2008) which may also be an interesting avenue to further explore. There are also key questions that should be solved: how do we locate incorrect or too general axioms? How do we check property inheritance consistency?

The last question I would like to discuss is whether the Web can be used for ontology learning if deep semantic techniques such as the ones presented here are to be exploited. For a domain specific ontology, semantic analysis systems must require the use of a dedicated corpus for the initial ontological extraction. This should avoid the risk of having false information and should provide a solid ground for the ontology. A specialized corpus is also more likely to have correct grammatical sentences which should be better handled by syntactic parsers. However, the idea of exploiting the Web should not be put aside. Definitely, semantic analysis systems should use the Web coupled with statistical and machine learning methods, as a way to ascertain the reliability of their patterns, learn new patterns, filter the extracted representations, cope with the data-sparseness problem and provide statistical evidences. The Web can also be of great interest for the kind of approaches described in the shallow semantic analysis section. In fact, it is worth noting that, if statistical NLP-based approaches are to be considered, then the Web seems to be a perfect ground for powerful language models and information extraction (Wilks & Brewster, 2009).

7. CONCLUSION

This chapter presented a quick overview over NLP methods for ontology learning, ranging from very shallow techniques to deep analysis methods. It also focused on lexico-syntactic patterns based on dependency grammars that should be considered as attempts towards deeper semantic analysis. Computational semantics is built around efforts from computational linguistics, knowledge representation and knowledge reasoning. Knowledge representations such as Discourse Representation Structures should certainly be of great interest for a better handling of text meaning. This should be useful not only in the context of the Semantic Web and ontology acquisition, but also as a general framework for text understanding. Moreover, the reasoning capabilities of ontologies, which are a little neglected until now, should be further enhanced based on deeper analysis.

The NLP methods produce semantic representations that may be ultimately exported into a domain ontology. However, this implies that filtering and ranking are performed over the obtained representations to identify important concepts and relationships. This is the objective of the ontologization task, which should be considered as equally important as the NLP process. This ontologization should be based on statistical methods and metrics. In fact, NLP and statistical and machine learning are equally essential to ontology learning and may benefit to each step of the ontology learning stages, as has been shown in this paper. Finally, using the Web as a corpus for building language models, filtering

patterns, ascertaining the quality of the extracted representations and dealing with the data scarcity problem should certainly be considered as a plus. In fact, the Web is a huge resource for language usages. In this respect, it complements NLP-based approaches which are built on lexico-syntactic rules but may not be exhaustive.

Further efforts should be done to exploit the whole potential of NLP based on recent progress in the field and on the maturity of the available syntactic and semantic tools. Such efforts should certainly greatly benefit ontology learning in particular and the Semantic Web in general.

ACKNOWLEDGMENT

The author would like to thank Prof. Michel Gagnon for very interesting discussions on deep natural language processing techniques. My thanks also go to Prof. Dragan Gasevic for his comments on the paper and to anonymous reviewers. The author is supported by a postdoctoral grant from the FQRNT.

REFERENCES

Abney, S. P. (1991). Parsing by chunks. In S. P. Abney R. C. Berwick & C. Tenny (Eds.), *Principle-based parsing: Computation and psycholinguistics*, (pp. 257–278). Dordrecht, The Netherlands: Kluwer.

Baker, C. F., Fillmore, C. J., & Lowe, J. B. (1998). The Berkeley FrameNet project. In *Proceedings of the COLING-ACL*, Montreal, Canada

Banko, M., Cafarella, M. J., Soderland, S., Broadhead, M., & Etzioni, O. (2007). Open information extraction from the Web. In [ACM.]. *Proceedings of IJCAI, 2007*, 68–74.

Barker, K., Agashe, B., Chaw, S. Y., Fan, J., Glass, M., & Hobbs, J. … Yeh, P. (2007). Learning by reading: A prototype system, performance baseline and lessons learned. In *Proceedings of Twenty-Second National Conference on Artificial Intelligence*, (pp. 280-286). AAAI Press.

Basili, R., Pazienza, M. T., & Vindigni, M. (2000). Corpus-driven learning of event recognition rules. In *Proceedings of Workshop on Machine Learning for Information Extraction held in conjunction with the 14th European Conference on Artificial Intelligence (ECAI-00),* Berlin, Germany, 2000.

Bender, E. M., Sag, I. A., & Wasow, T. (2003). *Syntactic theory: A formal introduction, 2nd edition, instructor's manual.* CSLI Publications. Retrieved July 23rd, 2010, from http://hpsg.stanford.edu/book/slides/index.html

Bos, J. (2008a). Introduction to the shared task on comparing semantic representations. In J. Bos & R. Delmonte (Eds.), *Semantics in Text Processing. STEP 2008 Conference Proceedings, volume 1 of Research in Computational Semantics,* (pp. 257–261). College Publications.

Bos, J. (2008b). Wide-coverage semantic analysis with Boxer. In J. Bos & R. Delmonte (Eds.), *Semantics in Text Processing. STEP 2008 Conference Proceedings, volume 1 of Research in Computational Semantics,* (pp. 277–286). College Publications.

Bos, J. (2008c). Computational semantics and knowledge engineering. *Proceedings of EKAW, 2008,* 4–5.

Briscoe, E., & Carroll, J. (2006). Evaluating the accuracy of an unlexicalized statistical parser on the PARC DepBank. In *Proceedings of the COLING/ACL 2006 Main Conference Poster Sessions,* Sydney, Australia. (pp. 41-48).

Buitelaar, P., & Cimiano, P. (Eds.). (2008). *Ontology learning and population: Bridging the gap between text and knowledge. Frontiers in Artificial Intelligence and Applications Series (Vol. 167).* IOS Press.

Buitelaar, P., Cimiano, P., & Magnini, B. (2005). Ontology learning from text: An overview. In Buitelaar, P., Cimiano, P., & Magnini, B. (Eds.), *Ontology learning from text: Methods, applications and evaluation* (pp. 3–12). IOS Press.

Bunescu, R., & Mooney, R. (2005). A shortest path dependency kernel for relation extraction. In *Proceedings of the Human Language Technology Conference and Conference on Empirical Methods in Natural Language Processing,* (pp. 724–731). ACL.

Church, K. W., & Hanks, P. (1990). Word association norms, mutual information and lexicography. In *Proceedings of the 27th Annual Conference of the Association of Computational Linguistics,* (pp. 22-29). MIT Press.

Cimiano, P., Pivk, A., Schmidt-Thieme, L., & Staab, S. (2005). Learning taxonomic relations from heterogeneous sources of evidence. In Buitelaar, P., Cimiano, P., & Magnini, B. (Eds.), *Ontology learning from text: Methods, evaluation and applications* (pp. 59–73). IOS Press.

Cimiano, P., & Völker, J. (2005). Text2Onto. *NLDB, 2005,* 227–238.

De Marneffe, M.-C., MacCartney, B., & Manning, C. D. (2006). Generating typed dependency parses from phrase structure parses. In *Proceedings of LREC,* (pp. 449-454). ELRA.

English, J., & Nirenburg, S. (2007). Ontology learning from text using automatic ontological-semantic text annotation and the Web as the corpus. *Proceedings of the AAAI 2007 Spring Symposium Series on Machine Reading.* Retrieved from http://www.aaai.org/Papers/Symposia/Spring/2007/SS-07-06/SS07-06-008.pdf

Etzioni, O., Cafarella, M. J., Downey, D., Kok, S., Popescu, A., & Shaked, T. … Yates, A. (2004). Web-scale information extraction in Knowitall: Preliminary results. In *Proceedings of WWW* (pp. 100-110).

Fellbaum, C. (1998). *WordNet: An electronic lexical database*. MIT Press.

Gildea, D., & Jurafsky, D. (2002). Automatic labeling of semantic roles. *Computational Linguistics*, *28*(3), 245–288. doi:10.1162/089120102760275983

Girju, R., Badulescu, A., & Moldovan, D. (2006). Automatic discovery of part-whole relations. *Computational Linguistics*, *32*(1), 83–135.

Giuglea, A., & Moschitti, A. (2006). Shallow semantic parsing based on FrameNet, VerbNet and PropBank. In *Proceedings of 17th European Conference on Artificial intelligence*, (pp. 563-567). IOS Press.

Greenwood, M. A., Stevenson, M., Guo, Y., Harkema, H., & Roberts, A. (2005). Automatically acquiring a linguistically motivated genic interaction extraction system. In *Proceedings of the 4th Learning Language in Logic workshop* (LLL05), Bonn, Germany.

Gruber, T. (1993). A translation approach to portable ontology specifications. *Knowledge Acquisition*, *5*(2), 199–220. doi:10.1006/knac.1993.1008

Guarino, N. (1998). *Formal ontology in Information Systems*. IOS Press.

Haase, P., & Völker, J. (2008). Ontology learning and reasoning - dealing with uncertainty and inconsistency. In *Proceedings of the Workshop on Uncertainty Reasoning for the Semantic Web*, (pp. 366-384). Berlin/Heidelberg, Germany: Springer.

Hearst, M. A. (1992). Automatic acquisition of hyponyms from large text corpora. In *Proceedings of COLING*, (pp. 539-545).

Jurafsky, D., & James, H. M. (2009). *Speech and language processing: An introduction to natural language processing, speech recognition, and computational linguistics* (2nd ed.). Prentice-Hall.

Kamp, H., & Reyle, U. (1993). From discourse to logic. In *Model-theoretic semantics of natural language, formal logic and discourse representation theory, studies in linguistics and philosophy*.

Kim, D., Barker, K., & Porter, B. (2009). Knowledge integration across multiple texts. In *Proceedings of the Fifth International Conference on Knowledge Capture (KCAP2009)*, (pp. 49-56). ACM.

Klein, D., & Manning, C. D. (2003). Accurate unlexicalized parsing. *Proceedings of the 41st Meeting of the Association for Computational Linguistics*, (pp. 423-430).

Kübler, S., McDonald, R. T., & Nivre, J. (2009). *Dependency parsing*. Morgan & Claypool Publishers.

Li, X., & Roth, D. (2001). Exploring evidence for shallow parsing. In *Proceedings of the 2001 Workshop on Computational Natural Language Learning - Volume 7. Annual Meeting of the ACL*, (pp.1-7). ACL.

Lin, D., & Pantel, P. (2001). Induction of semantic classes from natural language text. In *Proceedings of ACM Conference on Knowledge Discovery and Data Mining*, (pp. 317-322). ACM.

Lin, D., Zhao, S., Qin, L., & Zhou, M. (2003). Identifying synonyms among distributionally similar words. In. *Proceedings of, IJCAI-03*, 1492–1493.

Maedche, A., & Staab, S. (2001). Ontology learning for the Semantic Web. *IEEE Journal on Intelligent Systems*, *16*(2), 72–79. doi:10.1109/5254.920602

Maedche, A., & Volz, R. (2001). The ontology extraction maintenance framework Text-To-Onto. In *Proceedings of the Workshop on Integrating Data Mining and Knowledge Management.*

McDowell, L., & Cafarella, M. J. (2008). Ontology-driven, unsupervised instance population. *Journal of Web Semantics, 6*(3), 218–236. doi:10.1016/j.websem.2008.04.002

Mihalcea, R., Chklovski, T., & Kilgarriff, A. (2004). The Senseval-3 English Lexical Sample Task, in Proc. of Senseval-3, pp. 25--28, Spain.

Nanas, N., Uren, V., & de Roeck, A. (2003). *A comparative study of term weighting methods for information filtering.* KMi, (Technical report no. KMI-TR-128).

Nivre, J. (2005). *Dependency grammar and dependency parsing.* Last retrieved from http://stp.ling.uu.se/~nivre/docs/05133.pdf

Pantel, P., & Lin, D. (2002). Discovering word senses from text. In *Proceedings of ACM SIGKDD Conference on Knowledge Discovery and Data Mining,* 2002 (pp. 613-619). Edmonton, Canada.

Pantel, P., & Pennacchiotti, M. (2008). Automatically harvesting and ontologizing semantic relations. In Buitelaar, P., & Cimiano, P. (Eds.), *Ontology learning and population: Bridging the gap between text and knowledge* (pp. 171–195). IOS Press.

Pantel, P., & Ravichandran, D. (2004). Automatically labeling semantic classes. In *Proceedings of Human Language Technology- North American Association for Computational Linguistics,* (pp. 321-328). ACL.

Pease, A., Niles, I., & Li, J. (2002). *The suggested upper merged ontology: A large ontology for the Semantic Web and its applications.* In Working Notes of the AAAI-2002 Workshop on Ontologies and the Semantic Web, (pp. 7-10). AAAI Press.

Qi, G., Haase, P., Huang, Z., Ji, Q., Pan, J. Z., & Völker, J. (2008). A kernel revision operator for terminologies - algorithms and evaluation. In *Proceedings of the International Semantic Web Conference,* (pp. 419-434). Springer-Verlag.

Sag, I., Wasow, T., & Bender, E. (2003). *Syntactic theory: A formal introduction* (2nd ed.). CSLI.

Salton, G., & Buckley, C. (1988). Term-weighting approaches in automatic text retrieval. *Information Processing & Management, 24*(5), 515–523. doi:10.1016/0306-4573(88)90021-0

Snow, R., Jurafsky, D., & Ng, A. Y. (2004). Learning syntactic patterns for automatic hypernym discovery. *Advances in Neural Information Processing Systems, 17,* 1297–1304.

Steedman, M. (2001). *The syntactic process.* MIT Press.

Stevenson, M., & Greenwood, M. A. (2009). Dependency pattern models for information extraction. [Springer]. *Journal of Research on Language & Computation, 7*(1), 13–39. doi:10.1007/s11168-009-9061-2

Sudo, K., Sekine, S., & Grishman, R. (2001). Automatic pattern acquisition for Japanese information extraction. In *Proceedings of the Human Language Technology,* (pp. 1-7). ACL.

Sudo, K., Sekine, S., & Grishman, R. (2003). An improved extraction pattern representation model for automatic IE pattern acquisition. In *Proceedings of the 41st Annual Meeting of the Association for Computational Linguistics (ACL-03),* Sapporo, Japan, (pp. 224–231).

Velardi, P., Cucchiarelli, A., & Petit, M. (2007). A taxonomy learning method and its application to characterize a scientific Web community. *IEEE Transactions on Knowledge and Data Engineering, 19*(2), 180–191. doi:10.1109/TKDE.2007.21

Wilks, Y. (2008). The Semantic Web: Apotheosis of annotation, but what are its semantics? *IEEE Intelligent Systems, 23*(3), 41–49. doi:10.1109/MIS.2008.53

Wilks, Y., & Brewster, C. (2009). Natural language processing as a foundation of the Semantic Web. [Now Publishers Inc.]. *Foundations and Trends in Web Science, 1*(3-4), 199–327.

Yangarber, R. (2003). Counter-training in the discovery of semantic patterns. In *Proceedings of the 41st Annual Meeting of the Association for Computational Linguistics* (ACL-03), (pp. 343–350). ACL.

Zhang, Z., Iria, J., Brewster, C., & Ciravegna, F. (2008). A comparative evaluation of term recognition algorithms. *Proceedings of the Sixth International Language Resources and Evaluation*, (pp. 2108-2113). ELRA.

Zouaq, A. (2008). *An ontological engineering approach for the acquisition and exploitation of knowledge in texts.* PhD Thesis, University of Montreal (in French).

Zouaq, A., Gagnon, M., & Ozell, B. (2010). Semantic analysis using dependency-based grammars and upper-level ontologies. [Bahri Publications.]. *International Journal of Computational Linguistics and Applications, 1*(1-2), 85–101.

Zouaq, A., & Nkambou, R. (2009). Evaluating the generation of domain ontologies in the Knowledge Puzzle Project. *IEEE Transactions on Knowledge and Data Engineering, 21*(11), 1559–1572. doi:10.1109/TKDE.2009.25

ADDITIONAL READING

Brewster, C., Jupp, S., Luciano, J. S., Shotton, D., Stevens, R.D., Zhang. Z. (2009).

Cimiano, P., Reyle, U., & Šarić, J. (2005). Ontology-driven discourse analysis for information extraction. *Data & Knowledge Engineering, 55*(1), 59–83. doi:10.1016/j.datak.2004.11.009

Clark, P., & Harrison, P. (2008). Boeing's NLP System and the Challenges of Semantic Representation. In J. Bos & R. Delmonte (Eds.), *Semantics in Text Processing. STEP 2008 Conference Proceedings*, Volume 1 of Research in Computational Semantics, pp. 263–276. College Publications.

Copestake, A., Flickinger, D., Sag, I. A., & Pollard, C. (2005). Minimal Recursion Semantics: An introduction. *Journal of Research on Language and Computation, 3*(2–3), 281–332. doi:10.1007/s11168-006-6327-9

Davulcu, H., Vadrevu, S., Nagarajan, S., & Ramakrishnan, I. V. (2003). OntoMiner: Bootstrapping and Populating Ontologies from Domain-Specific Web Sites. *IEEE Intelligent Systems, 18*(5), 24–33. doi:10.1109/MIS.2003.1234766

Dellschaft, K., & Staab, S. (2008). Strategies for the Evaluation of Ontology Learning. In Proceeding of the 2008 Conference on ontology Learning and Population: Bridging the Gap between Text and Knowledge P. Buitelaar and P. Cimiano, Eds. Frontiers in Artificial Intelligence and Applications, vol. 167. IOS Press, pp. 253-272.

Flexible semantic composition with DUDES. In *Proceedings of the Eighth international Conference on Computational Semantics*, H. Bunt, V. Petukhova, and S. Wubben, Eds. ACL Workshops. Association for Computational Linguistics, Morristown, NJ, 272-276.

Issues in learning an ontology from text. *BMC Bioinformatics* 10(S-5). Callaway, C. B. (2008).

Navigli, R., Velardi, P., & Gangemi, A. (2003). Ontology Learning and Its Application to Automated Terminology Translation. *IEEE Intelligent Systems, 18*(1), 22–31. doi:10.1109/MIS.2003.1179190

Sánchez, D., & Moreno, A. (2008). Learning non-taxonomic relationships from web documents for domain ontology construction. *Data & Knowledge Engineering, 64*(3), 600–623. doi:10.1016/j. datak.2007.10.001

Stevenson, M., & Greenwood, M. A. (2005). A semantic approach to IE pattern induction. In *Proceedings of the 43rd Annual Meeting of the Association for Computational Linguistics*, pp. 379–386, ACL.

The TextCap Semantic Interpreter. In J. Bos & R. Delmonte (Eds.), *Semantics in Text Processing. STEP 2008 Conference Proceedings*, Volume 1 of Research in Computational Semantics, pp. 327–342. College Publications. Cimiano, P. (2009).

Völker, J., Hitzler, P., & Cimiano, P. (2007). Acquisition of OWL DL Axioms from Lexical Resources. In *Proceedings of the 4th European Semantic Web Conference*, pp. 670-685. Springer.

Wong, W. (2009), "Learning Lightweight Ontologies from Text across Different Domains using the Web as Background Knowledge". Doctor of Philosophy thesis, University of Western Australia.

Zouaq, A., & Nkambou, R. (2008). Building Domain Ontologies from Text for Educational Purposes. *IEEE Transactions on Learning Technologies, 1*(1), 49–62. doi:10.1109/TLT.2008.12

KEY TERMS AND DEFINITIONS

Ontology: an ontology is an explicit conceptualization which identifiers classes, taxonomical links, relationships and axioms.

Ontology Learning: designates the process of acquiring an ontology from a knowledge source.

Natural Language Processing: designates the various techniques that parse natural language to extract representations usable by machines.

Shallow Syntactic Analysis: includes shallow methods such as parts-of-speech tagging and phrase chunking.

Shallow Semantic Analysis: designates methods based on shallow methods for analyzing text meaning. These methods include simple patterns such as regular expressions.

Deep Semantic Analysis: is based on works from the computational semantics community which deal with complex linguistic phenomena such as co-reference resolution.

Lambda Calculus: can be considered as a glue language to combine semantic representations in a systematic way.

Discourse Representation Theory (DRT): is a theory which creates structures that deal with anaphora resolution in a discourse.

Discourse Representation Structures: are the structures that are the outputs in the DRT.

Computational Semantics: is a discipline that tries to produce deep formal semantic representations from natural language inputs.

Dependency Grammars: model the syntactic relationships of a sentence as grammatical relations between related pairs of words.

Lexicon: is a vocabulary in a given language. This vocabulary identifies how each word is used.

Chapter 3
Topic Extraction for Ontology Learning

Marian-Andrei Rizoiu
University Lumière Lyon 2, France

Julien Velcin
University Lumière Lyon 2, France

ABSTRACT

This chapter addresses the issue of topic extraction from text corpora for ontology learning. The first part provides an overview of some of the most significant solutions present today in the literature. These solutions deal mainly with the inferior layers of the Ontology Learning Layer Cake. They are related to the challenges of the Terms and Synonyms layers. The second part shows how these pieces can be bound together into an integrated system for extracting meaningful topics. While the extracted topics are not proper concepts as yet, they constitute a convincing approach towards concept building and therefore ontology learning. This chapter concludes by discussing the research undertaken for filling the gap between topics and concepts as well as perspectives that emerge today in the area of topic extraction.

INTRODUCTION

The last years have seen an increased interest in research on ontology learning, especially from *natural language texts*. Special attention has been given to texts found on the Web, as they have specific features that we will present later in this chapter. Ontologies can be seen as collections of concepts linked together through relations. Therefore ontology learning is closely connected to concept learning. Buitelaar, Cimiano, and Magnini

(2005) divide the process of ontology learning in a chain of different phases, the output of each phase being the input of the following one. An analysis of the state-of-the-art in terms of ontology learning at each of the various phases can be found in Cimiano, Völker, and Studer (2006).

In order to place topic extraction in the context of Ontology Learning process, we propose to take the reader into a descending overview of the inferior layers of the Ontology Learning Layer Cake (Bujtelaar et al. (2005)), highlighting the challenges at each step. Beginning from the observation that ontologies are dynamic, and that

DOI: 10.4018/978-1-60960-625-1.ch003

they keep evolving mainly by means of refining concepts or replacing old concepts with new ones, a special attention must be paid to the "concept" layer. Therefore, automated ontology learning is closely connected to concept learning. As shown in Cimiano et al. (2006), the main approach toward learning concepts and their taxonomy (the hierarchical relations between concepts) is Conceptual **clustering** (Michalsky and Stepp (1983)), an unsupervised machine learning technique closely connected to unsupervised hierarchical clustering. This approach generally outputs a concept tree, each level being more specific than the previous one. At each level, the collection of terms is partitioned around each concept, using clustering algorithms, thus obtaining partitions of different granularity levels: bigger under the root and smaller as we reach the leaves. Examples of algorithms developed for this purpose are the well-known COBWEB (Fisher (1987)) and the more recent WebDCC (Godoy and Amandi (2006)). While this approach is promising and has shown good results, the resulted hierarchy is still very noisy and dependent on both the quality of extracted terms and their frequency in the text collection. Therefore, researchers have tried to improve the quality by allowing the expert to validate and guide the process. Others touched the field of semi-supervised learning techniques by making the algorithm aware of external information,

Taking into consideration these preliminary observations about the dependency of the superior layers of the cake on the quality of terms, we descend another step into the ontology layer cake. At the *terms* and *synonyms* layers, new challenges arise, such as extracting pertinent, non-ambiguous terms and dealing with disambiguation. Term extraction literature proposes solutions, out of which we mention some recent ones such as Wong, Liu, and Bennamoun (2009) and Wong, Liu, and Bennamoun (2008). The purpose of the lower layers of the cake is to extract terms and regroup synonyms under the same concept and

finally defining the concepts, both in intention and in extension.

There are other approaches that pass though topics on the way towards concepts. Just like the later (see concept definition in Buitelaar et al. (2005)), topic definition is controversial. While some researchers consider a topic being just a cluster of documents that share a thematic, others consider topics as an abstraction of the regrouped texts that needs a linguistic materialisation: a word, a phrase or a sentence that summarises the idea emerging from the texts. Figure 1 presents an example of the topics that can be extracted from text. More details about some experimentation made with this system will be presented later, in section "Combining the two phases into an integrated system for extracting topics".

A topic is not a concept since it is an abstraction of the idea behind a group of texts rather than a notion in itself. While the difference between the two is subtle, evolving a topic into a fully fledged concept is still to be achieved and the reader will find a couple of ideas in the section "Conclusions and Perspectives".

In this chapter we propose to present a method of topic extraction from natural language texts, focusing on flat clustering techniques obtaining a partition of the documents at a single level. Basically, by means of Unsupervised Machine Learning, these algorithms divide the input set of texts into groups that are similar in terms of their thematics (politics, economics, informatics etc), meaning that all the texts in a group approach the same domain and there is a visible distinction between them and the texts from the other groups. We chose to present these approaches not only from the point of view of topic extraction, but also regarding their usage at the different layers in the Ontology Learning Cake.

Most of these clustering algorithms present at the output a central point for each of the created groups. This central point is often called a centroid and summarises the common part of all the documents in the cluster. The centroid can be

Figure 1. Example of output of the topic extraction system

Topic Name	Highest Rated Words	Docs covered	Text Excerpt
cocoa buffer stock	stock, cocoa, buffer, deleg, icco, consum, produc, rule, meet, council	66	The International Cocoa Organization (ICCO) Council reached agreement on rules to govern its buffer stock, the device it uses to keep cocoa off the market to stabilise prices, ICCO delegates said. The date on which the new rules will take effect has not been decided but delegates said they expected them to come into force early next week, after which the buffer stock manager can begin buying or selling cocoa. France is to provide Togo with 475 mln cfa francs of aid for a range of projects that include development of the coffee and cocoa industries and reafforestation in the south of the country, official sources said. The Coffee, Sugar and Cocoa Exchange amended regulations governing expanded trading limits on coffee, cocoa and sugar contracts to provide uniformity (...) Previously exchange rules required the first three limited months to move the limit in coffee and cocoa. It had required the first two limited sugar deliveries to make such moves for three consecutive sessions.
oil and gas company	oil, mln, ga, year, barrel, billion, lt, compani, reserv, natur	169	Kelley Oil and Gas Partners Ltd said it has agreed to purchase all of CF Industries Inc's oil and natural gas properties for about 5,500,000 dlrs, effective July 1. It said the Louisiana properties had proven reserves at year-end of 11 billion cubic feet of natural gas and 85,000 barrels of oil, condensate and natural gas liquids. Kelley said it currently owns working interests in some of the properties. Hamilton Oil Corp said reserves at the end of 1986 were 59.8 mln barrels of oil and 905.5 billion cubic feet of natural gas, or 211 mln barrels equivalent, up 10 mln equivalent barrels from a year before. Brazil will export 6,000 tonnes of poultry and 10,000 tonnes of frozen meat to Iraq in exchange for oil, Petrobras Commercial Director Carlos Sant'Anna said. Brazil has a barter deal with Iraq and currently imports 215,000 barrels per day of oil, of which 170,000 bpd are paid for with exports of Brazilian goods to that country.
tonnes of copper	tonn, copper, cent, price, mine, effect, beef, lb, meat, export	100	Mountain States Resources Corp said it acquired two properties to add to its strategic minerals holdings. The acquisitions include a total of 5,100 acres of titanium, zirconium and rare earth resources, the company said. (...)The company also announced the formation of Rare Tech Minerals Inc, a wholly-owned subsidiary. Magma Copper Co, a subsidiary of Newmont Mining Corp, said it is cutting its copper cathode price by 0.75 cent to 66 cents a lb, effective immediately. Newmont Mining Corp said Magma Copper Co anticipates being able to produce copper at a profit by 1991, assuming copper prices remain at their current levels. In an information statement distributed to Newmont shareholders explaining the dividend of Magma shares declared Tuesday ...
united food and commercial workers	unit, compani, plant, union, beef, lt, offer, contract, iowa, term	93	The United Food and Commercial Workers union, Local 222 said its members voted Sunday to strike the Iowa Beef Processors Inc Dakota City, Neb., plant, effective Tuesday. The company said it submitted its latest offer to the union at the same time announcing that on Tuesday it would end a lockout that started December 14. Union members unanimously rejected the latest company offer that was submitted to the union late last week, UFCW union spokesman Allen Zack said. Brazil will export 6,000 tonnes of poultry and 10,000 tonnes of frozen meat to Iraq in exchange for oil, Petrobras Commercial Director Carlos Sant'Anna said. Brazil has a barter deal with Iraq and currently imports 215,000 barrels per day of oil, of which 170,000 bpd are paid for with exports of Brazilian goods to that country. European Community agriculture ministers agreed to extend the 1986/87 milk and beef marketing years to the end of May, Belgian minister Paul de Keersmaeker told a news conference. He said the reason for the two-month extension of the only EC farm product marketing years which end during the spring months was that it would be impossible for ministers formally to agree 1987/88 farm price arrangements before May 12. This is when the European Parliament is due to deliver its opinion on price proposals from the EC Commission.

viewed as an abstract representation of the topic denoted by that group, a prototype. Even if highly rated features in this vector are correlated in the topic, the vector or the distribution itself rarely makes any sense to a human.

That is why it is more convenient to choose a name for it. There are multiple ways of naming a topic: choosing an arbitrary number of high rated words, selecting a document as the representative, assigning it a meaningful, human-readable expression(phrase) etc. In order to facilitate the passage between topics and concepts, we believe that the assigning phrases to the topics could prove to be the most useful, as they would serve later to construct the concepts intention. What makes a good topic name? Roche (2004) presents the problem in detail. One of the first things that must be taken into consideration is that words have the property of polysemy, meaning that the same word can have different meanings in different contexts. For example, each of the words "data" and "mining" have different meanings than the phrase "data mining". Seen from the light of these observations, we would like to allow groups of documents to overlap, authorising documents to be part of more than one group. In this way, a text that talks about the "economical outcomes of a political decision" can be part of both the "politics" groups, as well as the "economics" group.

This second phase gives the topic a linguistic materialisation. It allows to go from an abstract centroid, a prototype that summarises the common part of all documents in its group, to a human comprehensible topic.

STATE OF THE ART

Textual Clustering

Given the property of polysemy of terms, an important aspect of the synonyms layer is the identification of the appropriate sense of terms, which determines the set of synonyms that have to be extracted. Buitelaar et al. (2005) present the two main approaches towards finding synonyms:

- algorithms that rely on readily available synonym sets such as *WordNet* or *EuroWordNet* (Turcato et al. (2000); Kietz, Maedche, and Volz (2000));
- algorithms that directly discover synonyms by means of clustering.

The same authors state that "the second group of algorithms, which are based on statistical measures used mainly in Information Retrieval, start from the hypothesis that terms are similar in meaning to the extent in which they share syntactic contexts (Harris (1968))". Therefore, performing textual regrouping on the entire collection of texts, would place texts that share the same content into the same group. This would lead to synonyms to be placed in the same group.

In the following sections, we have divided the textual clustering algorithms into categories based on their ability to create overlapping groups. If terms can have different meaning depending on the context (polysemy) it is only natural to allow them to be part of more than one group. In this way, the clustering algorithm would not only find synonyms, but its output could also be used for disambiguation. It is worth mentioning that most of today's word sense disambiguation algorithms, like the one in Lesk (1986), rely on usage of synonym sets.

While some of the solutions presented below were created specifically for text mining (like LDA), others were designed for a general purpose clustering. They partition individuals into groups based on the similarity of their features. All of these methods can be used for textual clustering by representing the documents according to the Vector Space Model (as described in subsection "Vector Space Model")

Crisp solutions. Crisp clustering algorithms regroup the objects in a collection of disjointed classes forming a partition of the dataset (named "crisp" clustering). We present these three principally for didactical reasons. KMeans (Macqueen (1967)) is one of the most well-known clustering algorithms. Extensive work has been done and numerous papers proved its accuracy for various tasks. It To do this, the algorithm iteratively optimizes an objective criterion, typically the squared-error function. In the case of text mining and information retrieval, the cosinus distance can be used in order to calculate similarities between texts. Bisecting KMeans (Steinbach, Karypis, and Kumar (2000)) is a hierarchical variant of KMeans which has been proved to be more accurate than KM for the task of text clustering. It is based on a top-down algorithm that divides, at each step, the documents into two crisp sub-clusters. For instance, at the first level, the whole corpus is divided into two subsets according to multiple restarting 2-means. For the next level, one of the subsets is chosen (for example, the bigger one) and split: globally, we obtain three text clusters. The process is iterated until a stopping criterion is satisfied, e.g. a fixed number K of clusters. The final output of BKM can be seen as a truncated dendrogram. Hierarchical agglomerative clustering (HAC) in another hierarchical clustering technique used more frequently in Information Retrieval. It construct the hierarchy bottom-up and consists in merging at each step a pair of clusters.

Of course, there are many other systems offering clustering solutions, some of them even having topic extraction capabilities, like AGAPE (Velcin and Ganascia (2007)). Their main inconvenience is that they output a crisp partition, where each document can be part of only one group. While, from the point of view of the Ontology Learning Cake, they can be used for regrouping synonyms, they cannot be used for disambiguation. From the topic extraction point of view, they do not allow overlapping for the clusters, forcing a document to be associated with only one topic.

Fuzzy solutions. In fuzzy clustering, each document has a degree or a probability of belonging to all clusters, rather than belonging completely to just one or several clusters. Thus, a document at the edge of a cluster, is associated with it in a lower degree than a document in the center of the cluster. For each document d, we have a coefficient giving the degree (similar to the probability) of being in the kth cluster $u_k(d)$. Still, fuzzy logic clustering algorithms can be adapted to output an overlapping partition by choosing a threshold θ and considering that if $u_k(x) > \theta$ then the document d is in the kth cluster.

Fuzzy KMeans (Dunn (1973)) is an adaptation of the KMeans algorithm to the fuzzy logic. The main differences between the Fuzzy KMeans and the original version are:

- the way the objective function is calculated - every document contributes to the update of the centroid according to the weight associated to that cluster;
- the output of the algorithm - a vector with the probabilities of membership to clusters.

Latent Semantic Indexing (Berry et al. (1995)) is a statistical topic discovery algorithm using Singular Value Decomposition (SVD) as the underlying mathematical ground. In LINGO (Osinski (2003)), LSI is used for the clustering purpose in conjunction with the Suffix Array (Manber and Myers (1990)) frequent phrase extraction algorithm, which will be detailed in section "Combining the two phases into an integrated system for extracting topics". The main idea of the algorithm is to decompose the term/document matrix in a product of three matrices: $A = USV^T$. U and V are orthogonal matrices, containing the left and right singular vector of A, and S a diagonal matrix, with the singular values of A ordered decreasingly. If we keep only the k highest ranking singular values and eliminate the rest, along with the corresponding columns in U and lines in V, the product $A_k = USV^T$ is also known as the k-approximation of A.

It is well-known that most clustering algorithms take the number of clusters as a parameter, which is arbitrarily set by an expert. The LSI approach allows an automatic approximation of the number of clusters, based on the value of singular values of the original matrix. This is known in literature as a dimension reducing technique. Hence, in LINGO, the Frobenius norm of the A and A_k matrices is used to calculate the percentage distance between the original term / document matrix and its approximation.

The columns in U corresponding to the k highest singular values create an orthogonal basis for the document space. According to the mathematical vectorial space theory, every component of the space, in our case every document, can be expressed as a weighted sum of the elements of the base.

$$d_i = \alpha_1 e_1 + \alpha_2 e_2 + . + \alpha_k e_k$$

The elements $e_l, l \in \{1k\}$ of the base can be considered as the centers of the classes and the formula above is highly similar to the fuzzy approach described earlier, the document d_i having the probability α_j of belonging to the jth cluster.

Latent Dirichlet Allocation (LDA) (D. M. Blei, Ng, Jordan, and Lafferty (2003)) is a probabilistic generative model designed to extract topics from text corpora. It considers documents as collections of words and models each word in a document as a sample from a mixture model: each component of the mixture can be seen as a "topic". Thus each word is generated from a single topic, but different words in a document are generally generated from different topics. Each document is represented as a list of mixing proportions of these mixture components and thereby reduced to a probability distribution on a fixed set of topics.

LDA is highly related to probabilistic Latent Semantic Analysis (pLSA), except that in LDA the topic distribution is assumed to have a *Dirichlet*

Figure 2. Schema of Latent Dirichlet Allocation

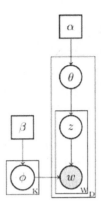

prior. This point is highly important because it permits to go beyond the main limitations of pLSA: overfitting and the impossibility of making true inferences on new documents (see (D. M. Blei et al., 2003) for details). More precisely, LDA is based on the hierarchical generative process illustrated in Figure 2.

The hyperparameters α and β are the basis of two Dirichlet distributions. The first Dirichlet distribution deals with the generation of the topic mixture for each of the $|D|$ documents. The second Dirichlet distribution regards the generation of the word mixture for each of the K topics. Each topic is then a distribution over the W word of the vocabulary. The generative process is the following: for each word $w_{d,i}$ of the corpus, draw a topic z depending on the mixture θ associated to the document d and then draw a word from the topic z.

Note that words without special relevance, like articles and prepositions, will have roughly even probability between classes (or they can be placed into a separate category). As each document is a mixture of different topics, in the clustering process, the same document can be placed into more that one group, though resulting in a (kind of) Overlapping Clustering Process. Learning the parameters θ and z, and sometimes the hyper-parameters α and β, is rather difficult because the posterior $p(\theta, z / D, \alpha, \beta, K)$ cannot be fully calculated, because of an infinite sum in the denominator. Therefore various approximation algorithms must be used, such as variational EM, Monte-Carlo Markov processes, etc.

This probabilistic approach presents advantages and disadvantages:

- The theoretical framework is well-known in bayesian statistics and well-grounded. It has led to many fruitful researches (see below).

- It is designed to make inferences on new documents: what are the associated topics and with which proportions? What part of the document is associated to which topic? Depending on the likelihood $p(d / \Theta)$, does a new document describe an original mixture of topics or a new, never seen before topic?

- LDA is a complex mathematical model, which considers each document as a combination of possibly many topics. While this may be interesting for describing the documents, in the case of clustering, it could lead to a situation where each document belongs, more or less, to many clusters (similar to a fuzzy approach). An issue is therefore to be able to choose a finite (and hopefully short) list of topics to be associated to the document, beyond setting a simple threshold parameter.

- This method does not present a center for each cluster, but a distribution of the document over the topics. This could make it difficult to associate a readable name to the cluster. Note that recent works relative to LDA are seeking to find useful names using n-grams (X. Wang, McCallum, and Wei (2007)).

- As in the other presented methods, this probabilistic approach does not solve the classical problem of finding the global op-

timum and choosing the number K of topics. For the latter, some methods are proposed inspired by the works in model selection (Rodrì guez (2005)).

Numerous works have followed the way designed by Blei et al. to deal with various related issues: extracting topic trees (hLDA) (D. Blei, Griffiths, Jordan, and Tenenbaum (2004)), inducing a correlation structure between topics (Lafferty (2006)), modeling topics through time (D. Blei and Lafferty (2006)), finding n-grams instead of single words to describe topics (X. Wang et al. (2007)), etc.

Overlapping solutions. Overlapping K-Means (OKM) (Cleuziou (2007)) is a recent extension of the well-known K-Means. It shares the general outline of the algorithm, trying to minimize an objective function. It does so by initially choosing randomly k centroids (centers) from the data set, and then iterating in two steps:

1. Assigning the documents to the clusters;
2. Recalculating the clusters, based on the new configuration; until the objective value reaches a local minimum.

The main difference of the OKM algorithm compared to the K-Means is that a document can be assigned to multiple clusters. If in K-Means each document was assigned to the centroid that was closest to it, in terms of cosine distance (detailed in subsection "Vector Space Model"), OKM calculates an image of the centroids, adding each document to clusters so that the distance between the centroid and its image is minimal. This image is the *Gravity Center* of the assigned centroids.

Therefore, the function that OKM tries to minimize is the distortion in the dataset:

$$distorsion\left(\Pi\right) = \frac{1}{NK} \sum_{i=1}^{N} d\left(X^{(i)}, Z^{(i)}\right)^2$$

where $Z^{(i)}$ represents the image of document $X^{(i)}$, N the number of documents and K the number of desired clusters.

OKM inherits from K-Means most of its drawbacks (its powerful dependence on the initialization and the number of clusters that must be arbitrarily specified by the expert) and its advantages (linear execution time, good performance when working with texts). Nevertheless, it outputs directly an *overlapping partition* of the data set, without the need of setting a threshold parameter necessary for fuzzy approaches as those presented before. This is the main reason why it was chosen for the clustering task in the topic extraction algorithm that will be presented in detail in section "Combining the two phases into an integrated system for extracting topics". This threshold, necessary for transforming fuzzy into overlapping, is highly dependent on the chosen data set.

As stated in the beginning of this section, using an overlapping solution solves 2 problems at the same time:

- synonym terms are grouped together in the same cluster ;
- it addresses the disambiguation problem, allowing terms to be in more than one cluster. This way, terms that have different meanings depending on the context can be regrouped together with their synonyms for each meaning.

Cleuziou (2009) presents wOKM, a weighted version of OKM, that uses weights internally and achieves even better performance in terms of precision, recall and FScore. At the same time, it limits the overlapping in the clusters issued by OKM, which in certain cases can be significant. WOKM is a kind of subspace clustering approach, a review of which can be found in Parsons, Haque, and Liu (2004).

Keyphrase Extraction

The first level of the Ontology Layer Cake is the *Terms Layer*. This layer is a prerequisite for all aspects of ontology learning from text (Buitelaar et al. (2005)). Its purpose is to extract relevant terms that unambiguously refer to a domain-specific concept (Cimiano et al. (2006)). Buitelaar et al. (2005) observe that although "the literature provides many examples of term extraction methods that could be used as a first step in ontology learning from text", still "much of the research on this layer in ontology learning has remained rather restricted". Cimiano et al. (2006) also considers that automatic term extraction techniques have not yet reached their maturity, since the "resulting list of relevant terms will for sure need to be filtered by a domain expert."

Topic extraction, on the other hand, shares the same need for relevant, unambiguous terms or phrases to synthesize the thematic of the group of documents associated to the topic. The algorithm presented in the section "Combining the two phases into an integrated system for extracting topics" has 3 phases for extracting topics: overlapping document clustering, term/keyphrase extraction and cluster-name association. Such a topic name is a complete phrase, that contains all the words that have a special meaning together (like "data mining") and all the prepositions and articles that make sense to the human reader ("of" in "Ministry of Internal Affairs"). A keyphrase is "a sequence of one or more words that is considered highly relevant as a whole", while a keyword is "a single word that is highly relevant" Hammouda, Matute, and Kamel (2005).

The literature presents several ways of classifying the term extraction algorithms. Hammouda et al. (2005) divides the approaches into two categories, based on the learning paradigm they employ:

- The approaches that construct the keyphrases, which is usually a *supervised learning* task, often regarded as a more intelligent way of summarizing the text. These approaches make use of the knowledge of the field expert, demanding him to validate, at each step for the incremental algorithms, the extracted phrases. While in this way the results are less noisy - only interesting collocations will be extracted -, involving a human supervisor can make the whole process slow, expensive and biased towards the specific field (e.g. microbiology). These approaches face problems when demanded to process large datasets of general purpose texts. Examples: *ESATEC*Biskri, Meunier, and Joyal (2004), *EXIT*Roche (2004), *XTRACT*Smadja (1991)

- The approaches that extract the keyphrases from a set of documents, which is an *unsupervised learning* technique, trying to discover the topics, rather than learn from examples. Not depending on a human expert makes this kind of approaches scale well to large datasets. Still, their major drawback is the almost exponential quantity of extracted phrases, most of them having no real interest for the specific domain of the application, leading to a noisy output. However, there are techniques to ameliorate their precision, some of them presented later in this section. Examples: *CorePhrase*Hammouda et al. (2005), *Armil*Geraci, Pellegrini, Maggini, and Sebastiani (2006), *SuffixTree Extraction*Osinski (2003).

Other researchers (Roche (2004); Buitelaar et al. (2005); Cimiano et al. (2006)) divide topic extraction algorithms into 3 categories, according to their employed methods: linguistic, numeric and hybrid.

Linguistic approaches. These algorithms take inspiration from terminology and *Natural Language Processing* research. They employ linguistic

processing like phrase analysis or dependency structure analysis.

In Roche (2004), three linguistic systems are presented: TERMINO, LEXTER and INTEX & FASTR. All these systems make use of morphological and syntactic informations about the words in the texts. The POS tagger (Part-Of-Speech) tries to recognize whether the word is a noun, adjective, verb or adverb, and tries to characterize it morphologically (number, person, mode, time etc). Based on this information, the lemmatisation process extract the radix of the word (masculine single - for nouns, infinitive - for verbs). With the texts tagged, each system has its own approach toward discovering the keyprases. In TERMINO, a lexical-syntactic analyser is used to describe the sentences, and then certain patterns are used to uncover the keyphrases (ex: < Head > < Prepositional Group > < Adjectival Group >). LEXTER uses the morphological information to extract from the text nominal groups and then searches for dis-ambiguous maximal nominal groups.

Keyphrase extraction methods based on linguistic approaches do succeed in obtaining less noisy output, but they are also vulnerable to multilingual corpora and neologisms. They also have the tendency to adapt to stereotypical texts (texts from a specified narrow field) (Biskri et al. (2004)). In other words, they do not adapt or scale easily to new fields or datasets. This makes them particularly difficult to work with when dealing with term extraction from texts found on the internet. Documents on the internet do not necessarily have a scientific writing style, nor do they always respect the official spelling.

Also, the use of linguistic methods leads to an almost exponential explosion of the numbers of collocations extracted when the size of the corpus increases. That is why usage of methods based only on linguistic information could prove prohibitive. Nevertheless, this could be dealt with to a certain extent by use of statistical filters (see subsection "Hybrid approaches")

Numerical approaches. These algorithms are based on information retrieval methods for term indexing (Salton and Buckley (1988)) and make use of numerical (statistical) information in order to discover the topics. For each couple of words in the text, the statistical measure is calculated. This allows to quantify the dependency between the two words in the binary collocation, also called bigram. A well-known and used such measure is the *Mutual Information*, which is given by the formula:

$$IM(x,y) = \frac{P(x,y)}{P(x)P(y)}$$

where $P(x)$ and $P(y)$ are the probabilities that the word x and, respectively, y appear in the text, while $P(x,y)$ represents the probability of the words x and y appearing together as neighbours. This allows us to calculate the correlation between two words that are one next to the other or in a window of specified dimensions. In Anaya-Sánchez, Pons-Porrata, and Berlanga-Llavori (2008), a window of dimension 11 is considered around a word (5 words before + word + 5 words after). Once we have the tool for extracting bigrams from the text, some authors (EXIT Roche (2004), ESATEC Biskri et al. (2004)) propose ways of constructing ngrams, by combining iteratively the bigrams or adding to an existing (n-1)gram another word, trying to obtain longer collocations that have a higher *Mutual Information* score.

Of course, many statistical measures have been proposed to calculate the strength of the relationship between two words. In Anaya-Sánchez et al. (2008) the algorithm first identifies a set of terms that are frequent (over a minimum threshold). Then, a set of pairs of these terms is created, retaining only the ones that score a minimum frequency. The β-similarity is calculated just for these pairs, and the set of documents for which the pair is representative is constructed. In Silva,

Dias, Guilloré, and Pereira (1999), Dias, Guilloré, and Lopes (2000), the authors consider that a special "glue" exists between words that make them have a sense when they are placed together. LocalMaxs is used in conjuncture with the Symmetric ConditionalProbability (SCP) measure to extract Continuous Multiple Word Units and with the Mutual Expectation (ME) measure for extracting Non-Continuous Multiple Word Units. Thanopoulos, Fakotakis, and Kokkinakis (2002) start from the idea that all n-grams can be constructed from bigrams and it is important to know what measure to use. They study the impact of some of the most known and used measures on the algorithm's performance, judging their ability to identify lexically associated bigrams. The measures compared are: t-score, Pearson's χ-square test, log-likelihood ratio, pointwise mutual information and mutual dependency.

There are other approaches that do not rely on bigram detection and ngram construction. In CorePhrase Hammouda et al. (2005) keyphrases are considered to naturally lie at the intersection of the document cluster. The CorePhrase algorithm compares every pair of documents to extract matching phrases. It employs a document phrase indexing graph structure, known as the Document Index Graph (DIG). It keeps a cumulative graph representing currently processed documents. Upon introducing a new document, its subgraph is matched with the existing cumulative graph to extract the matching phrases between the new document and all previous documents. The graph maintains a complete phrase structure identifying the containing document and phrase location, so cycles can be uniquely identified. Simultaneously, it calculates some predefined phrase features that are used for later ranking.

In LINGO Osinski (2003), a Suffix Array (Manber and Myers (1990)) based keyphrase discovery is used. The algorithm tries to avoid extracting incomplete phrases (like "President Nicolas" instead of "President Nicolas Sarkozy")

which are often meaningless, it uses the notion of *phrase completeness*. A phrase is complete if and only if all of its components appear together in all occurrences of the phrase. For example, if the phrase "President Nicolas" is followed in all its occurrences by the term "Sarkozy", then it is not a complete phrase. Starting from this definition, right and left completeness can be defined (the example above is left complete, but not right complete). Using a Suffix Array data structure, the complete phrases can be detected and the ones that occur a minimum number of times (frequent keyphrases) populate the candidate set for the topics. A more detailed explanation of this approach is presented in section "Combining the two phases into an integrated system for extracting topics".

Hybrid approaches. An hybrid system is usually adding linguistic information to an essentially numerical system or adding numeric (statistical) information to an essentially linguistic system. This process usually ameliorates the results.

It is well-known that statistical systems (like those based on Bayesian networks) produce noisy results in the field of Information Retrieval (Biskri et al. (2004)), meaning that among the extracted candidates, most of them pass the frequency threshold and get good scores, but they are uninteresting from the topics point of view. Such expressions can be comprised of common words (articles, prepositions, certain verbs, etc) like "he responded that" or "the biggest part of the", and they bring no new information. Such phrases should be eliminated. For that, linguistic filters are very useful.

Some of the linguistic methods rely on certain keyphrase formats (like < Subject > < Verb > or < Verb > < Adverb >) to construct the result. A morphological and syntactic tagger could be used as a final phase to filter out the noise from the candidates set resulted from statistical extraction. From such a filter benefits the system XTRACT (Smadja (1991)) which is comprised of three phases. In the first phase, bigrams are extracted from a grammatically tagged corpus, using an

eleven words window. The next phase consists in extracting longer phrases if they are frequent in the text. These phrases are called *rigid noun phrases*. The third phase is the linguistic phase. It consists in associating a syntactic etiquette to the extracted bigrams (< Noun > < Verb >, < Adjective > < Noun >) and afterwards, for each bigram, it associates together longer phrases containing the n-grams obtained at the second phase.

COMBINING THE TWO PHASES INTO AN INTEGRATED SYSTEM FOR EXTRACTING TOPICS

The literature provides many examples of systems that can extract topics from texts. Mei, Shen, and Zhai (2007), for example, see the labeling problem "as an optimization problem involving minimizing Kullback-Leibler divergence between word distributions and maximizing mutual information between a label and a topic model". In this section we will present a topic extraction system constructed by using textual clustering and keyphrase extraction, proposed by Rizoiu, Velcin, and Chauchat (2010). We will follow phase by phase the chain of processing that starts with a collection of texts (on-line discussions, forums, chats, newspaper articles etc) and presents at the output on one hand the topics extracted from the collection, under the form of readable expressions, and, on the other hand, the partition of texts around the topics.

Figure 3 presents a streamlined schema of the topic extraction system. In a first phase, each of the documents in the data set are pre-processed (see subsection "Pre-processing") in order to eliminate words that do not bring any information about the thematic of the text, thus do not help in extracting the topics. At the same time different inflected forms are brought to their stem in order to increase their descriptive value. After this phase of pre-processing, the documents are represented

Figure 3. Streamlined schema of the topic extraction system

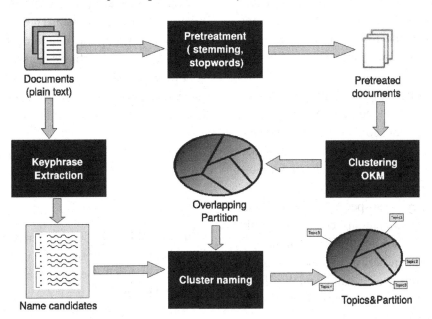

by the Vector Space Model (subsection "Vector Space Model") using one of the term weighting schemes, in order to render them compatible with the clustering algorithm.

Afterwards, the process of clustering starts, using the OKM algorithm (see subsection "Textual Regrouping"). Some of the reasons why Rizoiu et al. (2010) have chosen this algorithm will be discussed in the following subsections. With the documents now regrouped, we return to the original dataset in order to extract the complete frequent keyphrases, using the a Suffix Array based algorithm. The procedure will be detailed in the subsection "Keyphrase Extraction. Name candidates". The extracted phrases will be the candidates for the name of each topic. In the final phase (detailed in subsection "Associating names to clusters"), the best candidates are chosen to represent the topics, by means of reintroducing them into the Vector Space Model as pseudo-documents.

Pre-Processing

Pre-processing is an important part of the algorithm, as the quality of extracted topics is dependent on the quality of the input dataset and the pre-processing process. Its purpose it to augment the descriptive power of the words, limit the size of the vocabulary and eliminate certain words that are known to bring no useful information. It is traditionally composed of two elements: *stemming* and *stopwords removal*.

Stemming is the process through which inflection, prefixes and suffixes are removed from each term in the collection. It is extremely useful especially for languages that are heavily inflected (like the verbs in French) and reduces words to their stems. This guarantees that all inflected forms of a term are treated as one single term, which increases their descriptive power. At the same time, bare stems may be more difficult to be understood by the users, but since the stemmed version of the terms are never presented to the user, it will not hinder their usage. Stemming is dependent on language, but algorithms have been developed for most of the widely used languages. For English, the most used is Porter's stemmer (Porter (1980)), while for European languages one of the solutions can be that proposed by the CLEF Project[1].

Stopwords (articles, prepositions etc) do not present any descriptive value, as they are not connected to any thematic, so they are of no use for the clustering process. Even more, they only make the corpus dictionary bigger, so that computation is slower. Some term weighting schemes (such as Term Frequency) are especially vulnerable to stopwords, so their elimination is compulsory. This is done using stopword lists for each language.

Stemmed words are hard to read and stopwords improve the overall cluster names quality for a human reader. Therefore keyphrase discovery requires the texts to be in their natural form, so a non-treated version of the documents is also kept to be used for that phase. Pre-processing is the only part of the algorithm that is language dependent. Adding support for new languages is as easy as adding new stemming algorithms and stopwords lists.

Vector Space Model

As mentioned at the section "Textual Regrouping", most of the algorithms presented were not designed specifically for texts. That is why they require the text to be transformed into a specific format before it can be used. This problem has been addressed extensively in the *Information Retrieval* field and various models have been proposed: the *Boolean Model* compares True / False query statements with the word set that describes a document, the *Probabilistic Model* calculates the relevance probabilities for the documents in the set. The model that is most widely used in modern clustering algorithms is the *Vector Space Model* (Salton, Wong, and Yang (1975)).

In this model, each document is represented as a multidimensional vector. Each dimension is a keyword or a term and its value associated to a

document is directly proportional on the degree of relationship between them. There are four major ways of measuring this relationship degree, also known as term weighting schemes.

Presence / Absence. It is also known as binary weighting and it is the simplest way to measure the belonging of a word to a document. Its formula is:

$$a_{i,j} = \begin{cases} 1 & \text{if term } i \text{ is found in document } j; \\ 0 & \text{otherwise.} \end{cases}$$

In Osinski (2003), it is shown that this weighting scheme can only show if a word is related to a document, but it does not measure the *strength* of the relationship.

Term Frequency It is also known as term count. It is the number of times a given term appears in a document. While this is a better measure of the relationship between the term (word) and the document, this scheme has the tendency of favouring longer documents. In order to prevent that, normalization is usually used.

$$TF_{i,j} = \frac{n_{i,j}}{\sum_k n_{k,j}}$$

where $n_{i,j}$ is the number of occurrences of the considered term (t_i) in document d_j, and the denominator is the sum of number of occurrences of all terms in document d_j.

Inverse Document Frequency. It is a measure of the general importance of a term in the whole corpus. It expresses the idea that a word should be less important if it appears in many documents. In this way very common words, as prepositions, articles and certain verbs and adjectives could be filtered out or, at least, given less importance.

$$IDF_i = \log \frac{|D|}{|\{d \,|\, t_i \in d\}|}$$

where $|D|$ is the total number of documents in the collection and $|\{d \,|\, t_i \in d\}|$ is the total number of documents where the term t_i appears. In practice, IDF is never used alone, as it lacks the power to quantify the relationship between a word and a document. It also favourises the very rare words, which are most of the time just noise. Instead, IDF is used in conjunction with TF to bring dataset information in the TFxIDF weighting scheme.

TFxIDF. It is the most used scheme in Information Retrieval. It is the product of Term Frequency and Inverse Document Frequency.

$$TFxIDF_{i,j} = TF_{i,j} * IDF_i$$

This scheme aims at balancing local and global occurrences. A high weight in TFxIDF is reached by a high term frequency (in the given document) and a low frequency of the term in the whole collection of documents. This weighting scheme, hence, tends to filter out common terms.

Once documents are represented by the Vector Space Model using one of the schemes presented above, the similarity between two documents is usually calculated using the cosine distance.

$$similarity(a,b) = cos(\vec{a}, \vec{b}) = \frac{\sum_{i=1}^{t} a_i b_i}{\sqrt{\sum_{i=1}^{t} a_i^2} \sqrt{\sum_{i=1}^{t} b_i^2}}$$

which can be interpreted as the geometrical angle between the vectors in the multidimensional space.

Clustering

Having the documents pre-treated and represented by the Vector Space Model using one the the the four measures presented in subsection "Vector Space Model", the dataset is ready to be partitioned. At the beginning of this chapter, we have insisted on the importance of the polysemy of words and the need of term disambiguation for Ontology Learning. We have shown that one solution for addressing this problem would be the usage of an overlapping clustering solution that would allow documents to be part of more than one group. Therefore, the topic extraction system presented in Rizoiu et al. (2010) clusters the text documents using the OKM algorithm (presented in subsection "Textual Regrouping, Overlapping Solution").

The OKM implementation used by the authors Rizoiu et al. (2010) respects the original indications of Cleuziou (2007). The main difference is the stopping condition. In the original form, the iteration process comes to an end when the partition composition does not change any more - which means that a local minimum has been reached. While from the clustering's point of view the final result has been found, it does not necessarily mean that centroids do not evolve over the next iterations.

In K-Means, the centroid is computed depending only on cluster's composition. This means that if the clusters do not change between 2 iterations, neither do the centroids. In OKM the centroid update process is a little more complicated. In the documents - cluster assignment phase, OKM does not try to minimize the variance between a document and its centroid. It rather constructs *an image* of centroids to which the document is associated in such a way that the distance document - image is minimal. Therefore, in the phase of cluster update, the centroid is dependent not only on documents in their own group, but also on the other centroids resulted from the last iteration. The update formula for the centroids becomes:

$$c_{j,v} = \frac{1}{\displaystyle\sum_{x_i \in R_j} \frac{1}{\delta_i^2}} * \sum_{x_i \in R_j} \frac{1}{\delta_i^2}.\hat{x}_{i_v}^{j}$$

where $\hat{x}_{i_v}^{j}$ in the formula has the following expression $\hat{x}_{i_v}^{j} = \delta_i x_{i_v} - (\delta_i - 1)\bar{x}_{i,v}^{A\backslash\{c_j\}}$ while:

- A is the set of centroids to which the document x_i is assigned;
- R_j is the collection of documents associated to the centroid c_j;
- $\bar{x}_{i,v}^{A\backslash\{c_j\}}$ is the vth component of the image of the centroids to which x_i is assigned, except centroid j;
- $c_{j,v}$ is the vth component of the centroid to be updated.

This dependency means that centroids continue to change even if the cluster composition does not. In the process of general purpose clustering, the centroid is a by-product and the partition is the main result. But since the process of topic name assignment (presented in the next subsection) is dependent on the centroid quality, it is very important to have the centroids computed as exact as possible. That is why the iteration process should not stop when the clusters stop changing, but rather use a threshold ϵ. In this manner, the clustering process ends only when the variance of the objective function between two iterations drops under the threshold.

Keyphrase Extraction
Name Candidates

The next processing phase of the topic extraction system proposed in Rizoiu et al. (2010) employs a keyphrase extraction algorithm in order to build a topic name candidate set. Osinski (2003) presents the conditions that a collocation (or a term) must respect in order to be considered a name candidate:

- it appears in the text with a specified frequency. This is based on the assumption that the keyphrases that occur often in the text have the strongest descriptive power. Also, isolated appearances have high chances of being incorrect words (Roche (2004)).
- it does not cross the sentence boundary. Usually, meaningful keyphrases are contained into a sentence, because sentences represent markers of topical shift.
- it is a complete phrase. Complete phrases make more sense than incomplete ones (e.g. "President Nicolas" vs "President Nicolas Sarkozy").
- it does not begin or end with a stopword. Cluster name candidates will be stripped of leading or trailing stopwords, since this is likely to increase readability. Stopwords in the middle of the keyphrase will be preserved.

Both LINGO (Osinski (2003)) and the system presented in Rizoiu et al. (2010) chose the Suffix Array based (Manber and Myers (1990)) approach for the keyphrase extraction task. They motivated their choice by the approach's ability to extract the phrases from untreated text, its language independence, linear execution time and the power to extract humanly readable phrases. Also, both systems were designed to extract topics from texts found on the Internet, which requires a great flexibility and stability towards different writing styles - which can vary from informal discussions to scientific articles - and different languages. These two characteristics make dealing with texts that appear on the Web particularly difficult when using non-statistical approaches, like those presented in subsection "Keyphrase Extraction".

Suffix Array based makes use of the property of completeness (defined in subsection "Keyphrase Extraction, Numerical approaches"). The keyphrase discovery algorithm works in two steps: in the first step left and right complete expressions are found. In the second step, the two sets are intersected to obtain the set of complete expressions.

Suffix Array Construction. The algorithm of discovering right complete expressions relies on the usage of Suffix Array. A Suffix Array is an alphabetically ordered array of all suffixes of a string. We note here that in our case, the fundamental unit is not the letter (as in the case of classical strings), but the term / word. For example, having the phrase "we are having a reunion", the Suffix Array for it would be constructed as shown in Table 1.

One of the most important problems in the construction of the Suffix Array is the space-time and time-efficient sorting of the suffixes. In Larsson (1998), two approaches are presented: "Manber and Myers" and "Sadakane's algorithm". The paper also makes a comparison of the two, from both the theoretical and practical performance point of view. According to the test results of Larsson (1998), the second approach gives better results in terms of efficiency.

The only thing required for the algorithm is that the terms have a lexicographic order, so that they can be compared. If in the example in table 2, for the sake of clarity, we have used the alphabetical order, in real-case implementation, the criteria used is not important. The order of term arrival into the collection can also be used. The "Sadakane's sorting algorithm" is a modified bucket sorting, which takes into consideration the unequal dimensions of the suffixes. In Larsson (1998), it is shown that the sorting complexity is $O(n \log n)$, with n the number of suffixes. Considering that a keyphrase can not pass the boundary of a sentence, the implementation in Rizoiu et al. (2010) differs from that proposed in Osinski (2003) in that it constructs the Suffix Array on a sentence based approach, rather than the whole document approach found in the latter. Therefore a suffix identification is given not only by the beginning of the suffix, but also on the index of the sentence.

Table 1. Suffix Array construction for the phrase "we are having a reunion"

No	Suffix	Start Pos
1	a reunion	4
2	are having a reunion	2
3	having a reunion	3
4	reunion	5
5	we are having a reunion	1

Complete Phrase Discovery. The general idea behind the right complete keyphrase discovery algorithm is to linearly scan the suffix array in search for frequent prefixes, counting their occurrences meanwhile. Once such a prefix is identified, information about its position and frequency (initially the frequency is 2) is stored along with it.

Once the right complete phrases have been discovered, we also need to discover the left complete phrases. This can be achieved by applying the same algorithm as before to the inverse of the document - meaning that another version of the document is created, having the words in reverse order. While the algorithm finds the right complete phrases in lexicographic order, the left complete set needs another inversion to recover the right order.

Since both sets are in lexicographic order, they can be intersected in linear time. Name candidates are returned along with their frequency. We must note here that the extracted candidates can also be single terms, as sometimes a single word can be enough for explaining the content of the cluster (Osinski (2003)).

The last phase is filtering the candidate set. First, only phrases that appear in the texts with minimum frequency are kept, the rest are eliminated. In Osinski (2003), the value of this threshold is suggested to be between 2 and 5. The relatively low value for it can be explained by the fact that the most frequent expressions are not necessarily the most expressive, but usually they are meaningless expressions - noise in the output.

Afterwards, candidates are filtered based on one of the conditions that we enumerated at the beginning of this subsection: *not to begin or to end with a stopword*. Using the same methods as in the pre-processing phase, leading and trailing stopwords are recursively eliminated from the phrases. As a result some of the candidates disappeared completely (they were composed only from stopwords), while others reduced their form to another one (example: "the president" and "president of" become both "president").

Associating Names to Clusters

The clustering phase outputs a data partition that regroups documents relatively by their thematic similarity. At the same time, this phase outputs the centres of each class, also called centroids, which can be regarded as abstract representations of the topics. These centres are documents in the Vector Space Model, having a high weight for the terms that are specific to the group, i.e. the words that are characteristic for the specific topic.

On the other hand, the keyphrase extraction phase generates a list of name candidates for the topics. In this last phase, a suitable name is chosen for each centroid in order to label the topics. This 'centroid - name' association is done by taking all the name candidates and reintroducing them into the Vector Space Model document collection as "pseudo-documents". Initially, the same pre-processing as to the original documents is applied, because the keyphrases were extracted from natural language texts so they may contain inflected words and stopwords. Afterwards, they are translated into the Vector Space Model, using the same term weighting scheme as for the original documents of the collection. The last step is to calculate the similarity between each of these "pseudo-documents" and the centroid of the class. The one that scores the highest is chosen to be the cluster name.

This phase filters out the noise from the keyphrase candidate set. While centroids are

the essence of the documents in those classes, choosing the candidates that are closest to them naturally eliminates phrases that are too general. For example: in a document group that talks mainly about politics, the most important terms (measured with a *term weighting scheme*) should naturally be "parliament", "govern", "president", "party", "politics" etc. When calculating the similarity (cosine similarity) between this centroid and the phrase candidates, it is natural that a candidate that contains many of those words would be favoured. The phrase "presidential elections" would clearly score higher than the phrase "as a matter of fact the".

This candidate pruning side-effect resembles the hybrid approaches presented in the subsection "Keyphrase Extraction", without the actual linguistic filter. From such a linguistic-free approach, which is more suitable for text extracted from the Web, could surely benefit the Term Extraction layer from the Ontology Learning Layer Cake.

Experiments and Results

In this subsection we will briefly present some experiments and results that can be obtained with this system. The English dataset used in these tests is a sub-partition of the Reuters [2] corpus, composed of 262 documents. The writing style is journal article, containing between 21 and 1000 words. The authors also used in their experiments French forums, to test the performance of their systems with languages other than English and with different writing styles.

Experiments were performed to test both the clustering phase and keyphrase extraction phase. The behaviour of *OKM* in textual clustering is experimented with in Cleuziou (2007), Cleuziou (2009) and Rizoiu et al. (2010). The authors' main approach towards evaluating the quality of the resulted partition is to use the classical precision, recall and F-Measure indicators on a corpus that has been tagged a priori by human experts. They used a sub-collection of the Reuters corpus that had at least one tag associated with. Using this method of evaluation, the authors concluded that the overlapping approach indeed out-performs the classical crisp algorithms when being used for text clustering.

The evaluation of the topic names extracted with the *Suffix Array* approach is done in Osinski (2003) and Rizoiu et al. (2010). Here, the authors have used an expert based evaluation of cluster names, arguing that there are no widely accepted automatic topic quality measures (see next sub-section). Since topic names need to be humanly-readable and they need to synthesize the thematic of a group of texts, evaluating them is like trying to evaluate "human tastes". The experiments showed a rather good acceptance by the users of the extracted topics, especially when using the *Term Frequency* and the *Presence / Absence* term weighting schemes.

Table 1 presents an output example of extracted topics. The algorithm was run on the dataset presented at the beginning of this section. It was demanded to extract four topics. The first column shows the extracted topics: "cocoa buffer stock", "oil and gas company", "tonnes of copper" and "united food and commercial workers". The second column presents, for each topic, the ten words/terms in the texts that have achieved the highest scores. These words are the most important part of the centroid of each class. As they are output directly by the clustering algorithm, they are in their stemmed version. The next two columns present the number of documents covered and three examples of documents that are part of the clusters of each topic. Let's take as an example the most important topic of the dataset, the one that covers the maximum number of texts: "oil and gas company". The first two examples talk explicitly about the economical activities of companies that operate in the business of oil and natural gas (buying oil and natural gas proprieties in the first case and estimating reserves in the second case). On the other hand, the third document talks about the food-for-oil program between Brazil and Iraq.

Despite the fact that the text does not refer to an oil company, as in the first two cases, the document is still placed under this topic. This is because it still touches the thematic of "oil and gas", as it does with the thematic of food. That is why this document is also found under the topic "united food and commercial workers".

We can see in this example how important is the overlapping property of the clustering algorithm. With a crisp approach, this document would have been only under one topic, when in fact it talks about two topics. Still, the extracted topics are too specific. Topics like "food and gas" and "food" would have been more appropriate.

CONCLUSION AND PERSPECTIVES

Over the last ten years, several approaches have been proposed in order to regroup textual datasets into homogeneous clusters and, moreover, to label these clusters with topic names. Among these various approaches, some models are able to deal with the overlapping issue. That is an important point because it allows texts to be related to more than one unique topic. Here stands an important dichotomy between a "fuzzy" approach (each text is covered more or less by the topics) and a "crisp" approach (each text is exactly covered by one to several topics). Until now, the litterature does not present a rigorous comparison between different approaches for topic extraction (such as LDA, LSI, BKM, OKM etc.) in terms of assessment of topic names. The main reason is probably that the comparison criterion is difficult to set, which is highly linked to the question of the assessment of topic quality.

In this chapter, we present different approaches in order to extract useful topic names from texts. Even if some works try to avoid such an additional step (X. Wang et al. (2007)), these techniques seem to be an improvement which permits to go beyond a rough distribution over words. The extracted phrases are often more intelligible than series of single words. They may be a key to fill the gap between topics and concepts (the topic "data mining" is not far from the concept "data mining").

The "State of the Art" section must be read from two points of view. On the one hand, it provides the ingredients for the topic extraction system presented in the second part of the chapter. But on the other hand, all these algorithms can be used at the different layers of the Ontology Learning Layer Cake. The keyphrase extraction algorithms can be used for the term extraction at the Term Layer, while the clustering techniques can be employed at the synonym layer. Here the overlapping issue seems important in the disambiguation task. Allowing terms to be regrouped in more than one cluster means, in fact, letting the different meanings of a term be put together with their synonyms.

The chapter ends with the presentation of a whole integrated system. This system addresses the problem of topic extraction from textual data. The texts we are interested in present some rather challenging particularities, like being multilingual, having very different writing styles and purposes (from informal chats to academic microbiology articles). The main advantage of this system is that it allows overlapping between the clusters of texts, so that a text could be defined by more than one topic, which is an important aspect, especially giving the property of word polysemy.

For the concept learning, this system allows an extraction of terms and phrases involving a statistics-only approach. By means of transforming the name candidates (the extracted terms) into pseudo-documents and injecting them back into the Vector Space Model, the terms can be pruned, actually obtaining a less noisy list of terms. This has a similar effect as adding linguistic filters to statistic methods, but without their language and field dependency.

With the problem of topic extraction partly solved, there still remains the most strategic issue: filling the gap between topics and concepts. For the moment, the literature does not provide

any largely accepted solution. Of course, the simplest way to do it is to have a human expert manually evolving the topics into concepts by adding relations and building the structure of the ontology. But in the long term, the objective is to completely automatize the ontology building process. That is why relations need to be found in a human-independent way. Some of the recent topic extraction algorithms already provide the means. hLDA (D. Blei et al. (2004)) outputs an hierarchy of topics, which can provide, to a certain extent, the hierarchical relation between concepts. Other algorithms, like cLDA (Lafferty (2006)) obtain a correlation structure between topics by using the logistic normal distribution instead of the Dirichlet. Some authors consider that a hierarchy of topics can already be considered an ontology. Yeh and Yang (2008) extract the topics from the text, using LSA, LDA or pLSA. Then they regroup them into super-topics, using a hierarchical agglomerative clustering using the cosine distance. They consider that "because the latent topics contain semantics, so the clustering process is regarded as some kind of semantic clustering". In the end, they obtain an ontology in OWL. Topic to concept passage is also related to other perspectives, such as reconciling the similarity-based dendrograms built by traditional Hierarchical Agglomerative Clustering and the concept hierarchies used in Format Concept Analysis. The recent work of Estruch, Orallo, and Quintana (2008) proposes in this line an original framework to fill the gap between statistics and logic. Part of the solution is to make contributions relative to the assessment of topic quality. Other works are precisely directed towards such issues (Boyd-Graber, Chang, Gerrish, Wang, and Blei (2009)).

Two other important perspectives are related to the question of granularity. The "horizontal" granularity deals with building hierarchies of topics: each level of the hierarchy presents topics which are more general than the topics of the level below. Recently, several works try to address this issue. For instance, D. Blei et al. (2004), C. Wang and Blei (2009) build topic hierarchies based on the nested chinese restaurant process. Such topic hierarchies seem to be more adapted than "flat" topics in the task of concept construction. At the same time, it brings topics closer and closer to concepts, as these hierarchies provide a relation of taxonomy. The "vertical" granularity deals with the evolution of topics through time. Several probabilistic models have recently been proposed (D. Blei and Lafferty (2006), C. Wang, Blei, and Heckerman (2008)). It would be of high interest to relate such dynamic models to other works in the field of concept learning, such as those presented by Chen, Wang, and Zhou (2009). This kind of works will certainly help to address the question of automatic ontology evolution.

REFERENCES

Anaya-Sánchez, H., Pons-Porrata, A., & Berlanga-Llavori, R. (2008). A new document clustering algorithm for topic discovering and labeling. In *Ciarp '08: Proceedings of the 13th Ibero-American Congress on pattern recognition* (pp. 161–168). Berlin/Heidelberg, Germany: Springer-Verlag.

Berry, M. W., Dumais, S., O'Brien, G., Berry, M. W., & Dumais, S. T., & Gavin. (1995). Using linear algebra for intelligent information retrieval. *SIAM Review, 37*, 573–595. doi:10.1137/1037127

Biskri, I., Meunier, J. G., & Joyal, S. (2004). L'extraction des termes complexes: Une approche modulaire semiautomatique. In Purnelle, G., Fairon, C., & Dister, A. (Eds.), *Presses universitaires de louvain* (*Vol. 1*, pp. 192–201).

Blei, D., Griffiths, T., Jordan, M., & Tenenbaum, J. (2004). Hierarchical topic models and the nested Chinese restaurant process. *Advances in Neural Information Processing Systems, 16*, 106.

Blei, D., & Lafferty, J. (2006). Dynamic topic models. In *Proceedings of the 23rd International Conference on Machine Learning* (p. 120).

Blei, D. M., Ng, A. Y., Jordan, M. I., & Lafferty, J. (2003). Latent dirichlet allocation. *Journal of Machine Learning Research, 3*, 2003. doi:10.1162/jmlr.2003.3.4-5.993

Boyd-Graber, J., Chang, J., Gerrish, S., Wang, C., & Blei, D. (2009). Reading tea leaves: How humans interpret topic models. [NIPS]. *Advances in Neural Information Processing Systems, 31*.

Buitelaar, P., Cimiano, P., & Magnini, B. (2005). Ontology learning from texts: An overview. In Buitelaar, P., Cimiano, P., & Magnini, B. (Eds.), *Ontology learning from text: Methods, evaluation and applications* (*Vol. 123*). IOS Press.

Chen, S., Wang, H., & Zhou, S. (2009). *Concept clustering of evolving data*. In IEEE International Conference on Data Engineering (pp. 1327–1330).

Cimiano, P., Völker, J., & Studer, R. (2006). Ontologies on demand? A description of the state-of-the-art, applications, challenges and trends for ontology learning from text information. *Information, Wissenschaft und Praxis, 57*(6-7), 315-320. Retrieved from http://www.aifb.uni-karlsruhe.de/Publikationen/showPublikation?publ id=1282

Cleuziou, G. (2007). Okm: Une extension des k-moyennes pour la recherche de classes recouvrantes. In M. Noirhomme-Fraiture & G. Venturini (Eds.), *Egc* (Vol. RNTI-E-9, p. 691-702). Cépaduès-Éditions. Retrieved from http://dblp.uni-trier.de/db/conf/f-egc/egc2007.html#Cleuziou07

Cleuziou, G. (2009). Okmed et wokm: Deux variantes de okm pour la classification recouvrante. In J. G. Ganascia & P. Gancarski (Eds.), *Egc* (vol. RNTI-E-15, p. 31-42). Cépaduès-Éditions. Retrieved from http://dblp.uni-trier.de/db/conf/f-egc/egc2009.html#Cleuziou09

Dias, G., Guilloré, S., & Lopes, J. G. P. (2000). Extraction automatique d'associations textuelles à partir de corpora non traités. In M. Rajman & JC. Chapelier (Eds.), *Journées Internationales d'Analyse Statistique de Données Textuelles, 2*, 213-220. Lausanne, France: Ecole Polytechnique Fédérale de Lausanne.

Dunn, J. C. (1973). A fuzzy relative of the isodata process and its use in detecting compact well-separated clusters. *Journal of Systems and Cybernetics, 3*(3), 32–57. Retrieved from http://www.informaworld.com/10.1080/01969727308546046. doi:10.1080/01969727308546046

Estruch, V., Orallo, J., & Quintana, M. (2008). *Bridging the gap between distance and generalisation: Symbolic learning in metric spaces.* Unpublished doctoral dissertation, Universitat Politècnica de València.

Fisher, D. H. (1987). Knowledge acquisition via incremental conceptual clustering. *Machine Learning, 2*(2), 139–172. doi:10.1007/BF00114265

Geraci, F., Pellegrini, M., Maggini, M., & Sebastiani, F. (2006). *Cluster generation and cluster labelling for Web snippets: A fast and accurate hierarchical solution* (pp. 25–36). Retrieved from http://dx.doi.org/10.1007/11880561\ 3

Godoy, D., & Amandi, A. (2006). Modeling user interests by conceptual clustering. *Information Systems, 31*(4-5), 247–265. doi:10.1016/j. is.2005.02.008

Hammouda, K. M., Matute, D. N., & Kamel, M. S. (2005). Corephrase: Keyphrase extraction for document clustering. *MLDM, 2005,* 265–274.

Harris, Z. (1968). *Mathematical structures of language.* Wiley.

Kietz, J., Maedche, A., & Volz, R. (2000). *A method for semi-automatic ontology acquisition from a corporate intranet.* EKAW-2000 Workshop âœOntologies and Textâ, Juan-Les-Pins, France, October 2000.

Lafferty, D. (2006). Correlated topic models. In *Advances in neural information processing systems 18: Proceedings of the 2005 conference* (p. 147).

Larsson, N. J. (1998). *Notes on suffix sorting.* (LU-CS-TR:98-199, LUNDFD6/(NFCS-3130)/1–43/ (1998)).

Lesk, M. (1986). Automatic sense disambiguation using machine readable dictionaries: How to tell a pine cone from an ice cream cone. In *Sigdoc '86: Proceedings of the 5th annual international conference on systems documentation* (pp. 24–26). New York, NY: ACM.

Macqueen, J. B. (1967). Some methods of classification and analysis of multivariate observations. In *Proceedings of the fifth Berkeley Symposium on mathematical statistics and probability* (pp. 281–297).

Manber, U., & Myers, G. (1990). Suffix arrays: A new method for on-line string searches. In *Proceedings of the first annual ACM-SIAM Symposium on discrete algorithms* (pp. 319–327).

Mei, Q., Shen, X., & Zhai, C. (2007). Automatic labeling of multinomial topic models. In *Proceedings of the 13th ACM SIGKDD International Conference on knowledge discovery and data mining* (p. 499).

Michalsky, R., & Stepp, R. (1983). Learning from observation: Conceptual clustering. In In, R., Michalski, J. G. C., & Mitchell, T. M. (Eds.), *Machine learning: An artificial intelligence approach* (pp. 331–363). Morgan Kauffmann.

Osinski, S. (2003). *An algorithm for clustering of Web search results.* Unpublished Master's thesis, Poznań University of Technology, Poland.

Parsons, L., Haque, E., & Liu, H. (2004). Subspace clustering for high dimensional data: A review. *ACM SIGKDD Explorations Newsletter, 6*(1), 90–105. doi:10.1145/1007730.1007731

Porter, M. F. (1980). An algorithm for suffix stripping. *Program, 14*(3), 130–137. Retrieved from http://dx.doi.org/10.1007/11880561\ 3

Rizoiu, M. A., Velcin, J., & Chauchat, J. H. (2010). *Regrouper les donnèes textuelles et nommer les groupes à l'aide des classes recouvrantes*. In 10ème Conférence extraction et gestion des connaissances (egc 2010), hammamet, tunisie (Vol. E-19, p. 561-572).

Roche, M. (2004). *Intégration de la construction de la terminologie de domaines spécialisés dans un processus global de fouille de textes*. Unpublished doctoral dissertation, Université de Paris 11. Thèse de Doctorat Université de Paris 11.

Rodrìguez, C. (2005). The ABC of model selection: AIC, BIC and the New CIC. *Bayesian Inference and Maximum Entropy Methods in Science and Engineering, 803*, 80–87.

Salton, G., & Buckley, C. (1988). Term-weighting approaches in automatic text retrieval. *Information Processing & Management, 24*(5), 513–523. doi:10.1016/0306-4573(88)90021-0

Salton, G., Wong, A., & Yang, C. S. (1975). A vector space model for automatic indexing. *Communications of the ACM, 18*(11), 613–620. Retrieved from http://dx.doi.org/10.1145/361219.361220. doi:10.1145/361219.361220

Silva, J. da, Dias, G., Guilloré, S., & Pereira. (1999). Using localmaxs algorithm for the extraction of contiguous and non-contiguous multiword lexical units. *Progress in Artificial Intelligence*, 849. Retrieved from http://dx.doi.org/10.1007/3-540-48159-1\ 9

Smadja, F. A. (1991). From n-grams to collocations: An evaluation of xtract. In *Proceedings of the 29th Annual Meeting on association for computational linguistics* (pp. 279–284). Morristown, NJ: Association for Computational Linguistics.

Steinbach, M., Karypis, G., & Kumar, V. (2000). *A comparison of document clustering techniques.*

Thanopoulos, A. N., Fakotakis, N., & Kokkinakis, G. (2002). Comparative evaluation of collocation extraction metrics. In *Proceedings of the 3rd language resources evaluation Conference* (pp. 620–625).

Turcato, D., Popowich, F., Toole, J., Fass, D., Nicholson, D., & Tisher, G. (2000). Adapting a synonym database to specific domains. In *Proceedings of the ACL-2000 Workshop on recent advances in natural language processing and information retrieval* (pp. 1–11). Morristown, NJ: Association for Computational Linguistics.

Velcin, J., & Ganascia, J. G. (2007). *Topic extraction with agape* (pp. 377–388). In ADMA.

Wang, C., & Blei, D. (2009). *Variational inference for the Nested Chinese Restaurant Process.*

Wang, C., Blei, D., & Heckerman, D. (2008). *Continuous time dynamic topic models*. In The 23rd Conference on uncertainty in artificial intelligence.

Wang, X., McCallum, A., & Wei, X. (2007). Topical n-grams: Phrase and topic discovery, with an application to information retrieval. In *Proceedings of the 7th IEEE International Conference on data mining* (pp. 697–702).

Wong, W., Liu, W., & Bennamoun, M. (2008). *Determination of unithood and termhood for term recognition. Handbook of research on text and Web mining technologies*. Hershey, PA: IGI Global.

Wong, W., Liu, W., & Bennamoun, M. (2009). A probabilistic framework for automatic term recognition. *Intelligent Data Analysis, 13*(4), 499–539.

Yeh, J., & Yang, N. (2008). Ontology construction based on latent topic extraction in a digital library. *Digital Libraries: Universal and Ubiquitous Access to Information*, 93–103.

KEY TERMS AND DEFINITIONS

Topic: an abstraction of the idea behind a group of texts;

Topic Extraction System: an algorithm capable of finding the topics in a collection of texts and, eventually, the relations between them;

Clustering: a technique that allows regrouping documents based on the similarity of their features

Overlapping Clustering: a type of clustering that authorises a document to be part of more than one group;

Keyphrase: a sequence of one or more words that is considered highly relevant as a whole

ENDNOTES

[1]   http://www.clef-campaign.org/

[2]   http://mlr.cs.umass.edu/ml/datasets/Reuters-21578+Text+Categorization+Collection

Chapter 4
A Cognitive–Based Approach to Identify Topics in Text Using the Web as a Knowledge Source

Louis Massey
Royal Military College of Canada, Canada

Wilson Wong
The University of Western Australia, Australia

ABSTRACT

This chapter explores the problem of topic identification from text. It is first argued that the conventional representation of text as bag-of-words vectors will always have limited success in arriving at the underlying meaning of text until the more fundamental issues of feature independence in vector-space and ambiguity of natural language are addressed. Next, a groundbreaking approach to text representation and topic identification that deviates radically from current techniques used for document classification, text clustering, and concept discovery is proposed. This approach is inspired by human cognition, which allows 'meaning' to emerge naturally from the activation and decay of unstructured text information retrieved from the Web. This paradigm shift allows for the exploitation rather than avoidance of dependence between terms to derive meaning without the complexity introduced by conventional natural language processing techniques. Using the unstructured texts in Web pages as a source of knowledge alleviates the laborious handcrafting of formal knowledge bases and ontologies that are required by many existing techniques. Some initial experiments have been conducted, and the results are presented in this chapter to illustrate the power of this new approach.

INTRODUCTION

It has become somewhat of a cliché to say that a large quantity of human knowledge is stored as unstructured electronic text. This cliché is nevertheless a true representation of the reality in corporations, governments and even in our everyday life. Indeed, we are plagued by an increasing dependence on an ever-growing body of information on the Web. Some of the common means to date for managing this information explosion include online directory and automated search engines,

DOI: 10.4018/978-1-60960-625-1.ch004

all of which rely heavily on the notion of topics. In this chapter, topics are keywords that represent and convey the themes or concepts addressed in a text document. In this regard, topics can be seen as lexical manifestations of the general meaning of documents.

The main issues that prevent the application of existing computational means to generate content-representative topics for managing information on a Web-scale are: (1) computational inefficiency; (2) knowledge acquisition and training data bottleneck; and (3) inherent challenges of processing natural language such as handling ambiguity and metaphor. Existing computational methods fill this semantic gap by exploiting knowledge handcrafted by human experts. Natural language processing for example depends on language and encyclopedic knowledge for syntactic and semantic processing, while supervised learning techniques rely on human guidance to classify documents. The problem of acquisition bottleneck in turn leads to major scalability and robustness issues. Ideally, one would like a computational method that can identify topics in a way that is not dependent on any form of human intervention. In this regard, the desirable properties of such systems are autonomy and adaptability.

In this chapter, we present a computational method that is void of any dependence on expert-crafted knowledge resources or training data. This cognition-inspired paradigm of generating topics takes the stream of words from a single document and determines the main themes addressed in that document based on overlapping activations and decay of unstructured lexical information. The lexical information is retrieved from the Web by querying Web search engines. This approach exploits the information embedded in the ordering of words but without traditional syntactic processing.

The chapter is organized as follows. Section 2 presents a case study that illustrates some of the problems with existing topic identification methods and with vector-representation of documents. In Section 3, we introduce the fundamentals of

the proposed approach to represent text and to identify topics in documents. We then present and discuss the results obtained using a prototype computational model in Section 4. We conclude this chapter with an outlook to future work in Section 5.

ISSUES WITH EXISTING METHODS

A Case Study

The issues associated with the dependence on human intervention are well exemplified by document classification (also known as document categorization) (Sebastiani, 2002). Document classification aims at approximating a classifier function f: DxC $\rightarrow \{0,1\}$ given a document set $D = \{d_1, d_2, ..., d_R\}$ and a category (or class) set $C = \{C_1, C_2, ..., C_K\}$. The categories correspond to the topics predetermined by users or experts in the application domain. The goal is that the approximated function f' meets f with an acceptable error: $|f - f'| < \varepsilon$ ($\varepsilon > 0$). The learning process is guided by a set of training documents $D' = \{d_1, ..., d_R\}$ properly labeled by a human expert. The assemblage of the training set is a laborious activity that involves selecting a large set of archived documents, reading these documents, and then assigning one or several of the labels from the set C to each. Simply put, the next step consists of applying machine learning techniques to acquire the classifier function f' from the labeled data. Assuming that the training data is representative of future data (i.e. sampled from the same probability distribution), f' should classify new unseen cases well, i.e. it will generalize. However, the generalization capability of f' is limited by the additional assumption that the data distribution will not change. In reality, this is rarely the case. New documents can skew existing probability distributions, new important words can appear and new topics will need to be created. In such situations, the classifier must be re-trained using new samples that include documents responsible for the introduction of novelty.

Hence, document categorization incurs an important initial cost to first agree on a set of topics and then to label a training sample. Furthermore, a classifier may need to be retrained with a new labeled training set when novelty is suspected. In operational text categorization systems, automated integration of novelty and elimination of the need for labeling a training set would be very beneficial properties leading to more efficient and cost effective development and maintenance (Massey, 2005).

Another major issue with text classification is that it does not take into account the underlying 'meaning' of text. In general, text classification and other discriminatory methods like clustering (Jain, Murty & Flynn, 1999) are merely looking for patterns of similarity among a set of documents represented as vectors in lexical space (Salton & Lesk, 1968). The objective is to identify subcategories in the text data, which are then deemed to correspond to topics. In other words, the underlying meaning of text is entirely ignored. A popular way to deal with the problem of lack of access to underlying meaning is to add semantic information to the documents. However, there are instances in the literature reporting worse or unimproved results (Scott & Matwin, 1999) when using semantic information for document classification. Although others have reported positive progress (e.g., Bloehdorn & Hotho, 2004; Hotho, Staab, & Stumme, 2003), there is no conclusive evidence that using semantic information rather than just words will always improve the ability of topics identification systems to arrive at the underlying 'meaning' of text. This is rather troubling and counter intuitive since one would think that the more elaborate semantic representation would immediately improve clustering and classification in all cases compared to the simple use of words.

The problem can be partly traced to the statistical properties of large text collections. Indeed, the sheer quantity of words and their distribution among documents can be deemed to be a better indicator of the relative nature of content within the collection of documents than semantic features (Scott & Matwin, 1999). Although this is a clear possible explanation, it does not solve the problem of determining documents inherent 'meaning', thus leading to better topics identification. This is an important open problem that may only be solved with advanced natural language processing techniques. However, natural language processing is dependent on intense knowledge handcrafting and is computationally expensive. Hence, it tends to be restricted to smaller-scale, domain specific applications. If we are to be able to fully exploit the human knowledge stored in large text repositories like the Web, a better approach is needed. The idea of the Semantic Web (Berners-Lee, Hendler, & Lassila, 2001) is promising in that regard. However, it comes with its own set of problems, again related to the acquisition and crafting of knowledge for the ontologies required to drive semantically-based applications.

Hence it appears we have gone full circle. One first needs to acquire large quantities of knowledge to get to the inherent meaning of text. We argue that it is possible to break away from this dependence on knowledge handcrafting by considering that one of the fundamental issues with existing classification and clustering methods is the representation of documents as vectors, whether in lexical or semantic space. The second aspect of the solution we propose here is to use existing general-purpose knowledge, as what is available on the Web, instead of specialized handcrafted knowledge.

The Vector Representation of Documents

To make the representational issue clear, we now revisit in details how both categorization and clustering represent a document in computer memory as a high dimensional feature vector $d_i = (f_1, f_2, \ldots, f_V)$. A component f_p of the vector is not storing the word w_p itself, but rather is a placeholder for w_p. The index p in any vector always stand for the same word w_p. The vectors are of fixed size V determined by the number of words in the document collection. Hence there is a requirement to have prior access to the document collection or some suitable corpus of text to extract this information. However, this information is not always available, and the fact that a fixed vocabulary is used reduces adaptability.

This way of modeling documents is called bag-of-words because the vectors are assembled based on V distinct words from the collection of documents as a whole. This is completed irrespective of the order of words appearing in individual documents. The bag-of-words vector construction process can be described as follows. First, the document collection is scanned to extract all unique words. Stop words are also removed during this process. As this is taking place, statistical information on words such as their frequency of occurrence is collected. This information can be used later to establish the numerical value of each vector elements. Words can also be subjected to morphological normalization such as stemming. Simple stemming may for instance remove the s at the end of plural nouns and bring conjugated verbs to their infinitive form. More advanced stemming could perform suffix stripping that would bring words like explosion, explosive, exploded to their common stem explo. This is done to eliminate words of the same family from the representation. The goal and assumption in many pattern-matching techniques based on this vector representation is to eliminate dependence amongst features because it tends to cause anomalies in the subsequent analysis.

As words are extracted and counted, they can be stored in any suitable temporary data structure, e.g., a hash table. Words also need to be assigned consecutive and unique integer values that will be used later as the index p in vectors. This can be done with a counter incremented as words are read from each document in the collection.

Doing so, the order of words within a specific document is lost. Once all words have been collected, the words may be subjected to further filtering to reduce their number and eventually the dimensionality of the vectors. An effective yet simple strategy is to remove words that occur in very few documents and in a large number of documents, since these words would have little discriminatory power in identifying patterns in the data (either with categorization or with clustering). In the end, the number of remaining words that will be used as features to discriminate amongst document contents can still be very large, hence the high-dimensionality of vectors.

The above steps create an undesirable coupling with the data: one must have access to the whole text data prior to processing or to another collection of documents that is representative of the text data that will be processed in the future. In many real-life applications, such as real-time text mining of social media, streaming news reports and business or military intelligence, it is not possible to know in advance all words that might be meaningful in identifying topics, as well as their statistical properties across a yet unknown collection. Obviously, a training corpus of documents can be used for the purpose, with the hope that it is representative of words to come and of their distributional properties. Still, the assumption remains that such a corpus is available, or can be assembled at reasonable cost, and that it is representative of future data.

Once all words have been extracted from the document collection, individual document vectors can be assembled. This requires that each document now be re-examined to determine which words they contain. The values of the vector elements can be binary or real. In the binary case, a one at index p of the vector indicates that word p is present in this document (p being the unique consecutive integer assigned to each of the V unique words collected over the whole collection), and zero means it is not. In the real-valued case, the statistical information accumulated while previously scanning the document collection can be used conjointly with statistical information presently collected for a specific document to compute a numerical weight for each word. The number of words in a single document being much smaller than V, the resulting vectors will be sparse (i.e. with very few non-zero values).

Problems with the bag-of-words vector representation have generated an interest in research aiming at using conceptual representations based on the exploitation of background knowledge stored in lexical databases, dictionaries, ontologies or on the Web (e.g., Hu et al., 2008; Gabrilovich et al., 2009; Milne, Witten, & Nichols, 2007). However, when preparing a conceptual representation for documents, the concepts are determined from the words in the text and decision based on the ambiguity must be made. Concepts thus suffer from the same inherent natural language problem of polysemy as the original text. Hence, concepts can be flawed right from the start based on the quality of the word sense disambiguation process being applied. Words can either be replaced by concepts or concepts added to existing word features (Hotho, Staab, & Stumme, 2003). In the first case, compared to the lexical representation with words only, semantic representation looses information. For example, a series of animal related words may be replaced by the concept animal, in which case much discriminatory information may be lost. Indeed, information on the specific animal the text was discussing is lost. In the second case, adding the concepts to the words adds non-statistically viable information to the vector-space representation and increases dimensionality. Increased dimensionality makes metrics less trustworthy (Aggarwal, Hinneburg, & Keim, 2001; Weber, Schek, & Blott, 1998) and thus less accurate result may arise.

There is an underlying assumption by many classifiers that the dataset features are independent. Dependent features can lead to less acceptable results. The conceptual representations are not crafted as to ensure independence of features, thus once again faring no better than words. The word independence assumption is totally unrealistic since texts must be constructed cohesively (Halliday & Hasan, 1976; Harabagiu, 1999) to ensure meaning is created properly as a reader processes words sequentially. This implies that a text will include words that are semantically related to one another, and thus dependent features will inevitably be included.

This is where we introduce a key concept leading to a new text representation: the power of term dependence arising from a document lexical cohesion can be harnessed for topics identification. To achieve this aim, one must abandon the paradigm of vector-space bag-of-words modeling. Consequently, without vectors, there is no issue with vector dimensionality. We thus embark on a representation for text that is, in fact, representation-less, in the spirit of embodied Artificial Intelligence (Brooks, 1991). One may object that text must still somehow be represented. Indeed, text is represented as text itself, i.e. as a series of sequential words. There is no need to scan through a corpus to collect words statistics. There is no more loss of information related to the order of words within a document. In the framework we propose, a document text is preserved in its original form as a stream of words.

COGNITIVE-BASED TOPICS IDENTIFICATION

General Principles

We now discuss the general principles behind this representation-less paradigm as a basis to determine 'meaning'. First, we suggest exploiting to our advantage the dependence between terms rather than being defeated or negatively affected by it. We then present a radically different method to determine the topics of a document directly rather than relatively to other documents in a collection as is currently common in document classification (Sebastiani, 2002), text clustering (Berry & Castellanos, 2008) and corpus based approaches (e.g., Blei,Ng, & Jordan, 2003).

In this radically different approach, words are processed online in the order they are occurring in a document. Similarly to the way humans may process information when they read, each word triggers activation of lexical information related to the word. For a human reader, the equivalent would be neural activation of word-related knowledge stored in various regions of the brain. Overlapping of such activations over time indicates the degree of conceptual commonality. In the end, the lexical information items (or in the case of humans, the areas of the brain) with the strongest activation are deemed to be the ones with the most thematic importance.

Since there is no other document to relatively determine 'meaning' with or against, 'meaning' is determined incrementally based on the internal cohesiveness of the document being processed. The 'meaning' of the text is thus computed directly and absolutely using this new approach, which is very different from existing clustering or classification techniques that require determining similarity or pattern relative to other documents. 'Meaning' is derived compositionally based on sequential processing of words in the order they appear in text and on the individual meanings of words, but without formal syntax. The meanings of words are represented strictly as a list of words present in words definitions or on Web pages retrieved for words, without any particular representation formalism or linguistic processing. Hence, the general meaning of the text, which is its topics or main themes, is computationally derived strictly from unstructured lexical information.

We emphasize that the approach we propose is not attempting word sense disambiguation. Instead of choosing one single sense for a specific word, it implicitly looks for a small set of recurring word-related lexical information across the whole document. These repeating patterns of senses are then deemed to be strong thematic indicators.

Hence, we are not interested by the meaning of single words but rather by the global interaction of these meanings leading to the global theme of a document. Meaning determination in this context is macroscopic and is about identifying the main themes of a document directly from the content of a document and general-purpose lexical information rather than by comparing its similarity with other documents as in clustering or by words distribution patterns as in classification.

In the method of meaning determination we propose here, the topics are the answer to the question: what is the document about? This answer is presented as a list of evocative keywords. It is well understood that topics can shift along a document and that a document topic may not be unique, depending on application, context of use and perception of users (Zunde & Dexter, 1969). Indeed, topics can be determined on a paragraph-by-paragraph basis if required. In our context, the human user interpretation is complementary to the computational process, even an integral part of it. Topics exist in this symbiotic relation rather than in vacuum. Precisely, topics are keywords, which are usually alphabetic string labels that evoke the nature of a document and answer the question of what this document is generally about. There is thus no complex representational scheme involved. The key is the notion of *interpretability*, that is, labels generated as topics must be evocative in a human reader's mind of the main concepts or themes present in a document.

Algorithm

A document is an ordered sequence of words w_i, $i=1,2,3,\ldots,V$. To highlight the fact that this algorithm works on single documents in isolation from others, V here refers to the number of words in a specific document rather than in a collection of documents. A word w_i extracted from a document triggers the retrieval and activation of a set *related items* $I_i = \{I_j \mid j=1,2,3,\ldots,Q\}$ retrieved from an *information source*. The information source can be any data structure that can be queried with a word w_i and capable of returning information about that word. The knowledge source may for example be a dictionary with word definitions, a thesaurus containing synonyms or a search engine index. The related items (or items for short) are simply the words present respectively in the definitions, synonym sets or Web pages returned.

The overall algorithm consists of these steps:

1. Take a text document as input and extract words sequentially from it;
2. Query the information source with the current word to retrieve and incrementally activate the items related to the word;
3. Let items activation decay if they are infrequently retrieved from the information source;
4. Repeat steps 2 and 3 until all words in the input documents have been read;
5. Once all words have been read from the input text, output the most activated items.

More specifically in the first and second steps, as each word is read sequentially, a filter eliminates function words such as prepositions, articles, etc (based on a standard list of stop words). A word that passes this step is placed in working memory (WM). The word currently extracted from text immediately triggers retrieval and activation of related items from the information source. The items associated with each word are also placed in WM along with their activation value. The activation can be calculated as an incremental adaptation of TF-IDF weights (Spärck Jones, 1972) for each item, but other possibilities exist. TF-IDF is a commonly used measure of word importance in information retrieval, but we use it here to measure the importance (or activation level) of items related to words within a single document. This adaptation of TF-IDF has the advantage of balancing frequently occurring items against those that occur for too many words of the text and that may thus have little descriptive

power. The activation α_j of item j can thus be the product:

$$\alpha_j = tf \times idf \tag{1}$$

where: $tf = q_j / Q$ (originally in information retrieval, tf denotes term frequency, but here it is item frequency) q_j is the number of times item j is retrieved from the information source, and Q is the total number of items retrieved, for all words in the current document. $idf = \log(V/v_j)$ (inverse document frequency) V is the total number of words in the document and v_j is the number of words that trigger retrieval of item j.

In our currently implemented algorithm, retrieval from the information source takes the form of a query and access to Web pages content returned by the Yahoo™ search engine. Each non-stop word is used to initiate a query. The items retrieved are an amalgamated list of words that are present in the top Web pages returned. Filtering is applied to remove any word not part of the actual content of the Web pages, such as HTML tags and advertisement data. Stop words are also removed. There is no other linguistic processing taking place. The idea here is that Web pages returned by the search engine provide information about the queried word, i.e. explanation about the general meaning or usage of that word. The algorithm thus uses the unstructured and non-disambiguated amalgamated content of all Web pages, that is, lexical information, to determine the meaning of the query word. For example, if the document contains the word button, querying for that word may return Web pages about the Formula 1 racer, the GUI component and the clothing element. No attempt is made at analyzing the meaning of Web pages: all words from all Web pages less non-content and stop words are concatenated into a single list of items.

The third step is to allow for forgetting over time. Two types of forgetting occur. Similarly to limited WM capacity in humans (Miller, 1956), a new word read will interfere with the other words currently in WM. The oldest word read is thus eliminated from WM i.e. pushed out by a new word. The second type of forgetting is the decay of items activation. However, if another word is read that activates these same items, the activation accumulates. So, recurring items augment their activation, but memory also decays when not refreshed. The algorithm relies heavily on the assumption that the text is cohesive (Halliday & Hasan, 1976). Cohesion is the property of sentences to use related terms to unify text and provide information about the main topics of the document. Hence, as conceptually related words are read from the text, they will activate some of the same items repetitively, thus boosting their activation level. On the other hand, irrelevant words are expected to cause the retrieval and activation of infrequent items and consequently these items' activation will decay over time.

We note that WM can be seen as a sliding window over the text. It consists of a pre-determined number of word positions that may match the limited capacity of human WM. Each time a new word is read, the window slides to the right to include the next word while the left-most word is expulsed from WM. The size of the window also determines the duration for which item activation is protected from decay. Thus, the window width (i.e. WM capacity) defines the number of sequential words from the document that are under the focus of attention. When a word is pushed out of WM, the activation of items associated with the word starts to decrease. Hence, without focus of attention, decay is initiated. Among multiple different approaches, decay can be calculated as follows:

$$\alpha_j(t+1) = \alpha_j(t) - \alpha_j(t) / (\eta C) \qquad (2)$$

where C is the capacity of WM, $\alpha_j(t+1)$ is the activation of item j at the next discrete time increment (i.e. the next word read from the text) and $\alpha_j(t)$ is the current activation level. η is the decay rate, a larger value meaning a slower decay and a value of 1 meaning decay occurs entirely over the window width.

This process of gradual decay ensures that only the most active items retrieved from the information source, i.e. those retrieved throughout the document from beginning to end, have the most importance. Zero activation is reached only if an item is never encountered again. If it is retrieved again, due to extracting the same word from the document later on, or due to reading another word yielding the same item, the activation computed is added to the existing residual activation.

Thus, in step 5, the items in WM that are the most active are deemed to represent the most important concepts in a document. Since the items are words from the information source, they provide human readable and evocative labels that can be interpreted by a user, as per the notion of interpretability introduced above. The set of most active topics can be those with an activation exceeding a given threshold, or alternatively, a pre-determined number of items.

Examples

We now show some actual examples obtained when processing text documents with an implementation of the algorithm described above. The top three most activated items are selected as topics.

Document 1[1]

China Daily Says Vermin Eat 7-12 Pct Grain Stocks. A survey of 19 provinces and seven cities showed vermin consume between seven and 12 pct of China's grain stocks, the China Daily said. It also said that each year 1.575 mln tonnes, or 25 pct, of China's fruit output are left to rot, and 2.1 mln tonnes, or up to 30 pct, of its vegetables. The paper blamed the waste on inadequate storage and bad preservation methods. It said the government had launched a national programme to reduce waste, calling for improved technology in storage and preservation, and greater production of additives. The paper gave no further details.

Topic produced for document 1: food production processes

Document 2[2]

Although chutney is most widely known as a condiment originating in India, the concept has spread worldwide and mutated to suit local needs as most foods do. The term chutney comes from the East Indian chatni, meaning "strongly spiced," and is described as a condiment which usually consists of a mix of chopped fruits, vinegar, spices and sugar cooked into a chunky spread. Most chutneys are on the spicy-hot side, but it's easy to adjust the heat factor if you make your own.

Topics produced for document 2: recipes food Indian

Document 3[3]

Vaccine hope over lung infection. A virus that causes wheezing and pneumonia claims the lives of up to 200,000 children worldwide each year, a study has found. University of Edinburgh scientists found that about 3.4 million children were hospitalised after contracting respiratory syncytial virus (RSV). RSV is the single largest cause of lung infection in children. The scientists hope the research will help contribute to the development of a vaccine against the infection.[...] The team hopes that by identifying the numbers affected by the virus, it can contribute to the development of a vaccine against the infection.

Topics produced for document 3: virus respiratory baby

The topics generated by our algorithm appear to be good descriptions of what the documents are about. Although not necessarily precise in nature, they nevertheless express the general idea of the text content. As such, the labels used as topics would most likely evoke in a user's mind the general nature of the document (the interpretability

notion introduced earlier) and can help decide whether or not a document corresponds to the information need currently pursued.

We emphasize that the topics produced are not necessarily a reflection of statistical importance of words in the text. Indeed, the strings used as topics may occur with low frequency in the documents and some even do not appear at all. A good example is the word food in document 1: it is a topic yet this word is not in the text. The topic labels correspond to important concepts i.e. associated with multiple words of the text, but the labels themselves are actually obtained from the items retrieved from the information source, in this case Web pages returned by Yahoo™. Furthermore, to make this point clear, in the examples shown above each word queried with Yahoo™ was removed from the list of returned items. Hence, if a word present in the text is also found as a topic, it is not because it is in the text, but rather because it is often an item retrieved for other words.

EXPERIMENTAL EVALUATION

Method

Our experiments have two objectives: First, determine how well our new topics identification approach works, and second, to establish the value of using the Web as an unstructured knowledge source. In both cases, we aim at testing the new approach in its simplest and purest form to establish a baseline for future work.

The document collection employed in our experiments is the first 802 documents of the "ModApte split" test set of the Reuter-21578 Distribution 1.0[4] (hereafter called the Reuter™ text collection for short). The Reuter™ text collection is a benchmark text collection that has been extensively used in topics identification experiments, particularly clustering and classification. We use the test set to stress the point that there is no training required. It was not possible to use the whole 3,299 documents from the test set due to time constraints related to network access to the Yahoo™ search engine and also limits in the allowable number of queries.

Documents were not subjected to any pre-processing other than removal of stop words as well as simple stemming. There was no linguistic processing: no part-of-speech tagging, no named entity recognition, and no word sense disambiguation. Additionally, words in the documents used to query Yahoo™ were removed from their respective list of returned items to make sure they do not influence the choice of topics. This is not a necessary requirement of the method, just a way to experimentally demonstrate the power of the approach in that it does not depend on the words in the text themselves but rather on the items retrieved from the information source.

To meet our first experimental objective, we compared the topics generated by our approach with k-means clustering (MacQueen, 1967) and with topics extracted using the TF-IDF top-ranked words from the text. We consider these two approaches to provide valuable baselines due to their simplicity. The quality of the results obtained with each method was evaluated against the topics generated by human experts that came with the Reuter™ collection. The popular F1 quality measure (VanRijsbergen, 1979; Larsen & Aone, 1999) was used for that purpose. A value of 1 indicates maximal quality and 0 worst quality.

By comparing with clustering, we consider the basic discriminative ability of our method. This is an important potential application, as discriminative methods like classification and clustering allow for the identification of subclasses of documents for information retrieval tasks. Although our algorithm does not output clusters, its output can be treated as a clustering (i.e. a partition of the document set), namely a set of k topic labels attributed to documents, where documents sharing the same topic label are deemed to be in the same cluster. Therefore, the

same computation procedures for F1 can apply. The value of k for k-means was set to 93, which corresponds to the experts designated number of topics. K-means results are averaged over five runs because the results are non-deterministic due to random initialization. We also generate random clusters as a further baseline for all techniques tested here. There is crisp clustering if exactly one topic is generated for each document and multiple memberships clustering otherwise. In our experiments, we will only consider crisp clustering as a baseline evaluation.

By comparing with TF-IDF, we establish a baseline for topics identification using solely the statistics of the words presents in the set of documents. In this view, the topics are not discriminative among multiple documents but rather *descriptive* of the main concepts or themes in a single text. This descriptive view goes hand-in-hand with the notion of interpretability introduced earlier, which states that the topics must evoke something useful in the mind of the user performing an information seeking task. With TF-IDF, the themes identified are necessarily words in the documents. Since the output in this case is a list of words for each document, it can be treated the same as our algorithm, and thus evaluated with F1 for comparative purposes.

To establish the value of using the Web as an unstructured source of knowledge, we compared our algorithm under two conditions: a baseline case with WordNet (Fellbaum, 1998), a lexical database often used in knowledge based topics identification tasks and known to be incomplete, and with the top nine pages returned by the Yahoo™ search engine. The number of pages was arbitrarily determined to lower the quantity of items retrieved while aiming at obtaining a certain level of diversity of possible usage of a queried words. The textual contents of the Web pages were downloaded and extracted using the HERCULES tool (Wong, Liu, & Bennamoun, 2010). This tool removes HTML codes, advertisements and navigation panels from Web pages using a set of heuristics. All words left from all nine pages were then amalgamated into a single list of items. With WordNet, each word in the text was queried for all possible part-of-speech. The words present in the list of synonyms, definitions and example usage phrases were used as items. All words returned for all senses and all parts of speech were amalgamated in the same list of items. None of the other functionalities of WordNet such as hypernymy and other relations were exploited. For both WordNet and Yahoo™ items, no other linguistic pre-processing was applied.

The most activated item was selected as topic instead of an activation threshold. This allowed us to fully control this variable and to obtain crisp clustering for baseline comparison with k-means. Furthermore, selecting more items as topics would not be useful as it would only create more noise for the F1 evaluation procedure. Based on previous experiments, we found that setting the capacity C of WM to 7 and the decay rate η to 100 generally give good results, so we used these parameter values for all documents of this experiment. A full characterization of what parameter settings work best will be conducted in future work.

RESULTS AND DISCUSSION

The F1 quality results are shown in Table 1. Our method clearly exceeds both the TF-IDF and random baselines, while it performs about as well as k-means clustering. A quality similar to clustering is acceptable since it basically says that our method performs in the same general range as the well-established approach. Furthermore, our method offers advantages over clustering, for instance being able to generate evocative labeled topics for individual documents instead of mere groups relying on the presence of the whole set of documents. It also offers a more adaptive approach than clustering by eliminating the pre-selection of a fix vocabulary in a vector representation.

Table 1. Experimental results comparing our approach with WordNet and Yahoo™ as information sources vs. the top TF-IDF ranked words, k-means and random clustering as baselines. A higher F1 value indicates a better quality.

Method	total #topics	F1
Wordnet	249	0.25
Yahoo™	353	0.21
TF-IDF	620	0.16
k-means	93	0.23
random	245..360	0.12

An additional point to take into account is that k-means was evaluated in the ideal condition of $k=93$ clusters, that is the number of topics determined by human experts. Our method on the other hand has no such initial advantage. We therefore also ran k-means with the same number of topics generated by our method and obtained F1 = 0.18 for $k = 249$ and F1 = 0.17 for $k = 353$ given the number of topics respectively for Wordnet and Yahoo™. In this more equitable situation, k-means abilities are exceeded by our method. Note also that the random clustering results reported in Table 1 already took place with a range of topic similar to our method, that is $k = 245$ to 360.

A disappointing aspect was that Wordnet F1 quality exceeded Yahoo™. Our hypothesis was that the Web, with its richness of collaboratively provided information would yield better results than an incomplete source of information like Wordnet. One possible explanation for this lower quality is exactly the expected strength of the Web. Indeed, since the Web has so much more information provided in a mostly uncontrolled manner, it may contain more noisy information compared to Wordnet, which was built in a controlled manner with clear intentions. A possible evidence of this is the total number of topics generated (column 2 of Table 1). Wordnet results in 249 topics while Yahoo™ gives 353, hence topic assignments are less consistent with Yahoo™, i.e. documents on the same topic are less likely to be assigned the same topic label. More topics means added noise in the confusion matrix between the expert solution and the algorithmic solution when computing F1, and hence lower F1. Another potential issue is that, to limit the amount of data being processed, we have used only the top nine Web pages as source of information. This may miss important usages of the queried words and may impact the quality of the topics.

However, we must emphasize that F1 only captures how well the topics assigned algorithmically compare with human expert's assigned classes. This is fine for traditional methods like clustering and classification. In our case, F1 does not say anything about the ability of the words used as topics to identify the nature of the document content in a user's mind. This is, as we have mentioned earlier, the notion of interpretability of evocative topic labels. It is possible that Wordnet topics, although giving a better F1 value due to being less numerous and thus more consistent, are less evocative than those gathered from the Web. Human assessment thus appears to be an important additional step to conclusively establish what works best. An automated evaluation alternative could be to map the topics generated to the human expert ones and see which method maps the best.

During our experiments, we noticed that the difference in F1 values between Wordnet and Yahoo™ varied as the documents were being processed. This points to a very important methodological issue not only with this experiment but with any text and data mining evaluations, which is that the sample of the dataset used matters. In our case, we processed the first 802 documents of Reuter™. As shown on Figure 1, had we stopped the processing at documents between the low-300's to high-400's, the difference between Wordnet and Yahoo™ would have been less, varying between 0.02 and 0.03 in favor of Wordnet while in the results of Table 1, Wordnet

Figure 1. The quality varies as documents are processed. The F1 quality is computed on the result set after each document.

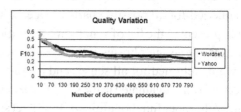

F1 results are 0.04 better than Yahoo's. This is not a major difference but it suggests that the average F1 quality over multiple points of the dataset is probably more representative than a quality evaluation performed at an arbitrary point of the dataset, be it on any sample, or at the actual end of the whole data. Furthermore, since the quality of small samples can be inflated, results from a small proportion of the total data should not be included in the average (as shown in Figure 1 for documents 1 to approximately 300).

From Figure 1, we can see that quality seems to be on a downward trend as the number of documents processed increases. From previous experiences with Wordnet, we know that this trend can change, supporting our recommendation to observe quality over time rather than at a unique arbitrary point. In the case of Wordnet, our experiment shows that F1 starts to increase around the 2,400[th] document. Due to the intense network access required, limited time and limited access to the Yahoo™ search engine, we could not complete a full processing of the 3,299 documents with the Web as a source of knowledge. As such we are unable to demonstrate if the downward trend will change in the case of using Yahoo™.

Another view of quality is precision, that is, to which degree documents labeled identically are actually of the same topic according to the human expert solution. Precision is defined as the ratio $p = a/(a + b)$, where a is the number of true positives and b is the number of false positives. The precision here is computed by considering

Figure 2. Precision is another way to look at topics quality and it also varies as documents are processed. A higher precision means better quality.

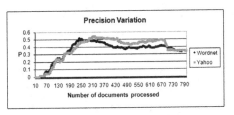

all pairs of documents as per Milligan, Soon, & Sokol (1983). As can be observed from Figure 2, precision also depends on the sample processed. However, contrary to F1, the topics obtained using Yahoo™ display a higher precision compared to those using Wordnet for a large portion, with an average difference of 0.02. However, precision may be inflated by the larger number of topics present in the Yahoo™ results. This is so because a perfect precision of 1 indicates that all documents of the same topic are indeed labeled as such, with no extraneous ones having wrongly been assigned the label. A trivial solution to achieve this aim is to assign a unique label to each document. With labels proliferation as we have here, there may be a tendency towards that triviality that causes an augmentation of the precision value. Note that this is counterbalanced in the F1 measure by recall, which also considers documents that are missing the correct labels, the so-called false negatives. This lack of reliability of automated quality evaluation reiterates the importance of complementing the evaluation with human assessors or developing other evaluation strategies.

There are many ways the results presented here can be improved upon. One area that requires exploration is the setting of parameters, such as decay rate and WM capacity since they can have a major impact on quality. Second, removing digits and other strings such as style, unit, set, put, etc that are currently not considered as stop words but that carry little useful information to evoke meaning in a user's mind might help to improve the quality of topics, at least from a human assessment point of view. Actually, preliminary experiments with Wordnet and an augmented list of 1,800 such non-evocative words resulted in a 17% increase of F1 quality. Furthermore, we have only performed crisp clustering for the sake of comparing with k-means, but it might be advantageous to assign more than one topic label to each document to better identify the nature of their content. This is a very easy thing for our method which has the potential to output as many topic labels as needed. As well, the Reuter™ expert's solution already contains multiple topics for some documents, and allowing this for our method might increase the F1 value by providing a better match with the expert's solution. From a purely dataset aspect, some documents in the Reuter™ collection had no topic assigned by the expert, which again can negatively affect the F1 evaluation. Other documents were very short with almost no intelligible words, which is impeding the ability of our method to find conceptual relations between words. It would be a good idea to remove these documents from the dataset in future work to obtain a better idea of topics quality.

Finally, we point out that in its current prototypical form, our system is slow because it relies on the query of the Yahoo™ search engine over the network. This should not be considered a major issue since an operational system could have its own crawler and local index.

FUTURE RESEARCH DIRECTIONS

We are continuing to test the ideas enunciated here on a larger scale and with other text collections to accumulate convincing and varied quantitative evidence on the power of this groundbreaking approach. We plan to conduct user assessments and comparison with conventional topics identification techniques. The current prototype implementation used here is simple and will serve as baseline for further work. For instance, it uses only single words from the text and single words extracted from Yahoo™ Web pages to determine topics: it is possible that hybrid systems, exploiting statistical and conventional linguistics techniques to identify named entity and part-of-speech could further enhance the groundbreaking method presented in this paper. However, a major issue in computational linguistics is the acquisition of knowledge or text data to support this sort analysis. Interestingly, our method could not only be supported by linguistics but it could also supplement linguistics processing of text by providing a general conceptual context for natural language processing.

There are many possible applications of our method that need to be investigated. A general idea of the theme of a document as expressed by our method can be very useful in search and other textual information management applications. One can for instance consider in particular the ability to organize search results by general themes or to automatically generate Web search engines indexes that are based on concepts or topics instead of only words. An area that has been lagging is search on small document sets such as corporate and desktop search. The lack of solid statistical data makes this kind of search less effective. Since the method we propose does not depend on the presence of large domain corpus statistics, it can handle small collections and situations where archived domain text is not available. A major advantage is that there is no need to have *a priori* knowledge of the vocabulary or topics: the method is therefore fully adaptable and language independent, the only requirement being to have access to some lexical information in the target language, something that may be universally available today with the Web.

Finally, the topics generated by our methods can be seen as the main concepts present in a document. One could also generate topics on segments of document (e.g., paragraphs) to get a larger variety of concepts or observe how topics shift within a document. These concepts could then be provided to an ontology learning system or integrated within an existing ontology by an ontology extension system. Since our method generates fairly general concepts, it can be expected that a domain corpus processed with our topic identification method could yield high-level concepts for a domain ontology or taxonomy. It is also possible to adjust the granularity of the concepts identified using various parameters or existing taxonomic information. A possibility is that instead of using only words from an information source, structural information such as Wordnet hypernyms could be exploited to adjust the level of abstractness of a concept. There are a multitude of other possibilities to explore and test. One is that since verbs and adjectives are possible items that can be outputted as topics, they could be utilized as relations and properties of concepts. Another is to use the unstructured content of the Web to extract concepts with our method and help assemble lightweight ontologies that can then be exploited to organize the Web and run semantically-based applications. This offers a very interesting prospect as a form of bootstrapping for knowledge acquisition in the context of the Semantic Web.

CONCLUSION

In this chapter, we explored the idea of identifying the topics of documents without the usual bag-of-words vector representation. The topics are keywords that evoke in a user mind, with the notion of interpretability, what the main concepts or themes present in a document are. The groundbreaking, human cognition-inspired approach we propose is radically different from existing techniques such as document classification, text clustering and corpus-based statistical methods. Our new topics generation paradigm takes the stream of words from a single document and determines the main themes addressed in the document based on overlapping activations and decay of unstructured lexical information. The lexical information is retrieved from the Web by querying the Yahoo™ search engine. This approach exploits the information contained in word order but without traditional syntactic processing.

Experimental results have shown that the method we proposed can successfully generate topic labels that identify the main concepts present in text documents. The implementation we tested was simple and established a baseline for future work aiming at improving the approach. At this point, it appears that the use of a dictionary instead of the Web yield slightly better quality topics based on F1 automated evaluation. This result needs further verification with human assessors because the F1 quality measure has many limitations in a semantic task like topics generation. The methodological issues related to evaluating topics quality is an important one that needs resolution in the short term to allow for real advances in the field.

The method we proposed has major practical advantages from an adaptability and autonomy point-of-view, namely, the absence of the need to handcraft a training set to initiate the system, no requirement for domain corpus to extract term co-occurrence data, no knowledge-intensive and computational expensive syntactic and semantic analysis is performed, and the method allows to process a single document in isolation. This new approach could potentially contribute to a major advancement in text mining and information retrieval technology by determining the general 'meaning' of documents (i.e. their topics) based solely on unstructured lexical information retrieved from the Web. In fact, our approach demonstrates that it may be possible to resolve an age-long problem in artificial intelligence, namely, computationally 'understanding' text without human intervention or large amount of handcrafted and formally structured knowledge. Certainly, this 'understanding' exists within the narrower sense of main theme or concept identification. Nevertheless, at least we know that making sense of textual information on a Web-scale by using only unstructured texts on the Web (i.e. understanding Web textual content using the Web) is now a definite possibility.

REFERENCES

Aggarwal, C., Hinneburg, A., & Keim, D. (2001). On the surprising behavior of distance metrics in high dimensional space. In *Proceedings of the 8th International Conference Database Theory* (pp. 420-434).

Berners-Lee, T., Hendler, J., & Lassila, O. (2001). The Semantic Web. *Scientific American, 284*(5), 34–43. doi:10.1038/scientificamerican0501-34

Berry, M. W., & Castellanos, M. (Eds.). (2008). *Survey of text mining II: Clustering, classification and retrieval.* Springer-Verlag.

Blei, D., Ng, A. Y., & Jordan, M. I. (2003). Latent dirichlet allocation. *Journal of Machine Learning Research, 3*, 993–1022. doi:10.1162/jmlr.2003.3.4-5.993

Bloehdorn, S., & Hotho, A. (2004). Boosting for text classification with semantic features. In *Proceedings of the Workshop on Mining for and from the Semantic Web at the 10th ACM SIGKDD Conference on Knowledge Discovery and Data Mining* (pp. 70-87).

Brooks, R. A. (1991). Intelligence without representation. *Artificial Intelligence, 47*, 139–159. doi:10.1016/0004-3702(91)90053-M

Fellbaum, C. (1998). *WordNet: An electronic lexical database.* Cambridge, MA: The MIT Press.

Gabrilovich, E., Broder, A., Fontoura, M., Joshi, A., Josifovski, V., Riedel, L., & Zhang, T. (2009). Classifying search queries using the Web as a source of knowledge. *ACM Transactions on the Web, 3*(2), 1–28. doi:10.1145/1513876.1513877

Halliday, M. A. K., & Hasan, R. (1976). *Cohesion in English*. Longman Pub Group.

Harabagiu, S. (1999). From lexical cohesion to textual coherence: A data driven perspective. *Journal of Pattern Recognition and Artificial Intelligence, 13*, 247–265. doi:10.1142/S0218001499000148

Hotho, A., Staab, S., & Stumme, G. (2003). Wordnet improves text document clustering. In *Proceedings of Semantic Web Workshop, the 26th annual International ACM SIGIR Conference* (pp. 541-544).

Hu, J., Fang, L., Cao, Y., Zeng, H., Li, H., Yang, Q., & Chen, Z. (2008). Enhancing text clustering by leveraging Wikipedia semantics. In *Proceedings of the 31st Annual international ACM SIGIR Conference on Research and Development in information Retrieval* (pp. 179-186).

Jain, A. K., Murty, M. N., & Flynn, P. J. (1999). Data clustering: A review. *ACM Computing Surveys, 31*(3), 264–323. doi:10.1145/331499.331504

Larsen, B., & Aone, C. (1999). Fast and effective text mining using linear-time document clustering. In *Proceedings of the fifth ACM SIGKDD International Conference on Knowledge discovery and data mining* (pp. 16-22).

MacQueen, J. (1967). Some methods for classification and analysis of multivariate observations. In *Proceedings of the 5th Berkeley Symposium on Mathematical Statistics and Probability - vol 1, Statistics*.

Massey, L. (2005). Real-world text clustering with adaptive resonance theory neural networks. In *Proceedings of 2005 International Joint Conference on Neural Networks*.

Miller, G. A. (1956). The magical number seven, plus or minus two: Some limits on our capacity for processing information. *Psychological Review, 63*, 81–97. doi:10.1037/h0043158

Milne, D. N., Witten, I. H., & Nichols, D. M. (2007). A knowledge-based search engine powered by Wikipedia. In *Proceedings of the Sixteenth ACM Conference on Conference on information and Knowledge Management* (pp. 445-454).

Salton, G., & Lesk, M. E. (1968). Computer evaluation of indexing and text processing. *Journal of the ACM, 15*(1), 8–36. doi:10.1145/321439.321441

Scott, S., & Matwin, S. (1999). Feature engineering for text classification. In *Proceedings of the 16th International Conference on Machine Learning* (pp. 379-388).

Sebastiani, F. (2002). Machine learning in automated text categorization. *ACM Computing Surveys, 34*(1), 1–47. doi:10.1145/505282.505283

Spärck Jones, K. (1972). A statistical interpretation of term specificity and its application in retrieval. *The Journal of Documentation, 28*(1), 11–21. doi:10.1108/eb026526

VanRijsbergen, C. J. (1979). *Information retrieval*. London, UK: Butterworths.

Weber, R., Schek, H., & Blott, S. (1998). A quantitative analysis and performance study for similarity-search methods in high-dimensional spaces. In *Proceedings of the 24rd international Conference on Very Large Databases* (pp.194-205).

Wong, W., Liu, W., & Bennamoun, M. (2010). Constructing specialised corpora through domain representativeness analysis of websites. *Language Resources and Evaluation*.

Zunde, P., & Dexter, M. E. (1969). Indexing consistency and quality. *American Documentation, 20*(3), 259–267. doi:10.1002/asi.4630200313

ADDITIONAL READING

Allan, J. (2002). *Topic Detection and Tracking: Event-Based Information Organization.* Norwell, MA: Kluwer Academic Publishers.

Chemudugunta, C., Smyth, P., & Steyvers, M. (2008). Combining concept hierarchies and statistical topic models. In *Proceeding of the 17th ACM Conference on information and Knowledge Management* (pp. 1469-1470).

Coursey, K., Mihalcea, R., & Moen, W. (2009). Using encyclopedic knowledge for automatic topic identification. In *Proceedings of the Thirteenth Conference on Computational Natural Language Learning* (pp. 210-218).

Duong, T. H., Jo, G. S., & Nguyen, N. T. (2008). A Method for Integration across Text Corpus and WordNet-Based Ontologies. In *Proceedings of the 2008 IEEE/WIC/ACM International Conference on Web Intelligence and Intelligent Agent Technology - Volume 03* (pp. 1-4).

Fanizzi, N., d'Amato, C., & Esposito, F. (2009). Metric-based stochastic conceptual clustering for ontologies. *Information Systems, 34*(8), 792–806. doi:10.1016/j.is.2009.03.008

Gabrilovich, E., & Markovitch, S. (2009). Wikipedia-based semantic interpretation for natural language processing. *Journal of Artificial Intelligence Research, 34*(1), 443–498.

Just, M. A., & Carpenter, P. A. (1992). A capacity theory of comprehension: Individual differences in working memory. *Psychological Review, 99*(1), 122–149. doi:10.1037/0033-295X.99.1.122

Lin, C. Y. (1995). Knowledge-based Automatic Topic Identification. In *the Proceeding of The 33rd Annual Meeting of the Association for Computational Linguistics*.

Massey, L. (2007). Contrast Learning for Conceptual Proximity Matching. In *Proceedings of the International Conference on Machine Learning And Cybernetics*.

McNamara, D. S. (in press). Computational methods to extract meaning from text and advance theories of human cognition. *Topics in Cognitive Science*.

Milligan, G. W., Soon, S. C., & Sokol, L. M. (1983). The Effect of Cluster Size, Dimensionality, and the number of Clusters on Recovery of True Cluster Structure. *IEEE Transactions on Pattern Analysis and Machine Intelligence, 5*(1). doi:10.1109/TPAMI.1983.4767342

Rocha, L., Mourão, F., Pereira, A., Gonçalves, M. A., & Meira, W. (2008). Exploiting temporal contexts in text classification. In *Proceeding of the 17th ACM Conference on information and Knowledge Management* (pp. 243-252).

Rypma, B., & Prabhakaran, V. (2009). When less is more and when more is more: The mediating roles of capacity and speed in brain-behavior efficiency. *Intelligence, 37*(2), 207–222. doi:10.1016/j.intell.2008.12.004

Schönhofen, P. (2008). Annotating Documents by Wikipedia Concepts. In *Proceedings of the 2008 IEEE/WIC/ACM international Conference on Web intelligence and intelligent Agent Technology - Volume 01* (pp. 461-467).

Wong, W., Liu, W., & Bennamoun, M. (2009). A Probabilistic Framework for Automatic Term Recognition. *Intelligent Data Analysis, 13*(4), 499–539.

KEY TERMS AND DEFINITIONS

Text: A series of words in an electronic file (a document) and written with the purpose of communicating with others. Examples of texts include news articles, Web pages, business letters, scientific papers and abstracts.

Topics: The main thematic content of a text document; what the text is about.

Term Extraction: The identification of key words present in a text document.

Topics Identification: The generation of words that identify the main thematic content or concepts in a document. The words are not necessarily present in the text.

Lexical Knowledge: Information about words, such as the definitions found in a dictionary. Excludes syntactic information such as grammatical rules, part-of-speech information, etc.

Text Clustering: The unsupervised learning task of grouping of text documents according to their similarity in content. The hypothesis is that documents in a same group (called a cluster) will be on the same topic.

Text Classification: The supervised learning task consisting in the identification of sub-classes within a set of documents. The labels for the sub-classes are pre-determined and are also called topics.

ENDNOTES

1   Reuters-21578 Distribution 1.0. article #14828

2   From http://homecooking.about.com/od/howtocookwithcondiments/a/chutney.htm

3   From http://news.bbc.co.uk/2/hi/uk_news/scotland/edinburgh_and_east/8623153.stm

4   Available from http://www.daviddlewis.com/resources/testcollections/reuters21578

Chapter 5

Named Entity Recognition for Ontology Population Using Background Knowledge from Wikipedia

Ziqi Zhang
University of Sheffield, UK

Fabio Ciravegna
University of Sheffield, UK

ABSTRACT

Named Entity Recognition (NER) deals with identifying and classifying atomic texts into pre-defined ontological classes. It is the enabling technique to many complex knowledge acquisition tasks. The recent flourish of Web resources has opened new opportunities and challenges for knowledge acquisition. In the domain of NER and its application in ontology population, considerable research work has been dedicated to exploiting background knowledge from Web resources to enhance the accuracy of the system. This chapter gives a review of existing literature in this domain with an emphasis on using background knowledge extracted from the Web resources. The authors discuss the benefits of using background knowledge and the inadequacies of existing work. They then propose a novel method that automatically creates domain-specific background knowledge by exploring the Wikipedia knowledge base in a domain- and language-independent way. The authors empirically show that the method can be adapted to ontology population, and generates high quality background knowledge that improves the accuracy of domain-specific NER.

INTRODUCTION

Ontology encompasses a set of terms or concepts and relations between the concepts, which collectively represent a domain-of-interest. It is the essential artifact for enabling Semantic Web. For this reason, ontology learning has attracted constant attention of researchers and practitioners from various domains. Automatic ontology learning consists of a number of different tasks, such

DOI: 10.4018/978-1-60960-625-1.ch005

as term extraction and normalization, synonym identification, concept and instance recognition, and relation extraction. Cimiano (2006) advocates that one of the most challenging tasks is ontology population, which addresses finding relevant instances of relations as well as of concepts, the latter being closely related to the task of named entity recognition (NER). On the other hand, NER is considered as one of the fundamental techniques towards ontology learning; and it has been studied extensively in this context, such as Guiliano (2009), and Weber and Buitelaar (2006).

The NER task originates from the sixth Message Understanding Conferences (MUC6) (Grishman & Sundheim, 1996), which defines the task as recognizing named entities and classifying them into proper concept classes. Despite the extensive research on this topic in the last fifteen years, the state-of-the-art solutions still suffer from lack of portability and extensibility, largely due to its dependence on domain-specific knowledge resources such as specialist lexicons and training corpus, and the cost of building and maintaining such resources. Recent years have witnessed the exponential growth of Web resources and the emergence of high-quality, large-scale collaboratively maintained knowledge resources such as Wikipedia and Wiktionary, which have proved useful in the application of knowledge discovery and acquisition. The abundance of such resources has created both opportunities and new challenges for the task of NER and ontology population. This has attracted significant attention from researchers, who have proposed new methods of mining useful background knowledge from these resources to enhance various knowledge discovery and acquisition tasks, such as NER and ontology population (Kazama & Torisawa, 2008, Guiliano & Gliozzo, 2008; Guiliano, 2009), computing semantic relatedness and similarity (Strube & Ponzetto, 2006; Gabrilovich & Markovitch, 2007; Zesch et al., 2008), and sense disambiguation (Cucerzan, 2007).

However, some issues remain unsolved; are there systematic ways of using a specific Web resource as background knowledge? Is there a generic method for exploiting domain-specific knowledge? How do we combine different Web resources into a coherent knowledge base for the task of entity recognition? This chapter aims to provide a review of existing work that address these issues, and propose a novel method of mining domain-specific background knowledge from Wikipedia and using the knowledge for NER and ontology population as an attempt to address these issues. The rest of the chapter is structured as follows. Firstly, we introduce the NER task and its relation to ontology population; next, we explain the importance of using background knowledge in NER, the new opportunities opened by the increasingly available Web resources, and review existing work carried out in this direction; then we introduce our novel method of exploiting the background knowledge from the most popular knowledge resource on the Web – the Wikipedia[1], and compare our approach with others; finally we discuss the advantages and the limitations of the proposed method and future trends of research, then concludes the chapter.

NAMED ENTITY RECOGNITION AND ONTOLOGY POPULATION

Defining the Task of Named Entity Recognition

The sixth Message Understanding Conference (MUC6) made the first attempt to define the NER as the task that involves "identifying the names of all the people, organisations and geographic locations in a text", as well as "time, currency and percentage expressions" (Grishman & Sundheim 1996). An example of such annotations is shown in Figure 1, in which names of entities are annotated using mark-up tags.

Figure 1. Example named entity annotation. Source article: "Google To Acquire YouTube for $1.65 Billion in Stock" (Google Press Center, 2006)

```
<ENAMEX:TYPE="LOCATION">MOUNTAIN VIEW, Calif. </ENAMEX>,

<ENAMEX:TYPE="DATE">October 9, 2006</ENAMEX>, -

<ENAMEX:TYPE="ORGNIZATION">Google Inc. </ENAMEX>, (NASDAQ: GOOG) announced

today that it has agreed to acquire <ENAMEX:TYPE="ORGNIZATION">YouTube</ENAMEX>,, the

consumer media company for people to watch and share original videos through a Web experience, for

<ENAMEX:TYPE="MONEY">$1.65 billion</ENAMEX>, in a stock-for-stock transaction.
```

Since MUC6 there has been increasing interest in this topic and extensive effort has been devoted into its research. Major computational linguistic conferences hosted special tracks for the task and there has been steady growth of publications throughout the years. Several events attempted to enrich the definition of the task by including more entity types to be recognised (MUC events, Chinchor 1999) or defining fine-grained structure of entity sub-types for recognition (Advanced Content Extraction or ACE, Doddington et al., 2004). The task has also been extended to specialised domains to recognise domain-specific entities, typically in the domain of bioinformatics to recognise domain-specific entities such as gene and protein names. Large amount of resources have been created for the purpose of evaluating biomedical entity recognition such as the Genia corpus (Ohta et al., 2002), and successive events such as the BioNLP/JNLPBA shared task on entity recognition (Kim et al., 2004) have been hosted to encourage the research. Other domain specific applications include archaeology (Byrne 2007), astronomy (Murphy et al., 2006), aerospace engineering (Iria 2009) and so on. Domain-specific entity recognition in these areas is much harder and results have been less satisfactory. This is due to the intrinsic complexity of terms in different domains because of multi-word expressions, spelling variations, acronyms, am-

biguities and so on (Roberts et al., 2008; Saha et al., 2009).

Common Techniques for Named Entity Recognition

The techniques for NER are most often divided into two main streams (Nadeau, 2007; Olsson 2008),: handcrafted rules for pattern matching – which we will refer to as rule-based systems – and machine learning based approaches although some combine the two approaches to complement the weakness of each other. Rule-based methods (such as Riloff & Jones, 1999) involve designing and implementing lexico-syntactic patterns and using existing information lists such as dictionaries that can frequently identify candidate entities. An example of such rules can be "a street name is a multi-word CamelCase phrase ends with the word X and proceeded by preposition Y", where X and Y are lists of common words that are suitable for this purpose. The major limitation of these systems is the language and domain dependency, the fact that they require considerable knowledge about the language and domain and existence of certain lexical resources. These knowledge and resources are often expensive to build and maintain and are not transferrable across domains. Consequently these approaches suffer from limited or no domain portability.

In contrast, Machine Learning is a way to automatically learn to recognise complex patterns or sequence labeling algorithms and make intelligent decisions based on data. Central to the machine learning paradigm is the idea of modeling distinctive features associated with existing positive and negative examples, and design algorithms that consume these features to automatically induce patterns for recognising similar information from unseen data. In the NER task, the target objects are tokens or sequences for recognition and classification, and example features of them may be capitalisation pattern, containment of digits or special tokens. In Machine Learning, usually we refer to the existing examples as labeled data, from which the system learns an inference model (training phase); on the other hand, we refer to the unseen data as unlabeled data, which is sometimes used to test the trained system (testing or validation phase). Although the automatic nature of machine learning delivers robustness and extensibility and it reduces the needs for human experts to manually study examples and deriving patterns or rules as in a rule-based system, it has been criticized for its dependence on labeled data, which prove to be equally expensive to build and maintain. The success of a machine learning system usually depends on the availability of large amount of labeled data, which requires human input. Studies have shown that the annotation process is costly, tedious and in fact error-prone (Ciravegna et al. 2002). For this reason, research has been carried out to reduce machine learning's dependence on labeled data using weakly supervised methods (Mohit & Hwa, 2005; Toral & Muñoz, 2006; Nadeau 2007); or improve the efficiency and effectiveness of the process for creating labeled data using Active Learning (Ciravegna et al., 2002; Olsson 2008); and even automatically generating labeled data for Machine Learning purposes (Nothman et al., 2008).

Named Entity Recognition and Ontology Population

NER plays a critical role in many complex knowledge discovery and acquisition tasks. For example, it is a pre-processing stage for relation extraction (Giuliano et al., 2006) that aims at identifying and classifying relations between entities. It is an important component in Question Answering (Mollá et al., 2006) systems, which relies on an entity recogniser to detect fact statements. According to Nadeau (2007), 80% of the evaluation questions ask for a named entity in the TREC-8 question answering competition. In information retrieval (Srihari & Peterson, 2008), domain-specific entities may be used for indexing documents and thus achieving high retrieval accuracy. In machine translation (Babych & Hartley, 2003), named entities often bear important information and must be recognised and translated properly. Also named entities are important types of lexicons for lexicon construction (Toral & Muñoz 2006).

In enabling the Semantic Web, entity recognition is a key technique for ontology learning, in particular, ontology population (Cimiano 2006). Typically, ontology elicitation produces ontologies at the conceptual level, i.e., defining concepts and relations among concepts in a domain. However, concepts and relations are abstractions of real world instances; they cannot be understood by a machine. Such ontologies need to be populated with instances of concepts and expressions of relations such that a machine can understand them. Ontology population is the task of automatically extracting such instances and expressions from various data sources and linking them to proper ontology concepts and relations. Essentially NER deals with identifying and classifying instances of concepts, which resembles the ontology population task. Therefore, the majority of solutions to ontology population have been developed based on the techniques of NER.

NER AND BACKGROUND KNOWLEDGE

Why Background Knowledge

The techniques for NER are essentially based on context modeling, comparison and classification, in which a named entity is represented by a vector space of its context and compared to others'. The idea is that similar types of entities tend to appear in similar contexts. Traditionally, context in the NER task often refers to a window of n tokens surrounding the target named entity and the characteristics of these tokens (features) (Nadeau 2007). In fact, many studies such as Jimeno et al. (2007), Mayfield et al. (2003), Klinger et al. (2007) only look at the problem at the sentence level, i.e., the contextual features are only derivable from tokens within the same sentence. Although these systems have performed reasonably well in experiments, they can be ineffective when such contexts are very limited. In case of very short sentences, typically in instructional texts or task descriptions such as recipes, sentence-level context is very limited, resulting in very sparse feature vector that can be ambiguous across different types of entities. In some extreme but practical scenarios such as entity recognition from image captions (Carvalho et al., 2008), the language is characterized by irregular use of punctuations and grammar, and very short phrases (1-2 words) on which pre-NER linguistic processing such as Part-of-Speech tagging will fail, which significantly decreases the accuracy of a learning system. Therefore, relying purely on the traditional "local" context is largely insufficient and additional domain knowledge is required for NER in these areas. Even for regular documents, researchers have proved the advantage of bringing additional information from an enlarged context and even external resources (Kazama & Torisawa, 2007; Ganti et al., 2008) in improving the accuracy of NER.

Another major challenge for NER is domain portability. Porting entity recognition systems to technical domains always introduces new problems due to the intrinsic complexity of domain-specific terms because of multi-word expressions, spelling variations, acronyms and ambiguities. Typically, the domain of biomedicine is characterised by enormous amounts of synonyms, acronyms, morphological, inflectional and derivational variants, which are often ambiguous (Ananiadou et al., 2004). Similar issues have been noted in the aerospace domain by Butters & Ciravegna (2008) and the archaeology domain by Byrne (2007). Significant drop in performance has been reported when an NER system is ported to technical domains. For example, systems tailored for bio-medical entity recognition (such as gene names, cell types, cell lines, proteins, DNAs and RNAs) typically obtain F-measure of 58 to 75 (BioBLP/JNLPBA 2004; Saha et al., 2009) on PubMed corpus as compared to over 90 F-measure reported in the general domain as reported in MUC7. It has been recognised that incorporating domain-specific knowledge from additional resources in the development of NER is critical to the success of domain portability.

To address these issues we introduce the notion of "background knowledge" for NER. We define the background knowledge of named entities as any information about the entity or its type, and that is available from additional resources (background) other than the target document in question, namely, the document from which the entity and its type is to be recognised and classified.

NER Using Background Knowledge: The Literature

Following the definition, the most commonly used source of background knowledge for NER is domain-specific lexicons, often in the form of gazetteers or lookup lists. A gazetteer is a dictionary or a directory, which contains important references about concepts. Such resources have been found crucial in improving NER accuracies, and particularly useful for porting systems to specialised domains and languages (Friedrich et al., 2006; Roberts et al, 2008). However, the major problem with such resources is their availability and cost of maintenance. Research has shown that it is difficult to create and maintain high quality lexical resources (Toral & Muñoz, 2006; Kazama & Torisawa, 2008). Certain well-curated domain-specific knowledge resources have been created and maintained in the past years, such as the Unified Medical Language System (UMLS)[2] for biomedical science, the Agravoc[3] thesaurus for agriculture related domains, and the Aquatic Sciences and Fisheries Abstracts (ASFA[4]) thesaurus. However, maintaining such resources require long-term dedicated investment. For example, the UMLS is the largest knowledge base containing large amount of controlled vocabularies in the biomedical science. The creation and maintenance of UMLS have required considerable effort and finance. In fact, UMLS was created in 1986 with support from US governments and has been maintained by the vigorous biomedical community.

Other major sources of background knowledge are domain-specific corpora. Usually, an additional set of documents similar to the corpus in question is selected for analysis and the extraction of additional domain-specific knowledge such as patterns (Riloff & Jones, 1999), gazetteers (Miller et al., 2004; Kazama & Torisawa, 2008) and terminology that are later used with the NER system on the target corpus.

Harvesting Background Knowledge from the General Web

In recent years, the exponential growth of the Web and the emergence and increasing popularity of Web 2.0 technologies have created enormous open data, which created new opportunities to knowledge discovery and acquisition and encouraged new methodologies to be developed. This has also attracted significant attention in the studies of NER and ontology population, in which researchers look for new ways of exploit-

ing background knowledge from Web resources to improve learning accuracy. Earlier studies explored the lexical resources in WordNet[5], a lexical database for English that groups words into sets of synonyms, which are called synsets. Each synset expresses a distinct concept. Each word is provided with a short definition, and synsets are interlinked by semantic and lexical relations. However, this chapter does not include a discussion of applications using WordNet, since it is not strictly a Web resource. Versions of WordNet are in fact published as standalone software available for download.

In the studies that explore the general Web, Evans (2003) studied the possibility of entity recognition in the open domain, which is concerned with recognition of any types of entity that may be useful to information extraction. Their approach started from identifying capitalised sequences that are likely to be named entities from a text, then compose search queries using these sequences together with Hearst patterns (Hearst 1992) and submit the queries to search engines to find hypernyms of the capitalised sequences from retrieved documents. For example, if a capitalised sequence is "Microsoft Inc.", the phrase "X such as Microsoft Inc." is submitted to search engines, and from the retrieved documents the word filling the position of "X" is considered to be the hypernyms of "Microsoft Inc.". Their method extracted large amount of triples which can be used to populate ontologies. However, this approach only extracts facts explicitly expressed in documents while in practice, knowledge is often implicit (Brewster et al., 2003). The method is also restricted by the limited availability of lexico-syntactic patterns. Guiliano & Gliozzo (2008) suggested that since terms that occur in similar contexts tend to have similar meanings, then given an instance in a particular context one can substitute it with another of the same ontological class and generate true statements. Following this hypothesis, given a new entity (question entity) to be classified, they query a search engine to obtain snippets of the entity.

Next, phrases including the question entity are extracted from the snippets, and the occurrences of question entity are substituted by some seed entities the types of which are already known to generate a list of hypothesis phrases. The phrases are submitted to search engine and a "plausibility" score of the phrases are computed using the search result counts. The scores are aggregated to indicate the substitutability of the question entity and a seed entity, upon which the class of the question entity is decided. They proved this method useful in a people ontology population task. Other approaches that exploit knowledge from the general Web data include Downey et al. (2007), who hypothesized that named entities are often Multi-Word Units (MWUs), and proposed using mutual information measures and frequency of words obtained based on a large collection of Web corpus to identify n-grams (where $n>1$) that are potential entities. The Web corpus is also created by querying search engines. The success of these systems in the general domain is largely due to the information redundancy on the Web, that the common facts are often repeated in large amount of resources. However in some specialised domains, new terms are constantly introduced at a high rate (Ananiadou et al., 2004; Roberts et al., 2008) and the composition of terms is much more complex than in the general domain. Due to these issues, information redundancy is less likely to exist for these domains. For example, searching for "AND CD11a gene promoter" (a term in the Genia corpus) returns no result from Google[6]. Also, typical search engines such as Google cannot disambiguate meanings from contexts and therefore, search results are found inaccurate in many cases (Goldschmidt & Krishnamoorthy, 2008).

Mining Structured Knowledge from Wikipedia

Another stream of research has focused on using well-curated knowledge resources from the Web, the best example being Wikipedia. Wikipedia is a multi-lingual, free online encyclopedia that is collaboratively created and maintained by voluntary contributors. Launched in 2001, throughout the years Wikipedia has gained vast popularity and exponential growth. As by June 2010, Wikipedia contains in total over 20 million articles in more than 250 languages. Wikipedia contains rich lexical semantic information and structured meta-data that are found useful to knowledge discovery and acquisition. Most articles in Wikipedia are about named entities, and they are heavily linked to each other and external resources. A folksonomy system, which is a mechanism supporting collaborative classification, is incorporated for adding semantic classification tags to articles and creating links between tags. This is usually called the category tree or the category graph (Zesch & Gurevych 2007). The redirection system in Wikipedia groups alternative names of an entity and point them to the same article. Disambiguation pages are used for listing names that refer to multiple entities. Another type of useful structured data in not all but many Wikipedia articles is the "infobox", which is a table-like summary of an entity's facts, often containing information generic to the class of the entity mentioned by the article.

Although the open and collaborative nature of Wikipedia has led to questions about quality and quantity of the knowledge, the report by Giles (2005) has shown that the quality of data is in fact about the same as that of Encyclopedia Britannica, a dedicated knowledge source that is written, validated and edited by experts. Another research by Holloway et al. (2007) focused on domain coverage by studying Wikipedia categories and category clusters and revealed that by 2005, there were already 78,977 unique categories divided into 1,069 disconnected category clusters, which can be considered as the number of domains.

The availability of knowledge and semi-structured nature of Wikipedia have created new opportunities for researchers. Within the last few years, large amount of studies have been carried out and proved the potential of using knowledge from Wikipedia for knowledge discovery and acquisition applications, such as in Named Entity Disambiguation (Bunescu & Pasca 2006; Cucerzan 2007), document classification (Gabrilovich & Markovitch 2006), information retrieval (Müller & Gurevych 2009) and question answering (Ferrández et al., 2009). In studies related to NER and ontology population, Toral & Muñoz (2006) used Wikipedia to build named entity gazetteers for location, person and organisation classes. They observe that the first sentence in a Wikipedia article usually defines the entity of mention and contains named entities of similar type. Therefore, they extract all noun phrases from the first sentences of Wikipedia articles, and then map the noun phrases to WordNet synsets. Next, starting from the identified synset, they follow the hypernymy hierarchy in WordNet until they reach a synset belonging to the entity class of interest. Kazama & Torisawa (2007) argued that the head noun of the first noun phrase after *be* in the first sentence of a Wikipedia article is often the hypernym of the mentioned entities. For example, the first sentence for the article "Sheffield" is "Sheffield is a city and metropolitan borough of South Yorkshire, England", in which the word "city" is a hypernym of "Sheffield". Following this hypothesis, they extracted hypernyms of candidate entities from Wikipedia as additional information to a supervised classifier and achieved good results. Sarmento et al. (2007) employed term co-occurrence statistics from a large corpus to expand a seed entity list by similarity. The assumption is that terms are similar if they co-occur frequently in lists. The method was applied to the Wikipedia exploiting the rich list structure embedded to expand seed entity sets of small sizes. Nothman et al. (2009) proposed a method to automatically create training corpus for entity recognition. They classify each article in a bootstrapping process using the head nouns extracted from its categories, definitional nouns from the first sentences (similar as Kazama & Torisawa, 2007), and title capitalisation. The process generates annotated Wikipedia corpus,

from which they selected sentences as training data for supervised NER. The trained systems obtained better results on cross-corpus (e.g., train a system on MUC corpus and test the system on CoNLL[7] corpus) evaluation than if trained on standard corpora published by MUC and CoNLL. Kliegr et al. (2008) used Wikipedia and WordNet in an unsupervised entity classification task for image caption analysis. Named entities that are not defined in WordNet are firstly looked up in Wikipedia. Once the corresponding article is found, the first paragraph is processed and lexico-syntactic patterns are used to identify the hypernym of the mentioned entity. For example, on the article about "Maradona", term "player" is extracted as its hypernym from the sentence "Maradona, born on October 30, 1960, is a former Argentine football player". The hypernym is then fed into a WordNet-based semantic similarity function to determine the closest candidate entity type from a pool of pre-defined labels, such as person, location, and organisation. A limitation of these studies is that they only extract background knowledge from small fractions of article contents, such as first paragraph, first sentence or categories. In contrast, we believe the full content body of the article bears equally useful knowledge. Also, these experiments have been restricted to the general domain. On the other hand, research by Milne et al. (2006) proved the usefulness of Wikipedia resources for domain-specific knowledge generation. Therefore, this work aims to test the method in named entity recognition from specialised domains.

Additionally, many researchers have studied methods of using knowledge in Wikipedia to compute semantic similarity or distance, which is often used as a technique for NER and ontology population. Strube & Ponzetto (2006) used path length measured by Wikipedia category structure and gloss overlap measured by the first paragraph of Wikipedia article to compute semantic similarity of two named entities. Turdakov & Velikhov (2008) analyzed different types of links (e.g., links in tables, lists) in Wikipedia and used those features with different weights for computing semantic similarity. Gabrilovich & Markovitch (2007) represented each Wikipedia concept using a weighted vector of words that occur in the corresponding article, and then build an inverted index that map each word into a list of concepts in which it appears. Thus to compute relatedness between two texts, a weighted vector of Wikipedia concepts is built for each text by aggregating the concept vectors of each word retrieved from the index. The vectors are then input to the cosine metric to derive a similarity score. Hassan & Mihalcea (2009) inherited from Gabrilovich and Markovitch's approach but introduced three modifications. Firstly they replaced the cosine similarity metric with a Lesk-like (Lesk 1986) metric, which places more emphasis on the overlap of two vectors rather than differences, thus better coping with sparse vectors. Secondly, they adapted the weighting schema to take into account the length of articles. Thirdly, they place more importance on category-type concepts in the weighting schema. The focus of these studies have been measuring similarity between named entities and concepts, and applying them to synonym identification and name disambiguation, but not on entity recognition.

A New Star: Wiktionary

Wiktionary is another project based on the idea of collaborative authoring by volunteer users. It is a multi-lingual free content dictionary, available in over 270 languages. Started in 2002, by 2010, it already contains over 5 million entries, of which 1.4 million belong to the English language. Entries in Wiktionary are accompanied with a wide range of lexical and semantic information such as part of speech, pronunciation, word sense, gloss, etymology, synonyms, antonyms, hypernyms, hyponyms, example usage, derived terms and references/quotations and so on. Compared to WordNet, the English Wiktionary provides addi-

tional information such as compounds, acronyms and abbreviations, common misspellings, simplified spellings, slangs, disputed usage words and so on (Zesch et al., 2008). Similar to Wikipedia, entries in Wiktionary are organized into semantic categories, and are linked to other entries in Wiktionary, as well as external resources.

Using Wiktionary in research is a relatively new direction. Among these, the majority of them apply knowledge in Wiktionary to compute semantic similarity of words, and adapt the technique to synonym detection, ontology matching and information retrieval. Zesch et al. (2008) used path-length by traversing semantic relations of words defined in Wiktionary and concept vector of words by aggregating the texts found in a Wiktionary entry of a word to compute semantic relatedness between two words. On seven test datasets, their method achieved better results than similar approaches that use WordNet and Wikipedia resources. Weale et al., (2009) applied a page rank based algorithm to compute relatedness of words using Wiktionary, and tested their method in a synonym detection task. Similarly, Navarro et al., (2009) used the semantic relations such as sub-senses, synonyms in Wiktionary to build networked synonyms. Müller & Gurevych (2009) used knowledge in Wiktionary to improve information retrieval systems. Essentially, the way they use Wiktionary is based on aggregating the semantic relatedness between each query and document term pair. Texts of Wiktionary entries of words are used to build representational concept vectors. Krizhanovsky & Lin (2009) used a variant of path-length based semantic similarity measure and applied it to ontology matching in Russian language.

However, studies by Navarro et al. (2009) have shown that Wiktionary has several disadvantages as a lexical knowledge resource; which include the incompleteness of many entries (some entries in Wiktionary are in fact empty), unbalanced coverage of different languages, and sparse synonym network. More importantly, it is a resource of words other than named entities, which are more important to knowledge discovery and acquisition (Strube & Ponzetto, 2006).

TACKLING THE ISSUES: A NOVEL METHOD

In this section, we propose a novel method for extracting and employing background knowledge from Web resources for the purpose of NER and ontology population. We show that the method can be applied to generate gazetteers, which are important sources of background knowledge for NER; and it can be also adapted to populate ontology and create ontology with hypernym-hyponym relations. In order to cope with the aforementioned challenges and limitations of existing work, the method is designed and implemented to be semi-automatic in a bootstrapping manner, language- and domain-independent, but capable of generating domain-specific knowledge in a scalable way. We choose Wikipedia as the source of background knowledge. This is based primarily on three reasons that have been introduced in the previous section; firstly, compared to the general Web, it provides easier access to structured and unstructured knowledge, and the quality of knowledge is considered better while the quantity of knowledge is reasonably good; secondly, compared to Wiktionary, Wikipedia provides knowledge based on named entities, which is more suitable to the task; thirdly, research on using Wikipedia is relatively mature compared to other resources, providing stronger referential cases for similar tasks. To prove the applicability of the method, we evaluate it in a domain-specific NER task for archaeology. In the following, we firstly describe the method for generating domain-specific gazetteers using knowledge from Wikipedia; next, we introduce the problem domain of archaeology; finally, we present experiments in which the domain-specific gazetteers generated using the method is used to

enhance domain-specific entity recognition for archeology.

The Methodology

Generally, starting with seed gazetteer lists of given types such as location, person, which we referred to as pre-defined coarse-grained class (CGC), our method explores Wikipedia networked resources and exploit various Wikipedia content information and structural elements including full article contents, hyperlinks, category structures, redirection links to discover similar terms, and extend the lists to more complete sets of same classes. The method is based on three hypotheses;

- Wikipedia contains articles about seed entities of a particular domain
- Articles about the seed entities contain fine-grained type labels for seed entities, which are referred to as fine-grained classes (FGC). Seed entities, FGCs and CGCs form a simple ontology with hypernymy relations
- Following the links on Wikipedia articles of a seed entity, we can reach a large collection of relevant named entities. If a relevant named entity's FGC (as extracted above) matches any of those extracted for seed entities, it can be added as an instance to that FGC, and therefore, an instance of the CGC

Following this logic, we divide our methods into three steps; firstly we match a seed entity to a Wikipedia article (the matching phase); next we extract information from the articles to label seed entities and build a pool of FGCs for the seed entities (the classification phase); finally we extract similar entities by following links in articles of seed entities (the expansion phase). The pseudo-algorithm is illustrated in Figure 2.

Figure 2. Pseudo algorithm

```
Input: seed entities SE of class (CGC) C
Output: new entities NE of class C
STEP 1 - the matching phase
    a. Initialize Set P to contain articles for SE;
    b. For each entity e: SE
    c.    Retrieve article p from Wikipedia for e;
    d.    Add p to P;
STEP 2 - the classification phase
    a. Initialize Set L
    b. For each p: P
    c.    Extract fine grained class labels (FGC) l;
    d.    Add l to L;
STEP 3 - the expansion phase
    a. Initialize Set HL;
    b. For each p: P
    c.    Add hyperlinks from p to HL;
    d. (optional) recursively crawl extracted hyperlinks and repeat b and c
    e. For each link hl: HL
    f.    Extract fine grained class labels (FGC) l';
    g.    If L contains l'
    h.        Add title of hl to NE;
    i.        Add titles of redirect links of hl to NE;
```

The Matching Phase

For a given seed entity, we search the exact phrase in Wikipedia to obtain the corresponding articles. If no articles are found, we use the leftmost longest match to retrieve articles that fuzzily match the seed entity. For example, for the phrase "Stone Age flint arrowhead", we search for the entire phrase, the reduced phrases "Age flint arrowhead", "flint arrowhead" and "arrowhead" in order until one phrase returns matching articles. In Wikipedia, searches for ambiguous phrases are redirected to a Disambiguation Page, from which users have to manually select a sense. We filter out any matches that are directed to disambiguation pages. This filtering strategy is also applied to the expansion phase (Step 3 in Figure 2) in extracting candidate entities.

The Classification Phase

Once Wikipedia articles are retrieved for all seed entities, we extract FGCs of seed entities from these articles. There are two types of information from Wikipedia that can be used as reliable labels. The first is based on Kazama and Torisawa (2007), who observed that the first sentence of an article is often a definitive sentence. Specifically, the head

noun of the noun phrase just after *be* is most likely the hypernym of the entity of interest. There are two issues in this approach. First, the head noun may be too generic to represent a domain-specific class. For example, following their approach the FGC extracted for the archaeological term "*Post-Classic Stage*" from the sentence "*The Post-Classic Stage is an archaeological term describing a particular developmental level.*" is "*term*", which is the head noun of "*archaeological term*". Clearly in such a case the phrase is more domain-specific than the head noun. For this reason we use the *first exact noun phrase* after *be* as FGC in our work. Second, their method ignores a correlative conjunction that often indicates equally useful FGCs. For example, the two noun phrases in italic in the sentence "*Leeds* is a *city* and *metropolitan borough* in West Yorkshire, England" are equally useful FGCs for the article "*Leeds*". For this reason, we also extract the noun phrase that is connected by a correlative conjunction as the FGC. For simplicity, we refer to this approach to classifying seed entities as *FirstSentenceLabeling*, and the FGCs created as FGC_s.

The second method for extracting FGC is based on the Wikipedia category structure. Many previous studies have suggested that although the structure does not follow strict taxonomic relations, in most cases, it resembles the tree-structure and the hypernymy-hyponymy relation remains valid for most categories. Following this observation, we extract category labels of articles as FGCs of entities, and refer to this method as *CategoryLabeling*, and denote the extracted FGCs by FGC_c.

There are three situations in which we need to refine the extracted FGCs by this method. Firstly, some articles have a category with the same title as the article itself. For example, the article about "Iron Age" has only one category, "Iron Age". To cope with this issue, we traverse the next level of the category tree by extracting categories of the category "Iron Age", including "1st Millennium BC", "2nd millennium BC", "Iron", "Periods and stages in Archaeology", and "Prehistory". Secondly, we discard arbitrary categories are created for management purposes, such as "Articles to be Merged since 2008", "Wikipedia Templates". Thirdly, we only keep FGCs that are extracted for at least 2 seed entities to reduce the noise caused by loose definition of the category structure.

The classification process generates a pool of FGCs which are hypernyms of seed entities but hyponyms of pre-defined CGCs. The process is equivalent to inserting another layer in the original ontology composed by the seed entities and the CGCs. For the purpose of gazetteer generation, in the next step use them as a control vocabulary to guide the expansion of similar entities.

The Expansion Phase

Next, expanding the seed entities involves identifying from Wikipedia the candidate entities that are related to the seed entities. This is done by following the hyperlinks from the full content of articles retrieved for the seed entities. The hyperlinks connect the main article of an entity (source entity) to other sets of entities (related entities). Therefore, by following these links we can reach a large set of related entities to the seed list. Next, the two approaches introduced in the previous section are used to identify the FGCs of candidate entities. If any candidates share one or more common FGCs with the seed entities (generated in the previous stage) and their FGCs are extracted using the same classification method, they are accepted into the extended gazetteers. That is, if the seed entity FGCs is built by *FirstSentenceLabeling* we only use *FirstSentenceLabeling* to classify the candidate related entities. The same applies to *CategoryLabeling*. This stage can be easily scaled by recursively crawling the hyperlinks contained in the retrieved pages if necessary.

In addition, for each qualifying Wikipedia page, we also keep its associated redirecting links, which groups several surface forms of a single entity. For example, the search for "army base" is redirected to the article "military base". From the ontology construction perspective, these surface forms can be considered as synonyms to each other and can be used to insert synonymy relations in the ontology. From the gazetteer generation perspective, we select all of them for the extended gazetteers.

After applying these processes, the original seed gazetteers are expanded by entities with which they share same FGCs, and therefore, pre-defined CGCs. The method can be easily repeated for a number of iterations, in which the newly added entities serve as seed entities and go through the three stages again. Depending on the size of seed entities and the desired scale of the output, one can customize the number of runs to build various sizes of gazetteers. From the ontology construction perspective, the first and the second phases insert a layer of fine-grained classes between seed entities and pre-defined entity classes. The third phase populates the ontology by adding in instances of this layer of FGCs. Similarly, by repeating the process, one can customize the ontology construction. In the following, we evaluate the methodology in an NER task for the archaeology domain.

The Archaeology Domain

The domain of modern archaeology is a discipline that has a long history of active fieldwork, which has generated a considerable amount of legacy data. Despite the existence of fast-growing large corpora, little has been done to develop high quality meta-data for efficient access to the information in these datasets, and there is a pressing need for knowledge acquisition technologies to bridge the gap (Jeffrey et al., 2009). NER in archaeology is a challenging task because of the complexity of language characterised by ambiguities, uncertainties, long and composite terms, changing language use, acronyms and so on. The Inter-Annotator-Agreement (IAA), which measures the extent to which human annotators agree on what and how to annotate in this task has been found very low (Byrne, 2007), indicating the difficulty of the task is high.

Our study deals with archaeological entity extraction from un-structured legacy data, which mostly consist of full-length archaeological reports archived by the Arts and Humanities Data Service (AHDS) and vary from 5 to over a hundred pages. According to Jeffrey et al. (2009), three types of entities are most useful to an archaeologist;

- **Subject:** a general class that containing heterogeneous topics that archaeological documents refer to, such as findings of artifacts and monuments. It covers various specialized domains such as warfare, agriculture, education, maritime, technology, and machinery. Examples belonging to this class contain "Roman pottery" and "arrowhead".
- **Temporal terms:** archaeological dates of interest, which are written in a number of ways, such as years "840 - 1066", "circa 400AD"; centuries "C3", "the 1st century"; concepts "Iron Age", "Dark Age"; and acronyms such as "IA" (Iron Age), "MED" (Medieval).
- **Location of interest:** place names of interest, such as site addresses and site types related to a finding or excavation. In our study, these refer to UK-specific places.

Experiment and Findings

We evaluate our method in an NER task to test its ability of enriching high quality domain-specific gazetteers. In order to build the NER system, we selected 30 full length UK archaeological reports archived by the Arts and Humanities Data Service (AHDS)[8]. These articles vary from 5 to 120 pages, with a total of 225,475 words. The corpus is then annotated by three domain experts. This corpus is then split into five equal parts for a five-fold cross validation experiment, in which annotations are randomly split to 5 complementary subsets, and the entity tagger learns from the annotations in four subsets and is then validated on the other one subset. The process is repeated for 5 iterations, in each time different subsets are used for training and validation. The final performance is the average of the performance figures obtained in all iterations.

We developed the NER tagger based on a Support Vector Machine (SVM)[9] classifier, which is a typical Machine Learning technique. The baseline features for the classifier include a context window of five tokens, morphological root of a token, exact token string, orthographic type (e.g., lowercase) and token kind (e.g., digit, letter). The performance measured in Precision, Recall and the harmonic F-measure (F1) of this baseline setting is shown in Table 1.

The results were found not very satisfactory by the domain experts, and therefore, a number of domain-specific gazetteers were provided to enhance the system performance. These include the MIDAS[10] Period list as the gazetteer for Temporal, the Thesaurus of Monuments Types (TMT2008) from English Heritage[11] and the Thesaurus of Archaeology Objects from the STAR[12] project as gazetteers for Subject, and the

Table 1. Baseline accuracy in the entity extraction task for each type of entities

	Location			Subject			Temporal		
	P	R	F1	P	R	F1	P	R	F1
Baseline (B)	69.4	67.4	68.4	69.6	62.3	65.7	82.3	81.4	81.8

Table 2. Baseline+gazetteer feature, System accuracy in the entity extraction task for each type of entities

	Location			Subject			Temporal		
	P	R	F1	P	R	F1	P	R	F1
Baseline + GAZ_original	69.0	72.1	70.5	69.7	65.4	67.5	82.3	82.7	82.5

Table 3. Number of unique entities in each gazetteer

	Number of unique entries in gazetteers		
	Location	Subject	Temporal
GAZ_original	11,786, 8,228 found in Wikipedia	5,725, 4,320 found in Wikipedia	61, 43 found in Wikipedia
$GAZ\_EXT_{firstsent}$	19,385, 7,599 new to gaz_original	11,182, 5,457 new to gaz_original	163, 102 new to gaz_original
$GAZ\_EXT_{category}$	18,861, 7,075 new to gaz_original	13,480, 7,745 new to gaz_original	305, 245 new to gaz_original

Table 4. Using extended gazetteers, System accuracy in the entity extraction task for each type of entities

	Location			Subject			Temporal		
	P	R	F1	P	R	F1	P	R	F1
B+ $GAZ\_EXT_{firstsent}$	69.9	76.7	73.1	70.0	68.3	69.1	82.6	84.6	83.6
B+ $GAZ\_EXT_{category}$	69.1	75.1	72.0	68.8	67.0	67.9	82.0	83.7	82.8

UK Government list of administrative areas as the gazetteer for Location. We will refer to these gazetteers as *GAZ_original*. We added a gazetteer membership feature using these lexical resources and re-trained the NER tagger. Results are shown in Table 2.

In order to further improve the system performance, we applied the gazetteer generation method using the provided gazetteers as seed lists to build more complete domain-specific gazetteers. Since we introduced two methods for classifying seed entities, which are also used separately for selecting related candidate entities, we use both methods to extend the seed gazetteers and compare them. Specifically for each entity type, $GAZ\_EXT_{firstsent}$ denotes the extended gazetteer built using *FirstSentenceLabeling* for classifying seed entities and selecting candidate entities; $GAZ\_EXT_{category}$ refers to the extended gazetteer built with *CategoryLabeling*. Table 3 lists statistics of the gazetteer expansion results.

Retraining the NER tagger produced improved performance as shown in Table 4.

Table 5. Number of unique entities in each gazetteer built by combining the two approaches

	Location	Subject	Temporal
GAZ_EXT_{union}	23,741 11,955 new to gaz_original	16,697 10,972 new to gaz_original	333, 272 new to gaz_original
$GAZ\_EXT_{intersect}$	14,022, 2,236 new to gaz_original	7,455, 1,730 new to gaz_original	133, 72 new to gaz_original

Table 6. NER performance using GAZ_EXT$_{union}$ and GAZ_EXT$_{intersect}$

	Location			Subject			Temporal		
	P	R	F1	P	R	F1	P	R	F1
B+ EXT$_{union}$	68.9	75.0	71.8	69.8	66.5	68.1	82.4	83.4	82.9
B+ EXT$_{intersect}$	69.3	76.2	72.6	69.7	67.6	68.6	82.6	84.3	83.4

The results so far have shown that, although the sizes of original gazetteers are relatively large as seed entity lists, these gazetteers are still incomplete and can be further enriched. Given the size of the original gazetteers, the gazetteer generation process was ran only once and not in an iterative manner. This still significantly increased the amount of domain-specific entities as indicated by the numbers in Table 3. Careful studies and comparison between the original and extended gazetteers reveal gaps between the document annotation and original gazetteers. For the Location gazetteer, many street names ("Blue Stone Heath Road", "A61"), place of interests ("Royal Armory Museum", "Abbey Village Reservoir") and alternative names are used in the corpus; however, these are largely missing in the original Location gazetteer, which only contains UK administrative areas. Similarly for Temporal, many alternative and new names are found in annotations but not included in the gazetteer. Examples include "renaissance", "Roman Republic", "Byzantine Empire". The problem is even more acute for Subject due to the heterogeneity of information in this class. The original gazetteers were initially divided into 44 sub-topics, which is equivalent to an average of roughly 130 entities per topic (total of 5,725 divided by 44). The gaz-

etteer generation process successfully doubled the size of Subject gazetteers. The quality of the generated gazetteers is considered to be good since they improved the performance from baseline with original gazetteers by 1 – 3 percent in F-measure.

Considering the similar nature of the two classification methods for seed and related candidate entities, we studied the effects of combining the two approaches. Specifically, two more sets of gazetteers were created and tested with the NER tagger. Firstly, GAZ_EXT_{union} merges gazetteers built using two different approaches; secondly, $GAZ\_EXT_{intersect}$ takes the intersection of $GAZ\_EXT_{firstsent}$ and $GAZ\_EXT_{category}$ i.e., only entities that are generated by both approaches. The sizes of the two new gazetteers are shown in Table 5. The NER performance using these gazetteers is shown in Table 6.

Interestingly, taking the intersection of gazetteers generated by the two approaches outperformed the union, but figures are still lower than the best results obtained with $GAZ\_EXT_{firstsent}$ as shown in Table 4. Also, system performance with $GAZ\_EXT_{category}$ is lower than with $GAZ\_EXT_{firstsent,}$ as indicated in Table 4. These observations suggest the quality of gazetteers generated using *CategoryLabeling* is worse than those by *FirstSen-*

Table 7. Number of FGCs and average instance per FGC generated by each approach

		# of FGCs	Size of final gazetteers	Avg instances per FGC
Location	*FirstSentenceLabeling*	597	19,385	32
	CategoryLabeling	779	18,861	24
Subject	*FirstSentenceLabeling*	1342	11,182	8
	CategoryLabeling	761	13,480	17
Temporal	*FirstSentenceLabeling*	11	163	14
	CategoryLabeling	10	305	30

Table 8. Top 5 most frequently extracted (by number of seed entities) FGCs for each entity type.

LOC		SUB		TEM	
FirstSentenceLabeling	*CategoryLabeling*	*FirstSentenceLabeling*	*CategoryLabeling*	*FirstSentenceLabeling*	*CategoryLabeling*
village, small village, place, town, civil parish	villages in north Yorkshire, north Yorkshire geography stubs, villages in Norfolk, villages in Somerset, English market towns	facility, building, ship, tool, device	ship types, monument types, gardening, fortification	period, archaeological period, era, century	Periods and stages in archaeology, Bronze age, middle ages, historical eras, centuries

tenceLabeling, therefore, merging the gazetteers included noisy entities from the low-quality gazetteer, while intersecting the gazetteers excluded valid entities from the high-quality gazetteer. After studying examples of the FGCs extracted by the two methods, we concluded that this is due to two reasons. First, the loose structure of the Wikipedia category graph does not always follow an *is-a* relationship. Although we have introduced and employed several heuristics to reduce noise, the FGCs extracted by this method are still noisier than those built by *FirstSentenceLabeling*. Such examples include "Bronze" for Temporal, "Units of force" for Location, and managerial categories that we failed to eliminate such as "uncategorized", "Wikify from December 2007". These noisy FGCs permitted invalid entries in the gazetteers. On the other hand, compared to Wikipedia categories, the FGCs extracted from the first sentences are sometimes very fine-grained

and restrictive. For example, the FGCs extracted for "Buckinghamshire" from the first sentence are "ceremonial Home County" and "Non-metropolitan County", both of which are UK-specific Location concepts. These fine-grained FGCs are believed to help control the gazetteer expansion to focus on the domain of interest. The better performance with *FirstSentenceLabeling* suggests that this has played a positive role in improving the quality of candidate entities.

From the ontology learning perspective, the experiment can be considered as enriching the ontology of Subject, Location and Temporal with *is-a* relation and populating the ontology. The method successfully inserted a layer of fine-grained concepts which bridge the three high level concepts and low level instances. As shown in Table 7 and Table 8, both approaches generated a large number of useful fine-grained concepts and populated instances.

DISCUSSION AND OUTLOOK

We have introduced a novel method for exploiting background knowledge from Web resources to generate domain-specific lexical and ontological knowledge that can be applied to gazetteer construction and adapted to ontology learning. The method has been evaluated in an NER task in a specialised domain – archaeology, and results have empirically proved its applicability in the relevant tasks. The method is designed to deliver good domain portability and scalability. It is language- and domain-independent, relying on the generic and rich information content and structural elements available from Wikipedia, which is a fast-growing, large scale, multi-lingual online knowledge base covering many specialised domains. It can be easily customized, and repeated in iterations to generate various sizes of knowledge resources depending on the size of the available input. Compared to existing works that employ other Web resources, Wikipedia provides the advantages of easier access to structured, better quality information, and good coverage of named entities and specialised domains, which are important to knowledge discovery and acquisition. The exponential growth of Wikipedia knowledge base ensures promising prospects for research of knowledge discovery and acquisition. Unlike other works that exploit knowledge from Wikipedia in similar tasks, our method explores multiple types of information content and structural elements and naturally integrates them. Also, to our best knowledge, we are the first to prove its applicability in a specialised domain rather than the general domain that has been extensively addressed.

Several questions remain to be answered in future research. Firstly, the current method explores only the named entities that have a page in Wikipedia. However, a vast amount of named entities exist in the articles of Wikipedia but they do not have a dedicated page. For example, "Dell Latitude D600" is a named entity that does not have a dedicated Wikipedia page but is mentioned on the page of "Dell Latitude". It may be beneficial to capture and include these entities in the learning process. Secondly, the scalability and domain portability are to be empirically verified by testing the method with minimally available seed resources and in more technical domains, such as aerospace engineering and computer science. Last but not least, more effort should be invested in combining multiple sources of knowledge and integrate the extracted knowledge in a coherent way. As described earlier, ever since the birth of the Internet, the amount of information and knowledge from the Web has been increasing at an extraordinary rate. The introduction of Web 2.0 invoked a revolution of knowledge creation and publication on the Web, in which individuals actively participate in the knowledge generation process and more structured and well-curated knowledge resources are created and maintained. Despite the two successful collaborative knowledge bases introduced in this chapter, i.e., Wikipedia and Wiktionary, other information sharing media such as blogs, forums (e.g., BBC news commenting service) and question answering websites (e.g., Yahoo! Answer) also provides useful knowledge. It is impossible to create an ultimate, complete knowledge base; however, different knowledge sources may complement each other. Therefore, it is desirable to have a way of interlinking knowledge from different sources and publishing them in a uniform way.

One interesting research in this direction is the DBpedia[13] project. DBpedia is a free online multi-million triple store initially created by extracting structured information from Wikipedia. It allows users to make complex queries against knowledge in Wikipedia and to link other datasets on the Web to Wikipedia data. The purpose of the project is to promote knowledge linking and sharing. Essentially, the idea of DBpedia is to extract the structured information from various sources and formalize them using a uniform representation, the RDF triples. These triples are stored in a triple store, which can be accessed by semantic query languages such as SPARQL. Initially, it was populated by extracting information from Wikipedia infobox, a table-like summary of an entity's facts, often containing information generic to the class of the entity mentioned by the article. For example, an infobox about an article of a politician may contain tabular information of the person's first name, last name, birth place and date, political party, roles and so on. These are naturally facts about the entity person and are turned into triples which can support complex semantic queries to allow seeking deep knowledge that is not directly available from any single knowledge resource, such as "show me all American politicians born after 1940".

The introduction of DBpedia is relatively new (first published in 2007), little research has explored the application of its data to computational linguistics. However, its power has been demonstrated in a number of pilot applications. Kobilarov et al. (2009) used DBpedia resource URIs as a controlled vocabulary to semanticize and interlink BBC news articles, which creates richly connected network of related articles to improve browsing and navigation. Becker & Bizer (2008) used geospatial data in DBpedia to build a recommender system for mobile phone platforms. The system requires a connection to DBpedia and GPS to work. The GPS constantly tracks the user's current geospatial coordinates, and the mobile phone is able to query DBpedia triple store for nearby place of interests by searching for geospatial coordinates within a radius of certain distance.

The concept behind DBpedia has gained broad recognition in the community such that as of November 2009, there are already 479 million triples and 3.7 million interlinks between DBpedia and other open data resources such as Freebase[14], OpenCyc[15], and GeoNames[16]. In future, we envisage interlinking knowledge from different resources and employing the interlinked knowledge will further enhance knowledge discovery and acquisition technologies.

CONCLUSION

This chapter reviewed the technique of Named Entity Recognition with a special focus on using background knowledge from the Web resources to enhance its performance. NER is an important enabling technique for ontology learning; in particular, it is often used for populating instances of concepts in ontology, which is part of the ontology population task. The important role of NER as a pre-processing step to many complex knowledge discovery and acquisition tasks has attracted extensive attention and significant effort from researchers for the last few decades. Earlier NER methods were based on the context-modeling approach, which models candidate entities using a vector space of features derived from a limited context (e.g., a few tokens) surrounding the candidate entities. This definition of context was found to be insufficient in many scenarios and research has advocated for including background knowledge about named entities from other resources. Using background knowledge also proves to be an effective approach to address the major challenge in NER, domain portability.

The recent astonishing growth of the Web and increasing popularity of collaborative knowledge resources have made abundant information and knowledge available on the Web. This has attracted researchers who explore methods of extracting domain-specific knowledge from the Web resources and employ the knowledge to enhance knowledge discovery and acquisition. The advance of NER has also benefited from this trend. New methods of NER using background knowledge harvested from the Web resources have been introduced and proved effective. We reviewed these works and discussed their inadequacies, and then proposed to address these limitations by a novel method of generating high-quality domain-specific background knowledge, which are then used to enhance NER in a specialised domain. We have shown that the method is domain- and language-independent, capable of generating domain-specific knowledge in a scalable and weakly supervised way. The method itself is also a process of ontology learning and population, in which hypernymy and hyponymy relations are inserted and instances of concepts are populated. We empirically proved the applicability of the method in a specialised domain, which has been rarely addressed in previous research on NER using background knowledge from Web resources.

With the vast amount of open data published on the Web and the fast growth of these resources, extracting knowledge from these resources for the purpose of knowledge discovery and acquisition will remain a major focus for the research community. What's more, interlinking data and integrating knowledge from diverse resources and making them available in a uniform way will bring further benefits to the research, and should become the major direction of future research in knowledge discovery and acquisition.

REFERENCES

Ananiadou, S., Friedman, C., & Tsujii, J. (2004). Introduction: Named entity recognition in biomedicine. *Journal of Biomedical Informatics*, *37*(6), 393–395. doi:10.1016/j.jbi.2004.08.011

Babych, B., & Hartley, A. (2003). Improving machine translation quality with automatic named entity recognition. *Proceedings of EAMT/EACL Workshop on MT, Budapest*.

Becker, C., & Bizer, C. (2008). DBpedia mobile: A location-aware Semantic Web client. *Proceedings of the Semantic Web Challenge*.

BioBLP/JNLPBA. (2004). *BioNLP/JNLPBA shared task on biomedical entity recognition.*

Brewster, C., Ciravegna, F., & Wilks, Y. (2003). Background and foreground knowledge in dynamic ontology construction: viewing text as knowledge maintenance. In *Proceedings of Conference Semantic Web Workshop, SIGIR03*: Association of Computing Machinery.

Bunescu, R., & Pasca, M. (2006). *Using encyclopedic knowledge for named entity disambiguation. ECAL-06*. The Association for Computer Linguistics.

Butters, J., & Ciravegna, F. (2008). Using similarity metrics for terminology recognition. *Proceedings in the sixth Language Resource Evaluation Conference*. European Language Resources Association (ELRA)

Byrne, K. (2007). Nested named entity recognition in historical archive text. *Proceedings of the International Conference on Semantic Computing*. (pp. 589-896). IEEE Computer Society

Carvalho, R., Chapman, S., & Ciravegna, F. (2008). Extracting semantic meaning from photographic annotations using a hybrid approach. *MMIU'08: Proceedings of the 1st International Workshop on Metadata Mining for Image Understanding*.

Chinchor, N. (1998). Overview of MUC-7/MET-2. *Proceedings of the Seventh Message Understanding Conference MUC-7*.

Cimiano, P. (2006). *Ontology learning and population from text: Algorithms, evaluation and applications. Springer Science+Business Media*. LLC.

Ciravegna, F., Dingli, A., Petrelli, D., & Wilks, Y. (2002). *Timely and non-intrusive active document annotation via adaptive information extraction*. In Semantic Authoring, Annotation & Knowledge Markup (SAAKM 2002), ECAI 2002 Workshop, (pp. 7-13)

Cucerzan, S. (2007). Large-scale named entity disambiguation based on Wikipedia data. *Proceedings of the 2007 Joint Conference on Empirical Methods in Natural Language Processing and Computational Natural Language Learning* (pp. 708-716)

Doddington, G., Mitchell, A., Przybocki, M., Ramshaw, L., Strassel, S., & Weischedel, R. (2004). The Automatic Content Extraction (ACE) program – tasks, data, and evaluation. *Proceedings of the fourth Conference on Language Resources and Evaluation (LREC)* (pp. 837-840). European Language Resources Association (ELRA).

Downey, D., Broadhead, M., & Etzioni, O. (2007). Locating complex named entities in Web text. *Proceedings of the 20th International Joint Conference on Artifical intelligence* (pp. 2733-2739). Morgan Kaufmann Publishers Inc.

Evans, R. (2003). A framework for named entity recognition in the open domain. In *Proceedings of Recent Advances in Natural Language Processing 2003*.

Ferrández, S., Toral, A., Ferrández, Í., & Ferrández, A. (2009). Exploiting Wikipedia and EuroWordNet to solve cross-lingual question answering. [Elsevier Science Inc.]. *Information Sciences: An International Journal*, *179*(20), 3473–3488.

Friedrich, C., Revillion, T., Hofmann, M., & Fluck, J. (2006). Biomedical and chemical named entity recognition with conditional random fields: The advantage of dictionary features. *Proceedings of the Second International Symposium on Semantic Mining in Biomedicine*.

Gabrilovich, E., & Markovitch, S. (2006). Overcoming the brittleness bottleneck using Wikipedia: Enhancing text categorization with encyclopedic knowledge. *Proceedings of the 21st National Conference on Artificial intelligence, vol. 2* (pp. 1301-1306). AAAI Press

Gabrilovich, E., & Markovitch, S. (2007). Computing semantic relatedness using Wikipedia-based explicit semantic analysis. *Proceedings of the 20th International Joint Conference on Artifical intelligence*. (pp. 1606-1611). Morgan Kaufmann Publishers Inc.

Ganti, V., Konig, A., & Vernica, R. (2008). Entity categorization over large document collections. *Proceeding of the 14th ACM SIGKDD International Conference on Knowledge discovery and data mining*. (pp. 274-282). Association for Computing Machinery

Giles, J. (2005). Internet encyclopedias go head to head. *Nature*, *438*, 900–901. doi:10.1038/438900a

Giuliano, C. (2009). Fine-grained classification of named entities exploiting latent semantic kernels. In [Morristown, NJ: Association for Computational Linguistics]. *Proceedings of CoNLL*, *09*, 201–209. doi:10.3115/1596374.1596406

Giuliano, C., Lavelli, A., & Romano, L. (2006). Exploiting shallow linguistic information for relation extraction from biomedical literature. In *Proceedings of the 11th Conference of the European Chapter of the Association for Computational Linguistics*.

Giullano, C., & Gliozzo, A. (2008). Instance-based ontology population exploiting named-entity substitution. In *Proceedings of the 22nd International Conference on Computational Linguistics, vol. 1* (pp. 265-272). Association for Computational Linguistics

Goldschmidt, D., & Krishnamoorthy, M. (2008). Comparing keyword search to semantic search: A case study in solving crossword puzzles using the Google™ API. [John Wiley & Sons Inc.]. *Software, Practice & Experience*, *38*(4), 417–445. doi:10.1002/spe.840

Google Press Center online. (2006). *Google to acquire YouTube for $1.65 billion in stock.* Retrieved from http://www.google.com/press/pressrel/google_youtube.html

Grishman, R., & Sundheim, B. (1996). Message understanding conference - 6: A brief history. *Proceedings of the 16th International Conference on Computational Linguistics,* vol. 1 (pp.466-471). Association for Computational Linguistics.

Hassan, S., & Mihalcea, R. (2009). Cross-lingual semantic relatedness using encyclopedic knowledge. *Proceedings of the 2009 Conference on Empirical Methods in Natural Language Processing* (pp.1192-1201). Association for Computational Linguisticts

Hearst, M. (1992). Automatic acquisition of hyponyms from large text corpora. *Proceedings of the 14th Conference on Computational linguistics,* vol. 2 (pp. 539-545). Association for Computational Linguistics.

Holloway, T., Bozicevic, M., & Börner, K. (2007). Analyzing and visualizing the semantic coverage of Wikipedia and its authors. *Journal of Complexity, Special issue on Understanding Complex Systems, 12*(3), 30-40.

Iria, J. (2009). Automating knowledge capture in the aerospace domain. *Proceedings of the fifth International Conference on Knowledge capture* (pp. 97-104). Association for Computing Machinery.

Jeffrey, S., Richards, J., Ciravegna, F., Chapman, S., & Zhang, Z. (2009). *The Archaeotools project: Faceted classification and natural language processing in an archaeological context. Special Theme Issues of the Philosophical Transactions of the Royal Society A, Crossing Boundaries: Computational Science.* E-Science and Global E-Infrastructures.

Jimeno, A., Ruiz, E., Lee, V., Gaudan, S., Berlanga, R., & Schuhmann, D. (2007). Assessment of disease named entity recognition on a corpus of annotated sentences. *Proceedings of the Second International Symposium on Languages in Biology and Medicine (LBM).* BMC Bioinformatics

Kazama, J., & Torisawa, K. (2007). Exploiting Wikipedia as external knowledge for named entity recognition. *Proceedings of the 2007 Joint Conference on Empirical Methods in Natural Language Processing and Computational Natural Language Learning (EMNLP-CoNLL).* (pp. 698-707). Association for Computational Linguistics.

Kazama, J., & Torisawa, K. (2008). Inducing gazetteers for named entity recognition by large-scale clustering of dependency relations. In *Proceedings of ACL-08: HLT.* (pp. 407-415). Association for Computational Linguistics.

Kim, J., Ohta, T., Tsuruoka, Y., Tateisi, Y., & Collier, N. (2004). Introduction to the bio-entity recognition task at JNLPBA. *Proceedings of the International Joint Workshop on Natural Language Processing in Biomedicine and its Applications (JNLPBA'04)* (pp. 70-75). Association for Computational Linguistics.

Kliegr, T., Chandramouli, K., Nemrava, J., Svatek, V., & Izquierdo, E. (2008). Combining image captions and visual analysis for image concept classification. *Proceedings of the 9th International Workshop on Multimedia Data Mining: held in conjunction with the ACM SIGKDD 2008* (pp. 8-17). Association for Computing Machinary.

Klinger, R., Friedrich, C., Fluck, J., & Hofmann-Apitius, M. (2007). Named entity recognition with combinations of conditional random fields. *Proceedings of the Second BioCreative Challenge Evaluation Workshop.*

Kobilarov, G., Scott, T., Raimond, Y., Oliver, S., Sizemore, C., & Smethurst, M. ... Lee, R. (2009). Media meets Semantic Web – how the BBC uses DBpedia and linked data to make connections. *Proceedings of the 6th European Semantic Web Conference on The Semantic Web: Research and Applications* (pp. 723-737). Springer-Verlag.

Krizhanovsky, A., & Lin, F. (2009). Related terms search based on WordNet / Wiktionary and its application in ontology matching. *Proceedings of the 11th Russian Conference on Digital Libraries RCDL.*

Lesk, M. (1986). Automatic sense disambiguation using machine readable dictionaries: How to tell a pine cone from an ice cream cone. *Proceedings of the 5th Annual International Conference on Systems documentation* (pp. 24-26). Association for Computing Machinary

Mayfield, J., McNamee, P., & Piatko, C. (2003). Named entity recognition using hundreds of thousands of features. *Proceedings of the seventh conference on Natural language learning at HLT-NAACL 2003*, vol. 4 (pp. 184-187). Association for Computational Linguistics.

Miller, S., Guinness, J., & Zamanian, A. (2004). Name tagging with word clusters and discriminative training. [Association for Computational Linguistics.]. *Proceedings of, HLT-04*, 337–342.

Mohit, B., & Hwa, R. (2005). Syntax-based semi-supervised named entity tagging. *Proceedings of ACL'05* (pp. 57-60). Association for Computational Linguistics.

Mollá, O., Zaanen, M., & Smith, D. (2006). Named entity recognition for question answering. *Proceedings of the 2006 Australasian Language Technology Workshop (ALTW2006).*

Müller, C., & Gurevych, I. (2009). Using Wikipedia and Wiktionary in domain-specific information retrieval. In *Evaluating Systems for Multilingual and Multimodal Information Access* (pp. 219–226). Berlin / Heidelberg, Germany: Springer. doi:10.1007/978-3-642-04447-2_28

Murphy, T., McIntosh, T., & Curran, J. (2006). *Named entity recognition for astronomy literature.* In Australasian Language Technology Workshop.

Nadeau, D. (2007). *Semi-supervised named entity recognition: Learning to recognize 100 entity types with little supervision.* Unpublished PhD thesis.

Navarro, E., Sajous, F., Gaume, B., Prévot, L., Shu Kai, H., & Tzu-Yi, K. ... Chu-Ren, H. (2009). Wiktionary and NLP: Improving synonymy networks. *Proceedings of the Workshop on the People's Web Meets NLP, ACL-IJCNLP.*

Nothman, J., Curran, J., & Murphy, T. (2008). *Transforming Wikipedia into named entity training data.* In ALTA-08.

Ohta, T., Tateisi, Y., Kim, J., Mima, H., & Tsuji, J. (2002). The GENIA corpus: An annotated research abstract corpus in molecular biology domain. *Proceedings of the Second International Conference on Human Language Technology Research* (pp. 82-86). Morgan Kaufmann Publishers Inc.

Olsson, F. (2008). Bootstrapping named entity annotation by means of active machine learning: A method for creating corpora. Unpublished PhD thesis.

Riloff, E., & Jones, R. (1999). Learning dictionaries for information extraction by multi-level bootstrapping. *Proceedings of the sixteenth National Conference on Artificial intelligence and the eleventh Innovative applications of artificial intelligence conference innovative applications of artificial intelligence* (pp. 474-479). American Association for Artificial Intelligence.

Roberts, A., Gaizauskas, R., Hepple, M., & Guo, Y. (2008). Combining terminology resources and statistical methods for entity recognition: An evaluation. In *Proceedings of the Sixth International Conference on Language Resources and Evaluation (LREC 2008)*. European Language Resources Association (ELRA).

Saha, S., Sarkar, S., & Mitra, P. (2009). Feature selection techniques for maximum entropy based biomedical named entity recognition. *Journal of Biomedical Informatics, 42*(5), 905–911. doi:10.1016/j.jbi.2008.12.012

Sarmento, L., Jijkoun, V., Rijke, M., & Oliveira, E. (2007). More like these: Growing entity classes from seeds. In *Proceedings of the sixteenth ACM Conference on information and knowledge management* (CIKM'07)

Srihari, R., & Peterson, E. (2008). Named entity recognition for improving retrieval and translation of Chinese documents. In *Proceedings of the 11th International Conference on Asian Digital Libraries: Universal and Ubiquitous Access to Information* (pp. 404-405). Springer-Verlag.

Strube, M., & Ponzetto, S. (2006). WikiRelate! Computing semantic relatedness using Wikipedia. *Proceedings of the 21st National Conference on Artificial intelligence,* vol. 2 (pp. 1419-1424). AAAI Press.

Toral, A., & Muñoz, R. (2006). A proposal to automatically build and maintain gazetteers for named entity recognition by using Wikipedia. *In Proceedings of the Workshop on NEW TEXT Wikis and blogs and other dynamic text sources in the 11th EACL.*

Turdakov, D., & Velikhov, P. (2008). *Semantic relatedness metric for Wikipedia concepts based on link analysis and its application to word sense disambiguation.* In Colloquium on Databases and Information Systems (SYRCoDIS).

Weale, T., Brew, C., & Fosler-Lussier, E. (2009). Using the Wiktionary graph structure for synonym detection. *Proceedings of the Workshop on the People's Web Meets NLP, ACL-IJCNLP.*

Weber, N., & Buitelaar, P. (2006). Web-based ontology learning with ISOLDE. In *Proceedings of the Workshop on Web Content Mining with Human Language, International Semantic Web Conference (ISWC).*

Zesch, T., & Gurevych, I. (2007). Analysis of the Wikipedia category graph for NLP applications. *Proceedings of the TextGraphs-2 Workshop (NAACL-HLT).*

Zesch, T., Müller, C., & Gurevych, I. (2008). Using Wiktionary for computing semantic relatedness. *Proceedings of the 23rd National Conference on Artificial intelligence* (pp. 861-866). AAAI Press.

Zhang, Z., & Iria, J. (2009). A novel approach to automatic gazetteer generation using Wikipedia. In *Proceedings of the ACL'09 Workshop on Collaboratively Constructed Semantic Resources,* Singapore, August 2009.

ADDITIONAL READING

Ananiadou, S., Friedman, C., & Tsujii, J. (2004). Introduction: named entity recognition in biomedicine. *Journal of Biomedical Informatics, 37*(6), 393–395. doi:10.1016/j.jbi.2004.08.011

BioBLP/JNLPBA (2004), BioNLP/JNLPBA shared task on biomedical entity recognition, *BioNLP/JNLPBA.*

Brewster, C., Iria, J., Zhang, Z., Ciravegna, F., Guthrie, L., & Wilks, Y. (2007). *2007 (RANLP-07).* Dynamic Iterative Ontology Learning. In Proceedings of Recent Advances in Natural Language Processing.

Brewster, C., Jupp, S., Luciano, J., Shotton, D., Stevens, R., & Zhang, Z. (2008). Issues in learning an ontology from text. *BMC Bioinformatics, 10*(5).

Bunescu, R., & Pasca, M. (2006). *Using Encyclopedic Knowledge for Named Entity Disambiguation. ECAL-06.* The Association for Computer Linguistics.

Cafarella, M., Downey, D., Soderland, S., & Etzioni, O. (2005). Knowitnow: Fast, scalable information extraction from the web, *Proceedings of the conference on Human Language Technology and Empirical Methods in Natural Language Processing.* (pp.563-570): Association for Computational Linguistics

Chinchor, N. (1998). Overview of MUC-7/MET-2, *Proceedings of the Seventh Message Understanding Conference MUC-7.*

Cimiano, P. (2006). *Ontology learning and population from text: algorithms, evaluation and applications: Springer Science+Business Media.* LLC.

Cimiano, P., & Völker, J. (2005). Towards large-scale, open-domain and ontology-based named entity classification. *Proceedings of RANLP'05.*

Doddington, G., Mitchell, A., Przybocki, M., Ramshaw, L., Strassel, S., & Weischedel, R. (2004). The Automatic Content Extraction (ACE) Program – Tasks, Data, and Evaluation, *Proceedings of the fourth Conference on Language Resources and Evaluation (LREC).* (pp.837-840): European Language Resources Association (ELRA)

2008 Extracting Lexical Semantic Knowledge from Wikipedia and Wiktionary. *Proceedings of the Sixth International Language Resources and Evaluation.*

Gabrilovich, E., & Markovitch, S. (2007). Computing semantic relatedness using Wikipedia-based explicit se-mantic analysis. *Proceedings of the 20th international joint conference on Artifical intelligence.* (pp.1606-1611): Morgan Kaufmann Publishers Inc.

Giles, J. (2005). Internet Encyclopedias Go Head to Head. *Nature, 438,* 900–901. doi:10.1038/438900a

Giullano, C., & Gliozzo, A. (2008). Instance-based ontology population exploiting named-entity substitution. In *Proceedings of the 22nd International Conference on Computational Linguistics.* Vol.1. (pp.265-272): Association for Computational Linguistics

Grishman, R., & Sundheim, B. (1996). Message understanding conference - 6: A brief history, *Proceedings of the 16th International Conference on Computational Linguistics.* Vol. 1. (pp.466-471).: Association for Computational Linguistics.

Holloway, T., Bozicevic, M., Börner, K. (2007). Analyzing and Visualizing the Semantic Coverage of Wikipedia and its Authors. *Journal of Complexity, Special issue on Understanding Complex Systems, 12(3), pp. 30-40*

Jentzsch, A. (2009). DBpedia – Extracting structured data from Wikipedia. *Semantic Web In Bibliotheken (SWIB2009)*

Kazama, J., & Torisawa, K. (2007). Exploiting Wikipedia as external knowledge for named entity recognition. *Proceedings of the 2007 Joint Conference on Empirical Methods in Natural Language Processing and Computational Natural Language Learning (EMNLP-CoNLL).* (pp.698-707): Association for Computational Linguistics

Milne, D., Medelyan, O., & Witten, I. (2006). Mining Domain-Specific Thesauri from Wikipedia: A Case Study. In *Proceedings of the 2006 IEEE/WIC/ACM International Conference on Web Intelligence*

Nadeau, D. (2007). PhD Thesis: Semi-Supervised Named Entity Recognition: Learning to Recognize 100 Entity Types with Little Supervision.

Nadeau, D. (2007). A survey of named entity recognition and classification [John Benjamins Publishing Company]. *Journal of Linguisticae Investigationes, 30*(1), 3–26. doi:10.1075/li.30.1.03nad

Nothman, J., Curran, J., & Murphy, T. (2008). Transforming Wikipedia into named entity training data. In *ALTA-08*

Pantel, P., Crestan, E., Borkovsky, A., Popescu, A., & Vyas, V. (2009). Web-Scale Distributional Similarity and Entity Set Expansion. In: *Proceedings of EMNLP Conference (EMNLP 2009)*

Ratinov, L., & Roth, D. (2009). Design Challenges and Misconceptions in Named Entity Recognition. *Proceedings of the Thirteenth Conference on Computational Natural Language Learning (CoNLL).* (pp.147-155): Association for Computational Linguistics

Richman, A., & Schone, P. (2008). Mining Wiki Resources for Multilingual Named Entity Recognition. *Proceedings of ACL-08: HLT.* (pp.1-9): Association for Computational Linguistics

Sarawagi, S. (2008). Information Extraction. [Now Publishers Inc.]. *Foundations and Trends in Databases, 1*(3), 261–377. doi:10.1561/1900000003

Sarmento, L., Jijkoun, V., Rijke, M., & Oliveira, E. (2007). More like these: Growing entity classes from seeds. In *Proceedings of the sixteenth ACM conference on Conference on information and knowledge management* (CIKM 2007)

Toral, A., & Muñoz, R. (2006). A Proposal to Automatically Build and Maintain Gazetteers for Named Entity Recognition by using Wikipedia, *In Proceedings of the workshop on NEW TEXT Wikis and blogs and other dynamic text sources in the 11th EACL.* Zesch, T., Müller, C., Gurevych, I.

KEY TERMS AND DEFINITIONS

Named Entity Recognition: The task of recognizing and classifying atomic text into pre-defined concept classes, often referred to as NER. NER is usually a pre-processing step for many complex information extraction and knowledge acquisition tasks.

Ontology Learning: a research task in Information Extraction that addresses automatically extracting relevant concepts and relations from given datasets to create an ontology.

Ontology Population: The task of automatically extracting instances of ontological concepts and expressions of ontological relations from various data sources.

Wikipedia: A multi-lingual, free online encyclopedia that is collaboratively created and maintained by voluntary contributors. Knowledge in Wikipedia are organised based on articles, which are often descriptions of named entities. Information can be accessed by semi-structured and structured way.

Wiktionary: A multi-lingual free content dictionary of words, currently available in over 270 languages.

Dbpedia: A free online multi-million triple store initially created by extracting structured information from Wikipedia. It allows users to make complex queries against knowledge in Wikipedia and to link other datasets on the web to Wikipedia data.

Machine Learning: Machine learning is a way to automatically learn to recognise complex patterns or sequence labelling algorithms and make intelligent decisions based on data.

Open Data: data that are freely available to everyone without restrictions from copyright, patents or other mechanisms of control (Wikipedia, 2010)

ENDNOTES

[1] http://www.wikipedia.org/

[2] Unified Medical Language System, http://www.nlm.nih.gov/pubs/factsheets/umls-meta.html

[3] http://www.fao.org/agrovoc/

[4] http://www4.fao.org/asfa/asfa.htm

[5] http://wordnet.princeton.edu/

[6] Google Feb, 2010

[7] CONLL - Computational Natural Language Learning

[8] http://ahds.ac.uk/

[9] Support Vector Machine,

[10] http://www.midas-heritage.info and http://www.fish-forum.info

[11] http://thesaurus.english-heritage.org.uk

[12] http://hypermedia.research.glam.ac.uk/kos/STAR/

[13] http://dbpedia.org/About

[14] http://www.freebase.com/

[15] http://www.cyc.com/cyc/opencyc/overview

[16] http://www.geonames.org/

Chapter 6
User–Centered Maintenance of Concept Hierarchies

Kai Eckert
University of Mannheim, Germany

Robert Meusel
University of Mannheim, Germany

Heiner Stuckenschmidt
University of Mannheim, Germany

ABSTRACT

Taxonomies are hierarchical concept representations that have numerous important applications from improved indexing of document collections to faceted browsing and semantic search applications. The maintenance of taxonomies includes the dynamic extension, analysis, and visualization of these representations. Instead of focusing on the construction of taxonomies from scratch, however, the authors describe several successful approaches to the semi-automatic maintenance of taxonomies. These approaches have in common that they incorporate the human expert as a central part of the system.

1 INTRODUCTION

Beside the full-fledged ontologies that are supposed to form the basis of the Semantic Web, other constructs exist to represent background knowledge. Many of them have a long tradition and history that goes back well before the birth of the Internet, including glossaries, dictionaries, vocabularies, gazetteers, taxonomies and thesauri, just to name a few. They all, including ontologies, have in common that they are used to represent and organize knowledge in a structured way to fulfill specific functions for different purposes, thus we refer to all of them as *Knowledge Organization Systems* (KOS). A subset of them have in common that they organize the concepts representing single units of knowledge in a hierarchical way, which we call concept hierarchies.

Concept hierarchies have numerous important applications from improved indexing of document collections to faceted browsing and semantic search applications. But the creation and maintenance of concept hierarchies is cumbersome and very time consuming. On the other hand, many

DOI: 10.4018/978-1-60960-625-1.ch006

concept hierarchies already exist and more and more of them become publicly available, ideally as *linked open data*, and can be reused for different purposes. If an existing concept hierarchy is to be reused, several tasks have to be performed, reaching from the proper selection of the source to start with to the adaptation for the desired purpose which includes deletion of unnecessary concepts, merging and splitting of concepts and especially the addition of missing concepts.

In this chapter, we describe several successful approaches to the semi-automatic creation and maintenance of different types of concept hierarchies. These approaches have in common that they incorporate the human expert as a central part of the system.

1.1 Concept Hierarchies

Contrary to full-fledged ontologies, concept hierarchies use only a limited set of semantic relations. Typically there is one main relation that leads to the hierarchical structure of the concepts. This relation is usually referred to as "broader than", respectively "narrower than", but can also have a very specific meaning, like "is a"/"has subclass" or "part of"/"has part". A common property of these semantic relations is transitivity which is essential for building a hierarchy: if A is broader than B and B is broader than C, A has also to be broader than C or the organization in a hierarchy would be counter-intuitive.

The most abstract and widely used representative of concept hierarchies are *taxonomies*. Taxonomies basically organize concepts by supertype-subtype or parent-child relations and according to this all concepts have to be as disjunct as possible. An example for a taxonomy is the Linnaean taxonomy:

Linnaean taxonomy *is one of the first appearance in science of taxonomies, which was used to classify concepts. In this special taxonomy Carolus Linnaeus classified the known and still*

existing concepts belonging into the imperium naturea into three different kingdoms: mineral, animal and vegetable. All in all his structure included four other classification levels beneath kingdom: class, order, genus and species. The work of Linnaeus was the starting point for the botanical nomenclature[1] as known today and is used to classify all kinds of animals and plants by biologists.

In comparison to taxonomies, *thesauri* basically extend the core functionality of taxonomies with additional accepted relations like *synonym*, *antonym* or *related term* to improve their ability to describe the world or a specific domain. The concepts in a thesaurus are not required to be disjunct. An example would be WordNet:

WordNet *is one of the largest living general English thesaurus[2]. The concepts are called synsets and include nouns, verbs, adjectives and adverbs which are cognitive synonyms describing the concept.*

The approaches in this chapter can be used in principle for both thesauri and taxonomies, as well as for other concept hierarchies. To avoid the long-winded term concept hierarchy, we refer to it often as thesaurus or taxonomy, usually depending on the current example dataset: the *Medical Subject Headings* (Section 3) are usually considered to be a thesaurus, while the *Indiana Philosophy Ontology* (Section 4) - despite the ontology in the name - is referred to as taxonomy on the project website. Here, we describe both concept hierarchies briefly:

Medical Subject Headings *(MeSH) is a medical thesaurus created and maintained by the National Library of Medicine (NLM). It includes over 25.000 concepts[3] which are arranged in an alphabetic and a hierarchical structure. This thesaurus is used by the NLM to index medical* articles which are searchable via the MEDLINE/ PubMED database.

Indiana Philosophie Ontology *(InPhO) is an semi-automatically created taxonomy which gives users the possibility to search and navigate through the Stanford Encyclopedia of Philosophy, Noesis, and Google Scholar. The creation process involves answers and evaluations of the user community and is described in Section 4. The project is held in trust by the Indiana University[4].*

1.2 Maintenance Approaches

Due to the fast growing number of novel concepts, manual maintenance of those structures is, if at all, only feasible for large central libraries. Moreover it is almost impossible to keep up with new topics that arise as a reaction to current events in the real world, quickly making their way into publications.

The recent past has provided us with a number of examples, two of which we want to mention here as motivation for our contribution. In economics, the financial crisis has led to a discussion of structured products finance and terms such as "CDO" (credit debt obligation) frequently occur in documents covering current events. Nevertheless, the very same term is not included in the leading German thesaurus on business and economics. In the area of medicine, the outbreak of the H1N1 pandemic has recently sparked numerous media and research reports about the so-called "swine flu." At that point the term "swine flu" was not included in any of the major medical thesauri because it was only recently coined by the media. The current version (2010) of the MeSH thesaurus lists the term "Swine-Origin Influenza A H1N1 Virus" as a synonym for "Influenza A Virus, H1N1 Subtype" but not the more commonly used term "swine flu."

This is just to get an idea what tasks might be required to maintain a concept hierarchy. As concept hierarchies are special kinds of ontologies, the creation and maintenance of concept hierarchies

can be seen as ontology learning. But the reduced complexity has implications for the extension process, as we give up some of the structure and formal power of an ontology. On the one hand, this can make our life easier: a very promising approach for the creation of taxonomies is the exploitation of the fact that they are usually restricted to only one relation between the concepts. Also for a thesaurus, the number of possible relations is strictly limited in contrast to ontologies. On the other hand, many techniques, especially reasoning and the identification of inconsistencies, are not available or only in a very limited form.

The remainder of this chapter is structured as follows: After an overview on related work in Section 2, we present two different approaches to maintain a concept hierarchy. The first approach (Section 3) is generally applicable and includes the identification of interesting terms in a set of documents that are candidates for the inclusion in the concept hierarchies and identifies appropriate adding locations for these terms. In Section 4, the creation process of the InPhO taxonomy is described which employs reasoning techniques on answers given by a user community to deduce relations between concepts that were automatically extracted from the Stanford Encyclopedia of Philosophy. Afterwards (Section 5), we introduce Semtinel, a research software that implements an interactive evaluation approach for concept hierarchies based on statistical analyses and appropriate visualizations.

2 RELATED WORK

Nguyen et al. (2007) used lexico-syntactic patterns mined from the online encyclopedia *wikipedia.org* to extract relations between terms. Gillam et al. (2005) describe a combination of term extraction, co-occurrence-based measures and predefined linguistic patterns to construct a thesaurus structure from domain-specific collections of texts. Another combination of these techniques using hidden markov random fields is presented by Kaji and Kitsuregawa (2008). Witschel (2005) employs a decision tree algorithm to insert novel concepts into a taxonomy. Katia Lida Kermanidis and Fakotakis (2008) present with Eksairesis a system for ontology building from unstructured text that is adaptable to different domains and languages. For the process of term extraction they use two corpora, a balanced corpus and a domain-specific corpus. The semantic relations are then learned from syntactic schemata, an approach that is applicable to corpora written in languages without strict sentence word ordering such as modern Greek. For most of these cases, pattern based approaches are hardly applicable.

Many methods focus only on the extraction of synonyms from text corpora: Turney (2001) computes the similarity between synonym candidates leveraging the number of hits returned for different combinations of search terms. Matsuo et al. (2006) apply co-occurrence measures on search engine results to cluster words. Curran (2002) combines several methods for synonym extraction and shows that the combination outperforms each of the single methods, including Grefenstette's approach (Grefenstette, 1994). In some cases, special resources such as bilingual corpora or dictionaries are available to support specialized methods for automatic thesaurus construction. Wu and Zhou (2003) describe a combination of such methods to extract synonyms. Other techniques using multilingual corpora are described by Plas and Tiedemann (2006) and Kageura et al. (2000).

A platform for automatic indexing with integrated thesaurus maintenance (IKEM platform) is presented by Vervenne (1999). The IKEM platform is a very promising and holistic approach to focus on the whole indexing process and not only on a subset. The maintenance is for example supported by providing the human expert with terms from the indexed documents that might be meaningful, but could not be assigned to existing thesaurus concepts.

Advanced methods that follow the same approach of identification of meaningful terms based on Latent Semantic Indexing and Multidimensional Scaling are presented by Weiner (2005).

3 EXTENSION USING WEB SEARCH ENGINES

In this section we describe an approach which could be used to extend concept hierarchies, no matter if they are more general or really specific. The approach assumes that a concept hierarchy, no matter what size (but not empty) or what degree of granularity, is already available and that new input is provided through new documents, as for example in libraries where a concept hierarchy is used to improve indexing and search of documents and new concepts arise out of new documents like books which are published all the time. For this approach it is not necessary to have specific topic knowledge in the first place. Therefore the different new concepts are extracted out of a document corpus using a tf-idf based method. In a second step possible locations in the existing concept hierarchies are identified with a Web search engine pattern based recognition approach similar to the method of Bollegala et al. (2007b) and finally suggestions about the relation between the locations and the new concepts are made. Additionally this section shows possibility to improve this approach and make it feasible for real-time extension of large-scale concept hierarchies.

Figure 1 depicts a typical instance of the thesaurus extension problem.

3.1 Method Description

The following section includes the different approaches which are necessary and needed to maintain a concept hierarchy in general. It is important to notice, that the presented approaches are not the only one which exists and also may

Figure 1. Fragment of the WordNet thesaurus

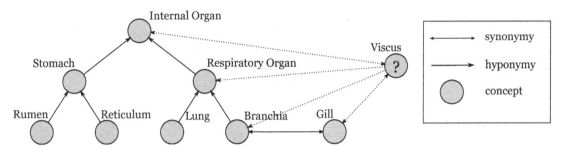

not fit to every specific case but give in general a good impression on how the issue can be handled.

Let us assume we are given a concept hierarchy H_1 that needs to be extended with novel concepts. The process of structural extension can be divided in two major phases. First, concept candidates have to be extracted from document collections and other textual content. In order to achieve satisfiable results it is necessary that the text corpora under consideration are semantically related to the concepts in H_1. For instance, if we want to extend a concept hierarchy of medical terms we would have to choose a document collection covering medical topics. Given a set of candidate terms, the second step of the structural extension involves the classification of these candidates according to the different available relations in H_1.

We propose a method supporting the knowledge modeler during both of these phases by (a) extracting terms from text corpora using a novel extraction method based on the well-known *tf-idf* measure and (b) by generating, for each of the extracted concept candidates, a reasonable sized set of suggestions for its position in H_1 (Salton & Buckley, 1988). For the latter, we distinguish between synonymy and hyponymy relationships if H_1 includes this relations. Figure 2 depicts a work-flow of the proposed thesauri extension support system. In the remainder of this section we describe the two components of the system in more detail.

Term Selection

Concept Extraction is the process of extracting terms that could serve as concepts in the concept hierarchy. This is usually done by applying statistical co-occurrence measures to a corpus of text documents. In order to quantify the importance of a term in a corpus we first compute the *tf-idf* value $w_{t,d}$ of term t in document d. We found that applying the *tf-idf* variant with (a) logarithmic term frequency weighting, (b) logarithmic document frequency weighting, and (c) cosine normalization yielded the best results. More formally, we computed the cosine normalized *tf-idf* value $w_{t,d}^{norm}$ for each term t and each document d according to Equation 1.

$$w_{t,d}^{norm} = \frac{w_{t,d}}{\sqrt{\sum_{t' \in d} w_{t',d}}} \; with \; w_{t,d} = \left(1 + \log\llbracket \left(tf_{t,d}\right)\right) * \log \frac{|D|}{df_t}\rrbracket$$

(1)

Since we want to assess the importance of a term t not only for a single document but the entire corpus, we compute the mean $\bar{w}_t$ of the *tf-idf* values over all documents in which term t occurs at least once.

$$\bar{w} = \frac{\sum_{d \in D} w_{t,d}^{norm}}{df_t}$$

(2)

Figure 2. The workflow of the thesaurus extension system

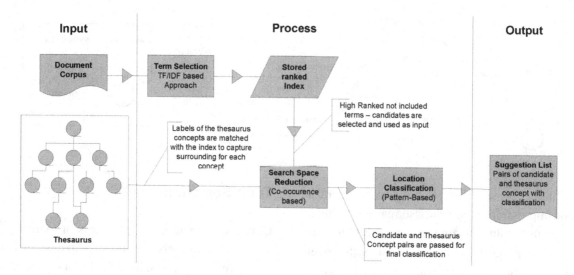

We finally assign the importance weight $\hat{w}_t$ to term $_t$ by multiplying the squared value $\bar{w}_t$ with the logarithm of the document frequency df_t.

$$\hat{w} = \log\left(df_{t=1}\right) \times \bar{w}_t^2 \qquad (3)$$

The intuition behind this approach is that terms that occur in more documents are more likely to be concept candidates for H_1 covering these documents. The presented importance measure $\hat{w}_t$, therefore, combines the average importance of a term relative to each document in the corpus with the importance of the term relative to the entire corpus.

It is to mention that this is only one possibility to extract corpus relevant terms which are not included in an existing concept hierachie. Another way to find relevant terms is presented by Wong et al. (2009) who use additional information to rank interesting concepts beside the pure usage of term frequency.

Concept Classification is the second step. The previously extracted concept candidates are *classified* in the existing concept hierarchy. In the

following we will always assume that this concept hierarchy is a thesaurus. Of course this method can also be adapted to other *light-weight ontologies*, therefore the different available relations between concepts have to be modified. Classification is the process of finding concepts in H_1 that are potential hypernyms and synonyms, respectively, for each of the candidate concepts. This process is also often referred to as *position extraction*. We apply established machine learning approaches to learn lexico-syntactic patterns from search engine results. Typical patterns for concepts and are, for instance, [*is a*] for hyponymy and [*is also a*] for synonymy relationships. Instead of only using a predefined set of patterns (Hearst, 1992), we learn these patterns from text snippets of search engines using existing thesauri as training data – similar to the approach presented by Bollegala et al. (2007b). The learned patterns are then used as features for the classification of the relationship between each concept candidate and existing thesaurus concepts. Since we are mainly interested in hyponymy and synonymy relationships, we need to train at least two different binary classifiers. Fortunately, the classifiers can be trained with concepts pairs contained in existing domain thesauri.

Figure 3. Yahoo Pattern Extraction Example

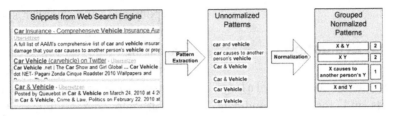

The pattern extraction approach of the proposed system is based on the method presented by Bollegala et al. (2007b). Instead of retrieving lexico-syntactic patterns to assess the semantic similarity of term pairs, however, we extract the patterns also for the purpose of classifying relationship types as either synonymy or hyponymy. For each pair of concepts (C_1, C_2) of which we know the relationship because it is contained in a training thesaurus, we send the query "$"C_1 + C_2"$" to a Web search engine. The returned text snippet is processed to extract all *n*-grams ($2 \leq n \leq 6$) that match the pattern "$C_1 X^* C_2$", where X can be any combination of up to four space-separated word or punctuation tokens. For instance, assume the training thesaurus contains the concepts "car" and "vehicle" with car being a hyponym of vehicle. The method would query a search engine with the string "car" +"vehicle". Let us assume that one of the returned text snippet is "every car is a vehicle." In this case, the method would extract the pattern "car is a vehicle". This pattern would be added to the list of potential hyponymy patterns with "car" and "vehicle" substituted with matching placeholders (cf. figure 3). Of course, the set of patterns extracted this way is too large to be used directly for machine learning algorithms. Therefore, we rank the patterns according to their ability to distinguish between the types of relationships we are interested in.

For all available relationships like synonymy and hyponymy relationship we rank the extracted patterns according to the chi-square statistic. For every pattern *v* we determine its frequency in

snippets for hyponymous (synonymous) word pairs and its frequency n_v in snippets for non-hyponymous (non-synonymous) word pairs. Let P denote the total frequency of all patterns in snippets for hyponymous (synonymous) word pairs and N the total frequency of all patterns in snippets for non-hyponymous (non-synonymous) word pairs. We calculate the chi-square value for each pattern as follows:

$$x_v^2 = \frac{(P+N)(p_v(N-n_v) - n_v(P-p_v))^2}{PN(p_v + n_v)(P + N - p_v - n_v)} \tag{4}$$

From the initially extracted set of patterns we kept only the 80 highest ranked patterns extracted with WordNet as training thesaurus and the 60 highest ranked patterns with the medical subject headings (MeSH) thesaurus as training thesaurus. The feature vector for the machine learning algorithms consists of the normalized frequencies for these top-ranked patterns. Finally, we learn a support vector machine with linear kernel, a support vector machine with radial basis function (RBF) kernel, and a decision tree algorithm (J48) using the generated feature vectors. Figure 1 depicts a typical instance of the thesaurus extension problem. The concept candidate "Viscus", which has been extracted from a text corpus, needs to be classified in the existing thesaurus. The thesaurus extension support system provides, for each candidate concept, a small ranked list of potential positions in the thesaurus. In the following section we report on the empirical evaluation of the presented approach.

3.2 Experimental Evaluation

Most concept hierarchies are comprised of a large number of concepts and, for every candidate concept, we would have to send a query to a Web search engine for every concept included in the hierarchy. Hence, we have to reduce the amount of potential positions for any given candidate concept. To achieve such a search space reduction we compute, for every candidate concept that needs to be classified, its similarity to each of the thesaurus concepts using the weighted Jaccard value of its surrounding words (Lin, 1998). Then, for each concept candidate, only the top-k most similar concepts are considered for the pattern based approach. In the following we call the concepts which are included in the top-k set the *similar concepts*. The concepts that share a hyponymy (or synonymy) relation with a candidate concept are referred to as *positional concepts*.

While the pattern extraction approach would work with any search engine, we decided to use the Yahoo search engine API[5] as it is less restrictive on the allowed number of queries per day. A single query with the API took up to three seconds. To evaluate and test our methods we used a thesauri extracted from the MeSH thesaurus of the year 2008[6]. The thesaurus was created by combining all concepts located under the top-level concept *anatomy* (1611 concepts) with all concept located under the top-level concept *humanity* (186 concepts). For each concept in these thesauri we retrieved the most relevant documents from PubMed[7] of the years between 2005 and 2008. The final document corpus included 13392 documents for the *anatomy* thesaurus and 1468 documents for the *humanity* thesaurus. We chose WordNet 3.0 as a second thesaurus for the experiments, primarily since this allows us to compare the results to those reported by Bollegala et al. (2007a).

For each of the three classes "synonymy", "hyponymy", and "neither synonymy nor hyponymy" we sampled 300 pairs of concepts belonging to the respective class. For the MeSH training set, these pairs were randomly sampled from the MeSH thesaurus excluding the previously constructed anatomy/humanity sub-thesaurus. Similarly, to create the WordNet training set, we randomly sampled 300 negative and positive training pairs for each class from WordNet. For testing, we isolated 100 concepts each from the anatomy/humanity sub-thesaurus and from Word-Net. These concepts serve as candidate concepts and the goal is to evaluate whether our approach can identify their correct positions. For both the 100 MeSH and WordNet candidate concepts we determined the top 100 most similar concepts in the MeSH and WordNet thesaurus, respectively, by applying the above-mentioned co-occurrence similarity measure. On average, 97 percent of the correct positions for each candidate concept were included in this set for WordNet and 90 percent for the MeSH thesaurus. This indicates that the Jaccard similarity measure is able to exclude the majority of all concept positions while retaining most of the correct positional concepts.

For each of the 100 concept candidates, we applied the trained classifiers on the set of the previously ranked 100 most similar concepts, resulting in 10000 classifications instances for each combination of thesaurus (MeSH or WordNet), classifier (linear SVM, RBF SVN, decision tree), and classification task. The accuracy values ((true positives + true negatives) / all instances) of these experiments are shown in Table 1. Evidently, the accuracy of the classifiers is strongly influenced by the properties of the thesauri. For instance, for the synonymy classification task, we achieved an accuracy of 86 percent with a linear SVM for WordNet but only an accuracy of 71 percent for the MeSH thesaurus. Not surprisingly, the three-class classification problem is more difficult and the approach is not as accurate as for the binary classification tasks. An additional observation is

Table 1. Accuracy results of the three machine learning approaches and two thesauri for different classification tasks

Training data	Classification task	SVM_{lin}	SVM_{RBF}	DT
WordNet	syn vs. no syn	86%	54%	98%
WordNet	hypo vs. no hypo	73%	63%	82%
WordNet	syn vs. hypo	70%	50%	71%
WordNet	syn vs. hypo vs. none	58%	47%	70%
MeSH	syn vs. no syn	71%	59%	85%
MeSH	hypo vs. no hypo	74%	60%	87%
MeSH	syno vs. no syn	53%	52%	68%
MeSH	syno vs. hypo vs. none	51%	40%	68%

Table 2. Percentage of candidate concepts wrongly classified as synonyms (hyponyms) by the linear support vector machine (SVM) and the decision tree algorithm

Training data	Classification task	SVM (linear)	Decision tree
WordNet	synonym vs. no synonym	7.8%	6.7%
WordNet	hyponym vs. no hyponym	10.6%	15.4%
MeSH	synonym vs. no synonym	3.6%	12.7%
MeSH	hyponym vs. no hyponym	6.1%	14.1%

that the classification results for the hyponymy vs. synonymy problem are rather poor pointing to the semantic similarity of the synonymy and hyponymy relations.

Furthermore, the results reveal that the decision tree algorithm (J48) leads to more accurate classification results for the majority of the tasks. The accuracy of the J48 classifier is on average 11.6 percent better than the linear SVM classifier and 24.1 percent more accurate than the radial basis function SVM. This is especially interesting because pattern based machine learning approaches mostly employ support vector machines for classification. Proper parameter tuning could close the performance gap between the two approaches, however, this is often not possible in real-world applications. While the decision tree approach is superior in accuracy the linear SVM classifier is more precise. Table 2 shows the percentage of false positives for the synonymy and hyponymy

classes for both the MeSH and WordNet thesaurus. Except for the synonymy vs. no synonymy classification problem the linear SVM algorithm results in fewer false positives. A thesaurus maintenance system should support the knowledge modeler by reducing the amount of novel concept/ position pairs without excluding correct ones. Therefore, we are especially interested in a high recall and moderate precision making the decision tree algorithm the preferred choice for the thesaurus maintenance setting.

For a librarian or knowledge modeler, the main application of the support system is to locate the correct position of the candidate concepts in the thesaurus. Let us assume we are given the concept candidate "tummy" and that we need to determine its position in the thesaurus fragment depicted in Figure 1. Now, two pieces of information will lead us to the correct location. The first one being that "tummy" is a hyponym of "internal organ" and the second being that "tummy" is a synonym of "stomach." In an additional experiment we evaluated, for each concept candidate, in how many cases we were able to determine the correct position in the target thesaurus. Hence, for each concept candidate, we looked at the set of concepts in the thesaurus which the pattern-based approach classified as either synonyms or hyponyms and checked whether at least one of these concepts led us to the correct position. The size of this set was 14 on average, meaning that, on average, the number of choices was reduced from 100 to 14. Figure 3 lists the percentage of cases for which we could determine the correct position for the MeSH thesaurus. We also widened the graph distance to the correct position from 1 to 4, where the graph distance 1 represents direct synonymy or hyponymy relations. The suggested position was at most 4 edges away from the correct one.

4 COLLABORATIVELY EXTENDING AND POPULATING CONCEPT HIERARCHIES

Ontology-based approaches to data organization and integration in specialized domains have produced significant successes, especially within bio- and medical informatics projects (such as the Gene Ontology) and in business applications. One of the major reasons hindering such approaches from being successfully applied to the Web at large, however, is the so-called "knowledge acquisition bottleneck", that is, the large amount of time and money needed to develop and maintain the formal ontologies. In addition, once elaborate and precise ontologies have been created they often lack users who employ and populate them. Since expertise in both ontology design and the relevant domain are required to populate and maintain ontologies, Semantic Web projects have faced the dilemma of either hiring expensive "double experts" highly-skilled in both ontology design and the relevant domain or face inevitable data and user sparseness

Table 3. Fraction of candidate concepts for which the correct position in the thesaurus could be inferred using the pattern-based classification results; and considering a graph distance of $1 \leq n \leq 4$

Graph distance	MeSH thesaurus
1	85%
2	95%
3	99%
4	100%

(Buckner et al., 2010). Several researchers have therefore begun to realize that the strength of both approaches could potentially provide a remedy for some of the mentioned weaknesses (Breslin et al., 2010, Ankolekar et al., 2008, Gruber, 2008) and have called for the development of the "social-semantic" Web, which would combine the social Web's ability to obtain large amounts of data from volunteer users with the Semantic Web's complex and interoperable data representations.

In previous works Niepert et al. (2007), Niepert et al. (2008) presented the InPhO project as one of the first that maintains a dynamically growing knowledge representation of the discipline of philosophy. The system is primarily developed to create and maintain a formal ontology for a well-established open-access reference work, the Stanford Encyclopedia of Philosophy (SEP). Three features of the SEP make it an ideal environment for developing and testing digital tools to learn and manage ontologies. First, it is substantial and complex: over 900 entries (>9 million words) of sophisticated humanities content that is beyond the comprehension of any one individual. Second, the SEP is dynamic: new and revised entries come online each month. Finally, it is expert-driven: more than 1,100 professional philosophers serve as its editors and authors. The feedback provided by SEP authors about their areas of expertise provides an overlapping mosaic of expert knowledge. We believe that many online reference works are well-positioned to address the mentioned

Figure 4. The flowchart of the Indiana Philosophy ontology system

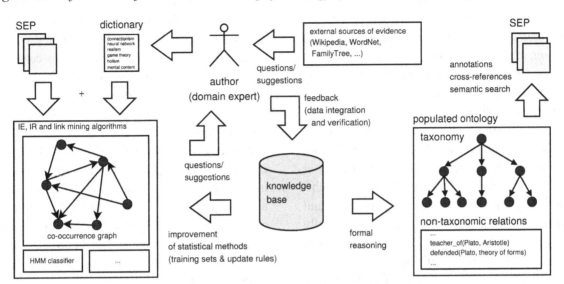

challenges by making use of their most valuable informational resource: the domain experts who serve as their editors and contributors. With care, expert feedback can be obtained to "approve" the recommendations of automated methods without presuming knowledge of ontology design or placing undue demands on the contributors' time. This feedback can give the modeler a window on the domain which is likely to be the most objective source of knowledge available. The InPhO project successfully maintains a dynamically growing taxonomy of philosophical ideas leveraging the feedback facts provided by a user community consisting of users ranging from interested amateurs to experts in the field.

The concepts in the InPhO taxonomy are related over *is-a* relations. Each of these concepts (e.g., *rationalism*) is referred to by a term in In-PhO's controlled vocabulary. The problem of determining hierarchical relationships between concepts can be reduced to that of finding hierarchical relationships between terms, that is, extracting hypernym and hyponym relations from text. A large number of measures for the semantic similarity between terms exist. Such measures of similarity and generality have been combined to

provide, for any given term, a ranking of possible hyponyms and hypernyms, respectively (Niepert et al., 2007). The ranking is then presented to InPhO's users to approve or falsify the estimates of semantic relatedness and relative generality of pairs of terms.

4.0.1 Method Description

As of now, the Indiana Philosophy Ontology contains four main categories: person (subclass of FOAF::person[8]), document (from AKT[9]), organization (from SUMO[10]), and philosophical idea, as well as an initial set of non-taxonomic relations. The idea category contains a taxonomic decomposition of the space of philosophical ideas according to the disciplinary relatedness of their *contents* rather than according to their structural roles. For example, instead of dividing *idea about philosophy* into *concept, distinction, argument, counterexample*, and so on, the InPhO decomposes it into subareas of philosophy – e.g. *idea about metaphysics, idea about epistemology, idea about logic, idea about ethics, idea about philosophy of mind*. Each subarea is in turn decomposed into a series of issues considered fundamental to work in that subarea; for example, *idea about philosophy of mind* is decomposed into *idea about consciousness*, *idea about intentionality*, *idea about mental content*, *idea about philosophy of artificial intelligence*, *idea about philosophy of psychology*, and *idea about metaphysics of mind*.

InPhO combines corpus-based measures of semantic similarity between words – for examples, see Manning and Schuetze (1999) – and a novel relative generality measure (Niepert et al., 2007), to provide, for any given philosophical idea, a ranking of possible hyponyms and hypernyms, respectively. Using these carefully designed interfaces, InPhO's users can validate or falsify the estimates of semantic relatedness and relative generality of pairs of philosophical ideas, using a predefined set of possible labels. The relatedness is scored on a five-point scale from highly related to unrelated, and the generality can be evaluated using four different options: same level of generality, *idea*1 is more general than *idea*2, *idea*1 is more specific than *idea*2, and the two are incomparable. The generality of two ideas is deemed incomparable if they are entirely unrelated or if one idea can be both more *and* less general than the other, depending on the context. Of course, users may skip idea pairs or provide only partial information. The feedback is stored as first-order facts in our knowledge base, together with provenance data. For example, when a user with id 45 provides the information that an idea about neural networks is more specific than an idea about connectionism, and that they are highly related, the facts *msp(neural network, connectionism, 45)* and *s4p(neural network, connectionism, 45)* are added to the knowledge base. For each user, automatically computed trust scores (see below) and levels of expertise are stored to evaluate her reliability. A non-monotonic answer set program with stable model semantics is used daily on the set of first-order facts to construct the global populated ontology (Niepert et al., 2008). The taxonomy can be browsed online[11].

Niepert et al. (2009) presented a general framework for the assignment of trust scores to individual users based on their deviation from other users' evaluations. A method to compute degrees of trustworthiness of users in a social network using semantic and social Web data sources was recently proposed by Heath et al. (2007). Here, we focus on trust scores that are computed using the users' evaluations of pairs of entities and their application to resolving feedback inconsistencies. Let U be the set of users, let A and B be two sets of individuals in the ontology, and let L be the set of possible *labels* that can be assigned to elements in $A \times B$. Let the *label distance* $dist : L \times L \rightarrow R^+$ be a function that assigns to each pair of labels a non-negative real number. Let $E = \{(a,b,\ell,u) \mid a \in A, b \in B, \ell \in L, u \in U\}$ be the set of 4-tuples representing the user evaluations, that is, the assignments of labels in L to elements in $A \times B$ by the users in U. We define the *evaluation deviation* measure $D : U \rightarrow R^+$ as

$$D(u) = \frac{1}{\mid N(u) \mid} \sum_{(a,b,\ell,u) \in E} \sum_{(a,b,\ell',u') \in E \, with \, u \neq u'} dist(\ell, \ell')$$

with $N(u) = \{(a,b,\ell',u') \in E \mid \exists (a,b,\ell,u) \in E$ with $u' \neq u\}$. Of course, the smaller the evaluation deviation, the higher the trust one can have in a particular user. The trust scores (some of which might be specialized to specific areas in philosophy) can then be used together with the users levels of expertise to enhance provenance information and settle feedback inconsistencies with increasing sophistication.

4.0.2 Experimental Results

As of March 25th 2010, InPhO (currently in beta testing) has 120 registered users, 43 of which provided one or more of the 4,800 evaluations of 2,969 distinct pairs of ideas. The set of users consists of volunteers who registered after the

Figure 5. Histogram of deviations of relatedness scores among InPhO users with overlap ≥ 10

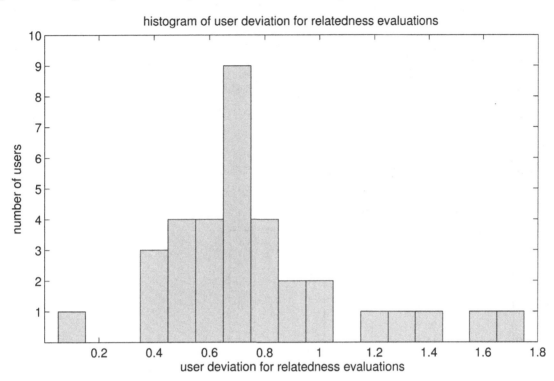

InPhO system had been announced on several e-mail newsletters and blogs. They will soon be joined by the authors and editors of the Stanford Encyclopedia of Philosophy. 39 out of the 92 users have the highest level of expertise (published in the area) and 37 finished a graduate class in the area. From the 47 subareas of philosophy that are currently specified in the InPhO, 31 were covered by at least one expert. The contribution incentives are twofold: (1) users have their own personal account that displays type and number of contributions and several agreement statistics and (2) the more feedback a SEP author provides the better is her entry embedded in browse and search applications. However, we consider the objective of providing sufficient incentives for user participation an ongoing research and interface design challenge.

We are specifically interested in the extent of user agreement on evaluations of idea pairs with semantic relatedness and relative generality labels.

Thus, in the remainder, *A* and *B* are the instances of the class *philosophical idea* in the ontology. Users can score the semantic relatedness of two philosophical ideas on a scale from 0 (unrelated) to 4 (highly related). Hence, for the relatedness score we have $L=\{0,1,2,3,4\}$ and $dist(\ell,\ell')=|\ell-\ell'|$. Figure 5 depicts the histogram of the *evaluation deviation* values for the 34 users who labeled the relatedness of one or more idea pairs that have also been evaluated by at least 10 other users (evaluation overlap ≥10). Except for some outliers, the majority of the users has a deviation of less than 0.8 where 4.0 is the possible maximum.

For the relative generality evaluations, $L=\{0,1,2,3\}$ with 0="more specific", 1="more general", 2="same generality," and 3="incomparable/either more or less general." Here, we can define *dist* as $dist(\ell,\ell')=1$ if $\ell\neq\ell'$ and $dist(\ell,\ell')=0$ otherwise. Figure 6 depicts the histogram of the *evaluation deviation* values for the 31 users who labeled the relative generality of one or more idea

Figure 6. Histogram of users' deviation on relative generality labels with evaluation overlap ≥ 10

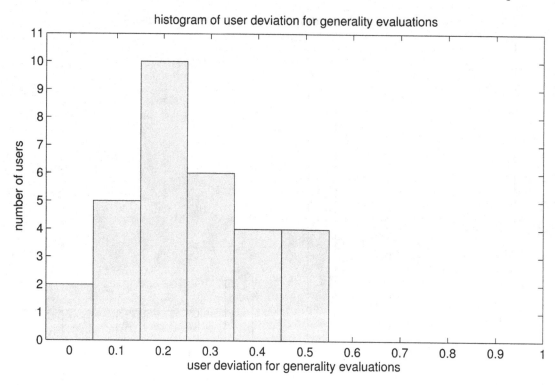

pairs that have also been evaluated by at least 10 other users. All users have a deviation of less than or equal to 0.5 where 1.0 is the possible maximum. These experiments illustrate that the approach delivers high-quality feedback that can be used to extend and populate the given taxonomy.

5 VISUAL EVALUATION

In this section, we describe a completely different approach to evaluate concept hierarchies, be they automatically or manually created. We use a sophisticated combination of statistical analyses and a graphical visualization that enables the user to get an in-depth view of the hierarchy in use.

A lot of measures exist to evaluate different aspects of a concept hierarchy, especially in the context of Information Retrieval (IR) systems. The performance of thesaurus-based IR systems can be evaluated and compared to systems without the support of an underlying thesaurus. Precision and Recall are commonly used in this case. Precision and Recall is also applicable to the results of automatic indexing with controlled concepts. Here, bad results can also indicate weaknesses in the concept hierarchy and are not necessarily caused by the indexer alone.

A general problems of such measures for the evaluation of a thesaurus is that they are designed to produce a number. Even in the case that the number suggests a bad result, the user still has no idea, where the weaknesses in the thesaurus reside. Another problem is, that these measures generally rely on the existence of a gold standard for some kind of comparison. This is useful to evaluate a specific technique, as demonstrated in section 3.2. Nevertheless, in practice, a user will face the problem to evaluate a concrete thesaurus, that was built (semi-) automatically by different techniques.

It is our belief that in this case only a graphical visualization with an intuitive, interactive interface can provide the necessary insights for the user to evaluate the result of the creation process by browsing and analyzing the thesaurus as a whole. This leads to the idea to put the concept hierarchy in the focus of the visualization and concentrate on a single concept as the subject of the analysis. This credo causes some fundamental changes in the design of a specific analysis. For example, if we want to analyze the results of an automatic indexing system, we would not be interested in the overall number of correct concept assignments, but more in the number of (correct) assignments of a specific concept. "Correct" is put in parentheses, as with this overall approach, the number of correct assignments (which requires a gold standard) is not required (but nevertheless valuable, if available), as shown below.

A second, more striking example is an analysis of some intrinsic property of the hierarchy, as balance. It is easy to imagine a measure that gives us a number for the degree of balance within the concept hierarchy. With our approach, you would not calculate the balance for the whole hierarchy, but for every single concept, representing the balance of the subtree below it. With a proper visualization, this directly shows the specific locations of the balance problems in the hierarchy.

The treemap visualization is one such visualization and described in the following section.

5.1 Visualization with Treemaps

To support our evaluation approach, we have to find a way to provide the user with a view on the thesaurus that encodes the overall structure of the thesaurus or selected parts of it and the evaluation results for the different concepts in the thesaurus. Ben Shneiderman tried to get an overview of disc usage of a particular hard drive and needed a compact representation of its directory structure, showing additional information like file size and file type in one view. He invented the treemap algorithm in the early 1990s (Shneiderman, 1992).

According to Shneiderman, treemaps are a representation designed for human visualization of complex traditional tree structures: arbitrary trees are shown with a 2-d space-filling representation. Consider a tree with weight or size information attached to each node and a 2-d space with corners (x_1, y_1) and (x_2, y_2). For each child of the root node, a partition of the space along the x-axis is calculated. For the first partition, this reads as

$$x_3 = x_1 + \left(\frac{|c_1|}{|r_1|} \right)(x_2 - x_1) \qquad (5)$$

with $|c_1|$ as the size of child node 1 and $|r_1|$ as the size of the root node. The size of a node is determined by an arbitrary metric and thus can be used to visualize some kind of analysis value for the node. A simple metric is the number of child nodes or descendants of a node, which is quite intuitive and represents the size of the subtree of the given node.

For the next level, the corresponding partition is partitioned again along the y-axis, then again on the x-axis and so on. Shneiderman called this approach the "slice-and-dice" algorithm. Since then, a lot of different implementations and optimizations were made by several people. One such optimization are so-called squarified treemaps, which try to avoid the long and thin rectangles resulting from small nodes. Other approaches are presented by Shneiderman and Wattenberg (2001), Bederson et al. (2002).

Figure 7 illustrates the principle of the creation of a squarified treemap of the following tree:

Figure 7: Creation of a treemap in four steps

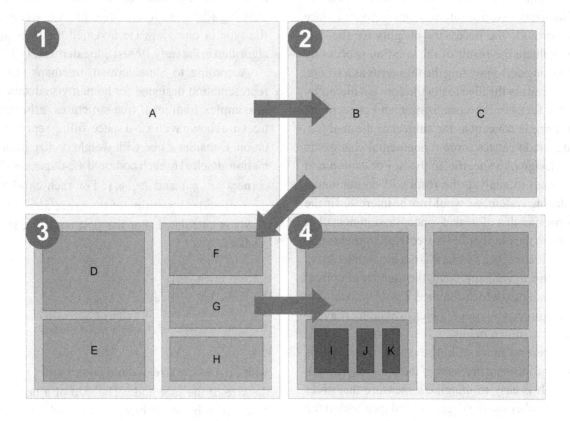

- A
  - ○ B
    - ▪ D
    - ▪ E
- I
- J
- K
  - ○ C
    - ▪ F
    - ▪ G
    - ▪ H

The algorithm recursively walks down the tree and subsequently divides the area of a node based on the size metric. Step 1 starts with the root node, which is divides in step 2 according to the sizes of B and C. Step 3 are actually two steps dividing B and C. In this case, D has a size other than E.

In step 4, only node E is further divided, as the other nodes have no further subnodes.

Beside the size metric, treemaps provide another way to visualize data: the color of the areas representing the nodes. The ability to visualize a whole tree from top up to a certain depth level with results of two simultaneous analyses is what makes treemaps so powerful. In the next section, we introduce the IC difference analysis, which is the main analysis approach that we use for the thesaurus evaluation.

5.2 IC Difference Analysis

IC stands for information content, also referred to as self-information, which originates from information theory according to Shannon. In this context, the information content of a probabilistic event is the higher the smaller the probability is that this event occurs. Resnik (1995) transfered the notion of an information content to the linguistics and used it to measure the generality of a concept in a concept hierarchy: The more general a concept is, the higher is its probability to occur in a given set of documents and consequently the lower is its information content. The information content of a concept is defined as:

$$IC_x(c) = -\log P_x(c) \qquad (6)$$

is determined by the frequency of documents contained in a set X that are annotated with concept c or one of its subconcepts.

The development of the IC Difference Analysis was originally motivated by the need to evaluate the results of an automatic indexer as described by Eckert et al. (2007). To compare the results of the automatic indexing process to the results of manual indexing, we calculated the difference of the information content for each concept, once using the automatic annotations and once the manual ones:

$$D_{IC}(c) = IC_s(c) - IC_R(c) \qquad (7)$$

where $IC_s(c)$ is the information content based on the subject of the analysis, in this case the annotations of the automatic indexer, and $IC_R(c)$ is the information content based on some reference, in this case the manual annotations.

This definition of IC Difference relies on the existence of some kind of reference, which in realistic scenarios is not always the case. In fact, as we will further elaborate in the next section, there are a lot of use cases where we have at most one set of documents that are annotated with concepts from the hierarchy. In these cases, we have to use a heuristic that can substitute the reference and is based only on the concept hierarchy itself: the intrinsic information content. This idea of an Intrinsic Information Content (IIC), i.e. an infor-

mation content that is determined only by means of the thesaurus structure itself, was introduced by Seco et al. (2004).

The IIC of a concept c denoted as $IIC(c)$ is defined as

$$IIC(c) = -\log\left(\frac{hypo(c) + 1}{\max}\right) \qquad (8)$$

with $hypo(c)$ as the number of hyponyms (i.e. child nodes) of a given concept c and max as the number of concepts in the whole thesaurus. $IIC(C)$ can always be used as a drop-in replacement for .

IC Difference is related to the *Kullback-Leibler Divergence* used in information theory which is defined as

$$D_{KL}\left(p \,||\, q\right) = \sum_i p(i) \log \frac{p(i)}{q(i)} \qquad (9)$$

The *KL Divergence* is a measure of the differences between two probability distributions p and q and can be used to get an overall measure of the thesaurus suitability, instead of evaluating a single concept. Examples for the evaluation of ontologies are presented by Calmet and Daemi (2004b), Calmet and Daemi (2004a).

Figure 8 shows the treemap visualization of the automatically generated InPhO taxonomy as explained in section 4. The size is calculated by the number of direct child concepts and the color represents the intrinsic information content, ranging from red (0, root concept) to blue (1, leaf concepts). This combination can be used to get an overview of the distribution of the concepts. The redder areas on top level denote the more populated subtrees, the bluer ones are rather shallow.

The treemap visualization requires some time for the user to get familiar with. A major drawback of treemaps is the possibility for the user to lose the orientation in the hierarchy as the visualization can not provide information about the environment

Figure 8. Treemap visualization of the InPhO taxonomy with IIC analysis

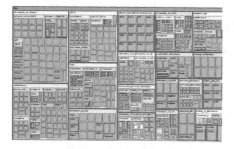

Figure 9. Treemap visualization of the InPhO taxonomy with IIC analysis

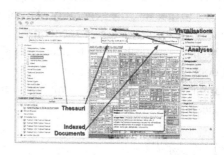

of the currently selected top concept. In the next section, we introduce Semtinel, the software we developed to make use of different kinds of visualizations and analyses, including the treemap visualization and IC Difference.

5.3 Semtinel

The statistical analysis and its proper visualization are only two building blocks for a complete system that enables the user to evaluate a concept hierarchy with respect to a specific criterion. Depending on the criterion, different visualizations and analyses have to be combined by the user and presented in an intuitive way that enables the user to browse and analyze the concept hierarchy and reach a decision about its suitability or the necessary steps how to further improve it.

Semtinel[12] is a research prototype that demonstrates how these requirements can be met. Figure 9 shows a screenshot of the interface. All locations of the elements of the application (experiments, visualizations and analyses palette, data sets, ...) can be arranged almost arbitrarily to meet the users needs and preferences. Usually, there are one or more visualization sections (so called experiments) that interactively present a visualization result for the desired data, visualization and analysis. In this screenshot, they are located in the center and in the top left area.

By means of drag and drop, the user configures the experiments. The available data is shown in

the Overview window in the lower left corner. It contains concept schemes ("thesauri"), document sets and annotation sets that contain the annotations of documents with concepts from the concept schemes ("indexed documents"). The actual visualization and the analysis that should be performed is taken from the palette, shown in the upper right corner. Semtinel automatically infers the data that is needed to calculate a given analysis. The treemap visualization of the IC Difference analysis in the center of the screen needs for example up to three inputs: one concept scheme and one or two annotation sets (one to calculate IC_S and the other to calculate IC_R. If IC_R is missing, the analysis automatically replaces it by *IIC*). On the other hand, the treeview visualization, as seen in the top left corner, only needs a concept scheme, as no analysis result is presented. It is just used to browse the hierarchy in an intuitive way.

This combination of a hierarchical common treeview with the treemap visualization turned out to be a very effective means to overcome the above mentioned weaknesses of the treemap visualization, allowing the interactive navigation through the thesaurus hierarchy without losing the orientation. By double-clicking on the treemap or by selecting a concept in the treeview, the user can zoom into the thesaurus structure.

5.4 Example Evaluations

The evaluation methodology as implemented in Semtinel was originally developed to evaluate a thesaurus based automatic indexing system. Specific examples for this use case is provided in more detail by Eckert et al. (2008). In this chapter, we focus on the description of analysis approaches that support the evaluation of concept hierarchies.

ANALYZING DOCUMENT ANNOTATIONS

Currently, thesauri are primarily designed and used for manual annotation of documents. So there are many bibliographic databases or document sets that have been meticulously annotated by domain experts. Analyzing such an annotated document base with the tool presented in this article can help finding problems with the thesaurus structure and its concepts.

In this case, the information content *IC* of the concepts can be compared to their intrinsic one (*IIC*). The intrinsic information content implicates that the thesaurus is hierarchically structured with child nodes being more specialized and parent nodes being more general and that a concept should occur less often in the document base, the more specialized it is.

By visualizing the IC Difference analysis in the treemap, concepts that occur more often or less often than expected can be identified. Both cases could be a cause for concern, as the thesaurus is not only used for annotation, but to facilitate searching the document base using its concepts. Usually, the query is refined by specializing and generalizing its keywords, until a satisfactory result set is achieved. For queries containing very often used concepts, whose corresponding thesaurus node have no children, the result set cannot be minimized in this way. The opposite holds true for rarely used concepts whose nodes have no parents.

ANALYZING AUTOMATIC ANNOTATIONS

When new document sets need to be annotated using existing thesauri, automatic processes are increasingly considered. Analyzing an automatically annotated document set with Semtinel can help finding concepts that unsettle the indexer. So if the concept hierarchy in question is to be used for automatic indexing, the same analysis as described above can be used. If manual annotations are available for comparison, they of course can be used as reference set to calculate IC_R which makes the identification of concepts with specific problems for the indexer easier, as other causes like problems in the hierarchical structure or an unbalanced focus of the documents are singled out.

Typical problems for automatic indexers that can lead to noticeable results in the visualization are:

- **Context Dependence** Concepts are sometimes homonyms of commonly used terms in a text. This preferably happens in highly specialized domains where special terminology is used. In this case there are two options. Either, advanced mechanisms for context detection can be used or in cases where these methods are too expensive, the corresponding term can be deleted from the thesaurus to avoid false annotations. This kind of problem normally causes a relatively low information content with respect to the automatic annotations.
- **Missing Definitions** Sometimes, concepts are not detected in documents because a certain synonym used in the text is not included in the thesaurus. In this case, the definition of the concept has to be refined adding the corresponding synonyms. This problem normally causes a relatively high

information content with respect to the automatic annotations.

- **Normalization Errors** In cases where rather simple linguistic tools are used for preprocessing the meaning of terms can be lost as ambiguity is introduced in the normalization step. In this case we either have to use more advanced preprocessing methods that are capable of eliminating the ambiguity introduced for instance by first detecting noun phrases and only using them as a basis for indexing. As above, if this approach is too expensive, we can also eliminate the corresponding terms from the thesaurus to avoid wrong annotations. This kind of problem normally causes a relatively low information content with respect to the automatic annotations.

- **Indexing Preferences** Human annotators sometimes show certain preferences in selecting index terms that cannot be reproduced in an automatic indexing process. A typical example is the use of check-tags, predefined lists of index terms that can more easily be assigned by selecting a check-box. These terms will be over-represented in manual annotations. These terms should be treated separately in the indexing process and special strategies need to be developed for this purpose. This problem normally causes a relatively high information content with respect to manual annotations.

REVIEW OF THE CONCEPT HIERARCHY

The most basic analysis is just a simple review of the hierarchy using *IIC*. As explained above (Figure 8), this way it is easy to determine, which parts of the hierarchy are more populated with concepts and provide more levels of depth than others.

DETERMINING THE FOCUS OF DOCUMENTS

Beside the specific problems a concept hierarchy might have according to the above described analysis approaches, it may be even more important for a user-centered approach for the maintenance of such hierarchies that it can be easily determined if the concepts fit to the documents that afterwards should be organized, indexed or classified.

This question is answered by Semtinel in two steps: First, a list of potential concepts is provided that are not already contained in the hierarchy, as explained in Section 3. The smaller the list the better, but scanning this list gives a pretty good impression, if important terms are missing in the thesaurus. But even if all meaningful terms would already exist as a concept, it still could be the case that the thesaurus is too broad and at least the main efforts for the maintenance could be concentrated on a subset. For this reason, Semtinel can be used in the second step to visualize the whole document set by means of the IC Difference analysis. This can be done with existing manual annotations, but it is also possible to use a simple automatic approach. Of course there might be a lot of mistakes, as explained above, but it is still easily possible to determine the focus of the documents. This enables the user to select an appropriate thesaurus at the beginning or to improve an existing one in the right direction.

6 CONCLUSION AND OUTLOOK

While ontologies form the base for the Semantic Web and a lot of research is concerned with the creation, merging, mapping and querying of ontologies, in practice, a lot more of the now called light-weight ontologies exist. These knowledge representations are widely used and will continue to provide the structural backbone of many important applications. For instance, data on the web is often linked using light-weight ontologies.

Taxonomies and ontologies no longer live in opposing worlds but rather complement each other as they become more widespread by means of Semantic Web technologies. With SKOS (Simple KOS) exists an W3C recommendation for the representation of light-weight ontologies in RDF and a lot of thesauri and taxonomies are already available in the SKOS format. Libraries publish their metadata in RDF and link it to the data of other libraries by means of these taxonomies. Hence, light-weight ontologies are already a crucial part of the Semantic Web and it is important to cope with the specifics of their (semi-)automatic and user-driven maintenance.

In this chapter, we presented four different building blocks for the creation and maintenance of lightweight ontologies, namely approaches for

1. the proper selection of new terms and concepts in a document corpus,
2. the placement of new terms and concepts in existing hierarchies,
3. the creation of a new hierarchy for given terms by means of crowdsourcing and
4. a proper visualisation to interpret and evaluate the resulting hierarchy.

We have shown that with these building blocks combined, it is possible to create, maintain and evaluate concept hierarchies in an efficient and semi-automatic way.

The approaches presented in this chapter are by no means exhaustive. Together with other ones, they have to be included in a commonly usable framework and application that can easily be used by interested individuals. With the publication of Semtinel as open source software (http://www.semtinel.org), we plan to extend it in this direction.

REFERENCES

Ankolekar, A., Krötzsch, M., Tran, D. T., & Vrandecic, D. (2008). The two cultures: Mashing up Web 2.0 and the Semantic Web. *Journal of Web Semantics*, *6*(1), 70–75.

Bederson, B. B., Shneiderman, B., & Wattenberg, M. (2002). Ordered and quantum treemaps: Making effective use of 2d space to display hierarchies. *ACM Transactions on Graphics*, *21*(4), 833–854. Retrieved from http://hcil.cs.umd.edu/trs/2001-18/2001-18.pdf. doi:10.1145/571647.571649

Bollegala, D., Matsuo, Y., & Ishizuka, M. (2007a). An integrated approach to measuring semantic similarity between words using information available on the Web. In *Proceedings of HLT-NAACL* (pp. 340-347).

Bollegala, D., Matsuo, Y., & Ishizuka, M. (2007b). Measuring semantic similarity between words using Web search engines. In *Proceedings of WWW* (pp. 757-766).

Breslin, J. G., Passant, A., & Decker, S. (2010). *The social Semantic Web*. Springer-Verlag.

Buckner, C., Niepert, M., & Allen, C. (2010). From encyclopedia to ontology: Toward dynamic representation of the discipline of philosophy. *Synthese*.

Calmet, J., & Daemi, A. (2004a). *Assessing conflicts in ontologies*. Tech. Rep., IAKS Calmet, University Karlsruhe (TH), Germany. Retrieved from http://avalon.ira.uka.de/iaks-calmet/papers/WSEAS 2004.pdf

Calmet, J., & Daemi, A. (2004b). *From entropy to ontology*. Tech. Rep., Institute for Algorithms and Cognitive Systems (IAKS), University of Karlsruhe (TH), Germany. Retrieved from http://iaks-www.ira.uka.de/calmet/papers/AT2AI4.pdf

Curran, J. R. (2002). Ensemble methods for automatic thesaurus extraction. In *Proceedings of ACL* (pp. 222–229).

Eckert, K., Pfeffer, M., & Stuckenschmidt, H. (2008). Assessing thesaurus-based annotations for semantic search applications. *International Journal on Metadata. Semantics and Ontologies, 3*(1), 53–67. doi:10.1504/IJMSO.2008.021205

Eckert, K., Stuckenschmidt, H., & Pfeffer, M. (2007). Interactive thesaurus assessment for automatic document annotation. In *Proceedings of the Fourth International Conference on knowledge capture (k-cap 2007),* Whistler, Canada.

Gillam, L., Tariq, M., & Ahmad, K. (2005). Terminology and the construction of ontology. *Terminology, 11,* 55–81. doi:10.1075/term.11.1.04gil

Grefenstette, G. (1994). *Explorations in automatic thesaurus discovery.* Heidelberg, Germany: Springer.

Gruber, T. (2008). Collective knowledge systems: Where the social web meets the Semantic Web. *Journal of Web Semantics, 6*(1), 4–13.

Hearst, M. A. (1992). Automatic acquisition of hyponyms from large text corpora. In *Proceedings of the fourteenth International Conference on computational linguistics,* Nantes, France.

Heath, T., Motta, E., & Petre, M. (2007). Computing word-of-mouth trust relationships in social networks from Semantic Web and Web 2.0 data sources. In *Proceedings of the Workshop on bridging the gap between Semantic Web and Web 2.0.*

Kageura, K., Tsuji, K., & Aizawa, A. N. (2000). Automatic thesaurus generation through multiple filtering. In *Proceedings Coling* (pp. 397–403).

Kaji, N., & Kitsuregawa, M. (2008). Using hidden Markov random fields to combine distributional and pattern-based word clustering. In *Proceedings of Coling* (pp. 401–408).

Katia Lida Kermanidis, M. M., Thanopoulos, A., & Fakotakis, N. (2008). Eksairesis: A domain-adaptable system for ontology building from unstructured text. In *Proceedings of LREC.*

Lin, D. (1998). An information-theoretic definition of similarity. In *Proceedings of ICML* (pp. 296–304).

Manning, C. D., & Schuetze, H. (1999). *Foundations of statistical natural language processing.* MIT Press.

Matsuo, Y., Sakaki, T., Uchiyama, K., & Ishizuka, M. (2006). Graph-based word clustering using a Web search engine. In *Proceedings of EMNLP* (pp. 542–550).

Nguyen, D. P. T., Matsuo, Y., & Ishizuka, M. (2007). *Exploiting syntactic and semantic information for relation extraction from Wikipedia.* In IJCAI07-TextlinkWS. Retrieved from http://citeseerx.ist.psu.edu/viewdoc/download?doi=10.1.1.73.9398&rep=rep1&type=pdf

Niepert, M., Buckner, C., & Allen, C. (2007). A dynamic ontology for a dynamic reference work. In *JCDL '07: Proceedings of the 7th ACM/IEEE-CS Joint Conference on digital libraries* (pp. 288–297). New York, NY: ACM.

Niepert, M., Buckner, C., & Allen, C. (2008). Answer set programming on expert feedback to populate and extend dynamic ontologies. In *Proceedings of the twenty-first international Florida artificial intelligence research society Conference, May 15-17, 2008, Coconut Grove, Florida, USA* (pp. 500-505).

Niepert, M., Buckner, C., & Allen, C. (2009). Working the crowd: Design principles and early lessons from the social- Semantic Web. In *Proceedings of the Workshop on Web 3.0: Merging Semantic Web and social Web at ACM Hypertext.*

Resnik, P. (1995). Using information content to evaluate semantic similarity in a taxonomy. In *Proceedings of the 14th International joint Conference on artificial intelligence (ijcai-95).* Retrieved from http://arxiv.org/pdf/cmp-lg/9511007

Salton, G., & Buckley, C. (1988). Term-weighting approaches in automatic text retrieval. In *Information processing and management* (pp. 513-523). Retrieved from http://citeseerx.ist.psu.edu/viewdoc/ download;jsessionid=1AAFE4AE3C28BA9C3DD59C416F8A6FEB?doi=10.1.1.101.9086&rep=rep1&type=pdf

Seco, N., Veale, T., & Hayes, J. (2004). An intrinsic information content metric for semantic similarity in wordnet. In *Proceedings of the 16th European Conference on artificial intelligence* (pp. 1089-1090). Valencia, Spain. Retrieved from http://eden.dei.uc.pt/~nseco/ecai2004b.pdf

Shneiderman, B. (1992). Tree visualization with tree-maps: 2-d space-filling approach. *ACM Transactions on Graphics*, *11*(1), 92–99. doi:10.1145/102377.115768

Shneiderman, B., & Wattenberg, M. (2001, 06). *Ordered treemap layouts.* Retrieved on February 19, 2007, from ftp://ftp.cs.umd.edu/pub/hcil/Reports-Abstracts-Bibliography/2001-06html/2001-06.htm

Turney, P. D. (2001). Mining the Web for synonyms: Pmi-ir versus lsa on toefl. In *Proceedings of EMCL* (pp. 491–502).

van der Plas, L., & Tiedemann, J. (2006). Finding synonyms using automatic word alignment and measures of distributional similarity. In *Proceedings of Coling* (pp. 866–873).

Vervenne, D. (1999). Advanced document management through thesaurus-based indexing: The IKEM platform. *CWI Quarterly*, *12*(2), 159–172.

Weiner, J. M. (2005). Differences in indexing term vocabularies and agreement with subject specialists. *Electronic Journal of Academic and Special Librarianship, 6*(1-2). Retrieved from http://southernlibrarianship.icaap.org/content/v06n01/weiner j01.htm

Witschel, H. F. (2005). Using decision trees and text mining techniques for extending taxonomies. In *Proceedings of the Workshop on learning and extending lexical ontologies by using machine learning methods.*

Wong, W., Liu, W., & Bennamoun, M. (2009). A probabilistic framework for automatic term recognition. *Intelligent Data Analysis*, *13*(4), 499–539.

Wu, H., & Zhou, M. (2003). Optimizing synonym extraction using monolingual and bilingual resources. In *Proceedings of the Second International Workshop on paraphrasing* (pp. 72–79).

KEY TERMS AND DEFINITIONS

Classification: A specific concept hierarchy. Classifications, as the name suggests, are used to classify ressources. The purpose is the organization of the resources, not necessarily the very accurate description of it.

Concept Hierarchy: The term "'concept hierarchy'" is used as an umbrella term for all kinds of background knowledge, vocabularies or glossaries. Concepts are units with a defined meaning, usually comprising more than a single term. The concepts are organized in an hierarchy, the hierarchical relationship may have different semantics, like broader/narrower concepts, subsumation or part-of relationships.

Crowdsourcing: Crowdsourcing means that a crowd of people contributes work for a common purpose, typically a small amount of work for each individual, but in the sum significant. Beside really creative work, like writing the Wikipedia, Crowdsourcing proved also to be very interesting for a lot of tedious work that yet can not be automated, like the tagging of websites.

Data Mining: Data Mining describes various approaches to find interesting correlations or additional information in – often unstructured or semi-structured – data.

Maintenance: Maintenance of a concept hierarchy, as opposed to creation, is the process of further editing and extending a once created concept hierarchy. Maintenance approaches can take advantage of the already existing hierarchy. That way, an approach can lead to good results in a maintenance setting, while it is not suitable for the creation of a hierarchy from scratch.

Ontology: Ontologies are formal representations of knowledge, with concepts and relationships between them. They can also contain rules and logic constraints that further describe the concepts and their relationships. Concept hierarchies can be seen as special ontologies. As their focus is often not as formal as for ontologies and they are somewhat limited in their ability to represent arbitrary knowledge, they are sometimes refered to as lightweight ontologies.

Thesaurus: A specific concept hierarchy. The core feature of a thesaurus is the availability of synonyms for each concept. They are typically used to define the concept. They often are not necessarily real synonyms, but also near or quasi-synonyms, which are summarized in one single concept. Thesauri are mainly used to describe resources with a controlled vocabulary, the hierarchy provides an easy access to the vocabulary for the users.

ENDNOTES

1 cf. http://www.bgbm.org/iapt/nomenclature/code/SaintLouis/0001ICSLContents.htm

2 cf. http://wordnet.princeton.edu/

3 In 2009 the MeSH includes 25,186 descriptors. cf. http://www.nlm.nih.gov/pubs/factsheets/mesh.html

4 http://inpho.cogs.indiana.edu/

5 http://developer.yahoo.com/

6 http://www.nlm.nih.gov/mesh/

7 http://www.ncbi.nlm.nih.gov/pubmed/

8 http://xmlns.com/foaf/spec/

9 http://www.aktors.org/publications/ontology/

10 http://www.ontologyportal.org/

11 http://inpho.cogs.indiana.edu/taxonomy/

12 http://www.semtinel.org

Chapter 7
Learning SKOS Relations for Terminological Ontologies from Text

Wei Wang
University of Nottingham Malaysia Campus, Malaysia

Payam M. Barnaghi
University of Surrey, UK

Andrzej Bargiela
University of Nottingham Jubilee Campus, UK

ABSTRACT

The problem of learning concept hierarchies and terminological ontologies can be divided into two sub-tasks: concept extraction and relation learning. The authors of this chapter describe a novel approach to learn relations automatically from unstructured text corpus based on probabilistic topic models. The authors provide definition (Information Theory Principle for Concept Relationship) and quantitative measure for establishing "broader" (or "narrower") and "related" relations between concepts. They present a relation learning algorithm to automatically interconnect concepts into concept hierarchies and terminological ontologies with the probabilistic topic models learned. In this experiment, around 7,000 ontology statements expressed in terms of "broader" and "related" relations are generated using different combination of model parameters. The ontology statements are evaluated by domain experts and the results show that the highest precision of the learned ontologies is around 86.6% and structures of learned ontologies remain stable when values of the parameters are changed in the ontology learning algorithm.

INTRODUCTION

Concept hierarchies used in most of the contemporary digital libraries are created and maintained manually. One of the most subtle problems with the manual approach is that the engineering and subsequent maintenance processes are time-consuming. The manually created hierarchies are also prone to suffer from obsolescence as research

DOI: 10.4018/978-1-60960-625-1.ch007

advances (e.g., invention of new techniques). Consequently, emergence of new terminologies in various research areas can not be easily reflected in such static concept hierarchies. It is also difficult to construct concept hierarchies with broader and deeper coverage, which can help users on query suggestion and expansion, browsing, and navigation. Unsupervised approaches for learning knowledge are perceived as promising approaches to alleviate these problems, minimising human involvement and effort.

The Semantic Web (Berners-Lee, Hendler, & Lassila, 2001) has been bringing more research attention towards knowledge acquisition using automated approaches. There have been a number of existing works that aim to learn different types of ontologies from unstructured text corpus using techniques from Natural Language Processing (Hearst, 1992, Cimiano & Staab, 2004, Cimiano, Pivk, Schmidt-Thieme, & Staab, 2005), Information Extraction (Cunningham, 2005, Cimiano & Völker, 2005, Kiryakov, Popov, Terziev, Manov, & Ognyanoff, 2004), and Machine Learning (clustering and classification) (Maedche, Pekar, & Staab, 2002, Biemann, 2005). An important and plausible assumption is that given sufficient amount of text in a domain, coverage of knowledge in that domain can be ensured (Cimiano, 2006). Although learned ontologies are less accurate than those created manually, the advantages of being inexpensive, time-saving, and resistant to obsolescence make the automated approaches attractive, especially in domains where semi-structured data is not available or cannot be directly transformed to structured form.

A concept hierarchy or topic hierarchy can be viewed as a simple form of a terminological ontology in which concepts are not only organised using more general/specific relations, but also other types of relations, such as "related" (introduction on the "related" and "broader" relations can be found in Section "SKOS Ontology Model" and "Information Theory Principle for Concept Relationship") defined in the SKOS ontology model[1].

In this chapter we explore a novel approach for learning terminological ontologies with respect to the SKOS model using Latent Dirichlet Allocation (Blei, Ng, & Jordan, 2003, Steyvers & Griffiths, 2005). The main objective is to establish "broader" and "related" relations between concepts using an unsupervised approach. The learned ontologies can be used to extend and expand existing topic hierarchies deployed in digital libraries and search engines, for different purposes such as facilitating search, browsing, query suggestion, and document annotation. The rest of the chapter is organised as follows. Section "Related Work" provides a short introduction on ontology categorisation and ontology learning tasks. It also gives an overview of existing methods for ontology learning from unstructured text. Section "Introduction to Latent Dirichlet Allocation" presents some background knowledge on the Latent Dirichlet Allocation, in particular the generative process, model representation and parameter estimation of the model. Section "Learning Relations in Terminological Ontologies" elaborates our approach for learning "broader" and "related" relations to construct terminological ontologies. We focus on the definition of concept relationship principle and an iterative algorithm for organising concepts into ontologies with the SKOS relations. Section "Experiment" describes the experiment conducted on a dataset which consists of abstracts of publications in the Semantic Web research area. Using the ontology learning algorithm with different parameters, around 7,000 ontology statements are generated. Results of evaluation in terms of recall, precision and F1 measures are demonstrated in Section "Evaluation". Section "Discussion and Future Work" concludes the chapter and describes the future work.

RELATED WORK

In this section we first provide some background knowledge on ontology categorisation and ontology learning processes in order to define the specific problem that our approach aims to solve. We briefly review prevailing ontology learning approaches which use techniques from Natural Language Processing (Hearst, 1992, Cimiano & Staab, 2004, Cimiano et al., 2005), Information Extraction (Cunningham, 2005, Cimiano & Völker, 2005, Kiryakov et al., 2004), Machine Learning (Maedche et al., 2002), and simple Data Co-occurrence Analysis (Sanderson & Croft, 1999, Diederich & Balke, 2007) (A detailed survey on ontology learning methods can also be found in (Biemann, 2005)).

ONTOLOGY CATEGORISATION

The philosophical word "ontology" is borrowed by computer science or more recently by the Semantic Web to denote a specification of conceptualisation (Gruber, 2003). The word has become one of the most fundamental concepts in the Semantic Web research. The following provides a taxonomy for types of ontology[2] which receives consensus.

1. **Formal Ontology**: a terminological ontology whose categories are distinguished by axioms and definitions stated in logic or in some computer-oriented language that could be automatically translated to logic.
2. **Prototype-based Ontology**: a terminological ontology whose categories are distinguished by typical instances or prototypes rather than by axioms and definitions in logic.
3. **Terminological Ontology**: an ontology whose categories are not fully specified by axioms and definitions.

A formal ontology explicitly defines mechanisms (i.e., axioms) for logical inference, whereas a prototype-based ontology consists of categories which are formed by collecting instances extensionally. In a terminological ontology, concepts

can be organised in a tree-like structure using subsumption or "broader" (or "narrower"[3]) relations as well as other types of relations (e.g., "related" in the SKOS model). The ACM classification tree[4] and Medical Subject Headings (MeSH)[5] are two well-known examples of concept hierarchy. One limitation with tree-based representation is that ("fuzzy") relations to more specific concepts cannot be modelled. The presence of the additional relations is one of the major differences between a terminological ontology and a concept hierarchy.

SKOS Ontology Model

SKOS (Simple Knowledge Organisation System) provides a model for expressing the basic structure and content of concept schemes such as thesauri, classification schemes, subject heading lists, taxonomies, folksonomies, and other types of controlled vocabulary. The SKOS is an ideal model for representing relations between concepts or topics (often in a form of noun-phrases) in scientific research, for example, advance in research accelerates co-operations between different disciplines: to solve a problem in one research area (e.g., ontology learning in Semantic Web) one often utilises techniques from others areas, such as natural language processing and machine learning. Another advantage of knowledge representation using SKOS ontology compared to traditional concept hierarchy is that it is able to represent emerging concepts and relations. This chapter shows how to learn SKOS relations based on probabilistic topic models which are originally developed for document modelling.

Ontology Learning Tasks

Cimiano (Cimiano, 2006) identifies six subtasks for learning ontologies. The subtasks are organised in a "layered cake" which is composed of learning terms, synonyms, concepts, concept hierarchies, relations, and rules, from bottom to top. Learning of terminological ontology can be divided to learning two sub-tasks, concepts or terms[6].

Ontology Learning from Text

Existing methods for learning ontologies of different types can be classified into four main categories as discussed in (Biemann, 2005): Lexico-syntatic based approach (Hearst, 1992, Cimiano & Staab, 2004, Cimiano et al., 2005), Information Extraction (Cimiano & Völker, 2005, Kiryakov et al., 2004), Clustering and Classification (Maedche et al., 2002), and Data Co-occurrence Analysis (Sanderson & Croft, 1999, Diederich & Balke, 2007).

Lexico-Syntatic Based Approach

Lexico-syntatic method uses natural language processing techniques to extract regular expressions that occur repeatedly in human languages, for example, the so-called Hearst-patterns (Hearst, 1992) are originally used to acquire hyponyms of some words from large text corpus. One of the limitations of this method is that the Hearst-patterns may not occur frequently in the text corpus which results in very low recall. Cimiano *et al* (Cimiano & Staab, 2004, Cimiano et al., 2005) attempt to explore the potential of large Web search engines to extract more occurrence of the language patterns, calling the method "Learning by Googling". In ontology learning, the technique is often used to learn instances of pre-defined concepts.

Information Extraction

Information Extraction (IE) (Cunningham, 2005) techniques, in particular, Named Entity Recognition (NER) is used to automatically populate knowledge base (Cimiano & Völker, 2005, Kiryakov et al., 2004). The most significant limitation is that the current NER technology is only effective for extracting instances of some general concepts such as "People", "Location", "Organisation" and their corresponding sub-concepts. This method, together with the Lexico-syntatic based approach have been primarily used for learning terms and concepts.

Clustering and Classification

Clustering is used to populate prototype-based ontology or to learn ontologies from scratch (corresponds to the learning concept hierarchies sub-task), whereas classification is used to augment a thesaurus (or extend concept hierarchies) with new lexical terms (Maedche et al., 2002). In methods based on these statistical learning techniques, terms are represented by vectors of terms in the vicinity. The representation is often based on an assumption called Harris' distributional hypothesis, which states that similar words tend to occur in similar contexts (Harris, 1968). Similarity or dissimilarity functions are then used to determine to which clusters or classes a new term or object is assigned.

Data Co-Occurrence Analysis

Data Co-occurrence Analysis is a simple while effective approach for learning concept hierarchies by exploiting first-order or high-order co-occurrence[7] of data. Sanderson *et al* (Sanderson & Croft, 1999) assume that "a term A subsumes B if the documents in which B occurs are (or nearly) a subset of the documents in which A occurs". Another method uses a variation of the PageRank algorithm (Brin & Page, 1998) called GrowBag (Diederich & Balke, 2007) to analyse high-order data co-occurrence for constructing concept hierarchies. The learned concept hierarchy has been deployed in the FacetedDBLP[8] browser to help users browsing and retrieving scientific publications.

INTRODUCTION TO LATENT DIRICHLET ALLOCATION

Latent Dirichlet Allocation (LDA) (Blei et al., 2003, Steyvers & Griffiths, 2005) is an instance of statistical topic models in which semantic properties of words and documents are represented with probabilistic (latent) topics. LDA, together with the probabilistic Latent Semantic Analysis (pLSA) (Hofmann, 1999a, 1999b), are originally developed as probabilistic extension of the Latent Semantic Analysis (LSA) (Deerwester, Dumais, Landauer, Furnas, & Harshman, 1990) for document modelling and topic extraction. Similar as its predecessors LSA and pLSA, LDA can also be used as an efficient dimension reduction technique. For example, in document clustering and classification, a document can be represented with a vector of topics in a low dimension space instead of vector of words in a high dimension to compute similarity with other documents. Before we elaborate the procedure of learning terminological ontologies using LDA, we provide some background knowledge of LDA in this section.

LATENT SEMANTIC ANALYSIS

The basic idea of LSA (Deerwester et al., 1990) is to reform document representation in high dimension word space to low dimension latent semantic space in order to capture implicit associations between words and documents. The low dimension latent space is obtained by decomposing a large term-document matrix using Singular Value Decomposition, a technique in linear algebra. An attractive characteristic of LSA is its capability to alleviate two classical Information Retrieval problems of synonymy (i.e., different words refer to the same meaning) and polysemy (i.e., one word has different meanings). One of the limitations of the technique is that although words and documents can be represented as points in the Euclidean space, the semantics of the model is difficult to be explicitly interpreted (Hofmann, 1999a, 1999b).

PROBABILISTIC LATENT SEMANTIC ANALYSIS

Probabilistic Latent Semantic Analysis (pLSA) (Hofmann, 1999a, 1999b) is a probabilistic extension of the LSA model. It is a statistical generative model for analysing general co-occurrence data using probabilistic theories. pLSA specifies a simple generative process for a word in a document:

1. choose a document d with a prior probability $P(d)$,
2. choose a latent class z from the document with probability $P(z \mid d)$,
3. choose a word w from the latent class distribution with probability $P(w \mid z)$.

Parameters (i.e., $P(w \mid z)$, $P(d \mid z)$ and $P(d)$[9]) in pLSA are estimated using the Expectation Maximisation (EM) algorithm (Hofmann, 1999a, 1999b).

LATENT DIRICHLET ALLOCATION

While pLSA is a significant step toward probabilistic modelling of text, it is incomplete in that it provides no probabilistic model at the level of documents, in other words, pLSA does not make any assumptions about how the mixture weights $p(z \mid d)$ are generated (Blei et al., 2003). Consequently, the number of parameters need to be estimated grows linearly with the size of the corpus, which leads to a serious problem of overfitting (Blei et al., 2003); and it is also difficult to test generalisability of the model to new documents (Steyvers & Griffiths, 2005).

In the original LDA model (Blei et al., 2003) a Dirichlet prior is introduced on document-topic distribution. As a conjugate prior for multinomial distributions (D'Agostini, 2003), Dirichlet prior simplifies the problem of statistical inference. Steyvers and Griffiths (Steyvers & Griffiths, 2005, T. L. Griffiths & Steyvers, 2004, T. Griffiths & Steyvers, 2002) modify the original LDA model by introducing another symmetric Dirichlet prior on topic-word distribution. They also show how to perform parameter estimation using Gibbs sampling, one form of the Markov Chain Monte Carlo (Andrieu, Freitas, Doucet, & Jordan, 2003).

Generative Process

In LDA, each word w in a document d is generated by sampling a topic z from topic distribution, and then sampling a word from topic-word distribution. The probability of any particular word token is defined by Equation (1):

$$P(w_i) = \sum_{j=1}^{T} P(w_i \mid z_i = j)P(z_i = j)$$

where $P(z_i = j)$ is the probability that jth topic is sampled for the ith word token, $P(w_i \mid z_i = j)$ is the probability of sampling w_i under topic j, and T is the number of hidden topics. Let $\phi^{(j)} = P(w \mid z = j)$ refer to multinomial distribution over words for the topic j, and $\theta^{(d)} = P(z)$ refer to multinomial distribution over topics in the document d. The complete generative process can be expressed as:

$$w_i \mid z_i, \phi^{(z_i)} \sim Discrete(\phi^{(z_i)})$$

$$\phi \sim Dirichlet(\beta)$$

$$z_i \mid \theta(d_i) \sim Discrete(\theta(d_i))$$

$$\theta \sim Dirichlet(\alpha)$$

Parameter Estimation

The original LDA paper (Blei et al., 2003) uses variational inference with EM algorithm to estimate parameters. In this work, we adopt the parameter estimation method using Gibbs sampling because of its simplicity as discussed in (Steyvers & Griffiths, 2005, T. L. Griffiths & Steyvers, 2004). In parameter estimation using Gibbs sampling, instead of directly estimating the topic-word $p(w \mid z)$ and document-topic $p(z \mid d)$ distributions, one estimates the posterior probability distribution over latent variable z given the observed data conditioned on topic assignment for all the other word tokens using Equation (2) (See (T. Griffiths & Steyvers, 2002, T. L. Griffiths & Steyvers, 2004, Steyvers & Griffiths, 2005) for details).

$$P(z_i = j \mid \mathbf{z}_{-i}, \mathbf{w}) \propto \frac{n_{-i,j}^{(w_i)} + \beta}{n_{-i,j}^{()} + W\beta} \frac{n_{-i,j}^{(d_i)} + \alpha}{n_{-i,\cdot}^{(d_i)} + T\alpha}$$

The first term in the right side of Equation (2) indicates the probability of a word w under topic j, whereas the second term indicates the probability of topic j in the document d. The intuition of this equation is that once many tokens of a word have been assigned to a topic j (across documents), it will increase the probability of assigning any particular token of that word to topic j; once a topic j has appeared many times in a document, it will increase the probability of any word tokens from that document will be assigned to topic j. Therefore, the assignment of a word to a topic depends on not only how likely the word is for a topic, but also how dominant a topic is in a document (Steyvers & Griffiths, 2005).

The Gibbs sampling algorithm starts with random assignment of word tokens to topics. Each Gibbs sample consists of topic assignments to all of the word tokens in the corpus. Samples before the "burn-in"[10] period are discarded due to poor estimates of the posterior probability. After the "burn-in" period, successive Gibbs samples start to approximate the posterior distributions over topic assignments. A number of Gibbs samples are preserved at regular intervals to prevent correlations between samples (T. Griffiths, 2002, T. L. Griffiths & Steyvers, 2004, Steyvers & Griffiths, 2005).

The word-topic ϕ and topic-document θ distribution can be obtained using Equation (3) and (4):

$$\hat{\phi}_j^{(w)} = \frac{n_j^{(w)} + \beta}{n_j^{()} + W\beta}$$

$$\hat{\theta}_j^{(d)} = \frac{n_j^{(d)} + \alpha}{n_{.}^{(d)} + T\alpha}$$

The values correspond to the predictive distributions of sampling a new word token w from a topic j, and sampling a new word token w from a topic j in a document d (For detailed derivation of the Equation (2), (3), and (4) refer to (T. Griffiths, 2002)).

LEARNING RELATIONS IN TERMINOLOGICAL ONTOLOGIES

The task of learning terminological ontology can be divided to two sub-tasks: learning concepts and relations. The problem of learning concepts in various domains has been well studied in existing work as discussed in Section "Related Work", whereas relation learning is less discussed. The main method for relation learning in existing work is the Data Co-occurrence Analysis: in (Sanderson & Croft, 1999) the method establishes subsumption relation based on a simple assumption to exploit first-order co-occurrence; in (Diederich & Balke, 2007) the method constructs concept hierarchies based on identifying high-order data co-occurrence. In a sense, both of the methods attempt to build concept hierarchies without content analysis and rely solely on the co-occurrence of data or concepts, making them ineffective in situations where desired concepts do not co-occur with each other frequently.

In contrast, our method first represents concepts (e.g., concepts in computer science literature) identified in the underlying corpus as documents[11] and then performs content analysis using Latent Dirichlet Allocation which has been proved as a superior model for document modelling. By using it as an effective dimension reduction technique, concept representation is reduced to a vector of topics extracted by LDA. Finally, the concepts are organised into terminological ontologies using an iterative algorithm based on the "broader" relation definition. The definition is named as "Information Theory Principle for Concept Relationship". The intuition is that by exploiting superior performance of topic models, semantic relations between words and documents can be captured in terms of probabilistic topics. Since concepts in our methods are represented as documents, semantic relations between concepts can then be captured based on modelling relations between topic distributions of the documents.

Throughout the paper, we limit the scope of our discussion to learning terminological ontologies in the domain of scientific research, and in particular, computer science, though it can be naturally applied to other research areas such as medical science. Differing from the work developed in (Diederich & Balke, 2007, Zavitsanos, Paliouras, Vouros, & Petridis, 2007) which exclusively learns concept hierarchies, our objective is to learn ontologies with respect to two SKOS relations (i.e., "broader" and "related").

CONCEPT REPRESENTATION

Concepts in various scientific research areas often have a form of noun-phrase in which several words together form a specific meaning that is often well understood by human. For example, we understand that "Support Vector Machines" and "Latent Dirichlet Allocation" are two specific techniques from Artificial Intelligence, where the former is widely adopted for classification and the latter for document modelling. However, the task of understanding meanings of these concepts and distinguishing between similar concepts is difficult for machines because they do not possess human cognition. Though the probabilistic topic models pLSA and LDA, as well as LSI, provide means for computing similarities between individual word tokens, they are not suitable to be applied to concepts in form of noun-phrases. Decomposing a noun-phrase representation of a concept into individual word tokens destroys the intentional meaning of that concept. The concept "Artificial Neural Network" denotes a specific technique in Artificial Intelligence, developed by computer scientists inspired by network of neurons which work together to perform some functions in human body. The word "Neural" means "relating to the nervous system", and "Network" is an ambiguous term (polysemy) and has different interpretations in different contexts such as Social Science, Computer Science, or Medical Science. The meaning of a concept is often completely different from the combined meanings of its constituents (i.e., individual tokens).

We represent concepts using the documents which are annotated by the concept mentions in the text corpus. Collectively, those word mentions (across documents) form a stable context which is able to explain the meaning of a concept. The idea is in line with the so-called "distributional hypothesis" (Harris, 1968) which states that similar words tend to appear in similar contexts. This is also similar to the idea of "Word Window" where words within a fixed size window centered on a particular word are used as "context" of that word.

In some applications using LDA, the learned topic-word distributions are directly interpreted as topics (T. L. Griffiths & Steyvers, 2004, Zavitsanos et al., 2007). For the purpose of learning ontology or concept hierarchy, the problem with direct interpretation is that one has to manually associate labels to those learned topics in order to provide meaningful interpretation. Some of the learned topics are expressed as distribution of intuitive word tokens, making the topic-label matching straightforward. While for other topics the label matching is difficult because the topics are expressed in distribution of general, non-sense, or even ambiguous word tokens. Intuitively, less latent topics generate more general concepts (and more topics generate more specific concepts), however, relations between topics learned using different number of latent classes can not be established in a precise way. Furthermore, the relations are often difficult to establish using automated approaches. On the contrary, representing concepts as documents does not suffer from these problems. Once the concepts are represented using documents, relations between them can be approximated by the relations between the representing documents in the low-dimension latent semantic space.

INFORMATION THEORY PRINCIPLE FOR CONCEPT RELATIONSHIP

As mentioned earlier, the SKOS model provides a convenient framework for expressing scientific terms in an ontological form, differing from traditional concept hierarchies in which concepts are organised in a tree-like structure. Our objective is to learn two relations: "broader" ("narrower" is the inverse property of "broader"), and "related" defined in SKOS. The "broader" relation can be interpreted as "more general than" ("narrower" as "more specific than") and is learned using a top-down approach. The mechanism for establishing "broader" relation between two concepts, called "Information Theory Principle for Concept Relationship" is defined based on Information Theory (MacKay, 2003). Before we give the definition of the principle, we provide some prerequisite definitions (for simplicity, these definitions are presented in mathematical form): Cosine similarity, Kullback-Leibler divergence (KL divergence, $D_{KL}(P \parallel Q)$) and Jason-Shannon Divergence (JS divergence, $D_{JS}(P \parallel Q)$) (MacKay, 2003). In the following definitions, P and Q are two probability distributions. The subscript i is used to denote the i th element in a distribution.

Definition: The Cosine similarity between two vectors with same dimension (could be probability distributions) is defined as:

$$COS(P,Q) = \frac{\sum_i P(i) \bullet Q(i)}{\sqrt{\sum_i P(i)^2} \bullet \sqrt{\sum_i Q(i)^2}}$$

Definition: The Kullback-Leibler divergence or relative entropy between two probability distributions $P(x)$ and $Q(x)$ is defined as:

$$D_{KL}(P \| Q) = \sum_i P(i) \log \frac{P(i)}{Q(i)}$$

The KL divergence is an asymmetric function, which means that $D_{KL}(P \| Q)$ is not equal to $D_{KL}(Q \| P)$. As such, the function is not a real metric and cannot be used as dissimilarity measures. Following the Gibbs inequity (MacKay, 2003), all values of KL divergence $D_{KL} > 0.0$

Definition: The Jason-Shannon divergence between two probability distributions $P(x)$ and $Q(x)$ is defined as:

$$D_{JS}(P \parallel Q) = \frac{1}{2} D_{KL}(P \parallel Q) + \frac{1}{2} D_{KL}(Q \parallel P)$$

The JS divergence is a symmetric function defined over the KL divergence and is a popular metric for calculating dissimilarity measures.

We define the "Information Theory Principle for Concept Relationship" as the following (Wang, Barnaghi, & Bargiela, 2009):

definition: A concept C_p is broader than a concept C_q if the following two conditions hold:

1. (Similarity condition) the similarity measure between them is greater than certain threshold TH_S (or divergence measure is less than certain threshold TH_D), and
2. (Divergence difference condition) the difference between Kullback-Leibler divergence measures
    $D_{KL}(P \parallel Q) - D_{KL}(Q \parallel P) < 0$.

In the context of this paper, P and Q stand for probabilistic distributions of latent topics for concepts C_p and C_q respectively. The similarity or divergence measures can be calculated using Cosine similarity or Jensen-Shannon divergence measures.

CONNECTION TO OTHER THEORIES

In most of the work reported in literature, the symmetric metric JS divergence is used for comparing dissimilarity between two vectors (or probability distributions) (Maedche et al., 2002, Biemann, 2005). Due to its asymmetry, KL divergence is less utilised for quantitative measures. One of explanations for the KL divergence $D_{KL}(P \parallel Q)$ is that P normally represents the "true" distribution of data, while Q represents a practical approximation of P. In other words, it is the average "surprise" of an incoming message drawn from distribution Q when it is expected that it comes from the true distribution P. The second condition or the divergence difference condition states that given the similarity condition holds, if the KL divergence $D_{KL}(P \| Q) - D_{KL}(Q \| P) < 0$, then the concept C_p is said to be a broader concept of C_q. An example would provide an intuitive explanation: a source transmits an message to a receiver who has been informed that the topic of the message is about "Ontology". The receiver is then expecting that the message is about the broad research topic "Ontology". However, after inspecting its content the receiver realises that exact topic is "Ontology Learning" (for example, ontology learning using Natural Language Processing techniques which is more related to Natural Language Processing rather than ontology). The receiver has an amount of "surprise", however, the quantity of the "surprise" is less than the amount after s/he observes that the paper is on "Ontology" while he has been told that the paper is about "Ontology Learning".

We exploit the asymmetry of KL divergence measure between two probability distributions to determine whether the "broader" relation holds between two concepts. Compared to the assumption made by Sanderson *et al* (Sanderson & Croft, 1999) in which "a term A subsumes B if the documents in which B occurs are (or nearly) a subset of the documents in which A occurs", our definition can be explained intuitively by the Information Theory (MacKay, 2003) and provides a probabilistic foundation for quantitative measure. Recently, the theory of "surprise" proposed in (Itti & Baldi, 2006) provides another method for measuring "surprise" of information. The quantity is defined as the KL divergence of prior and posterior distribution of a random variable. Our

definition is similar to the theory, while it measures the difference between two divergence values of "true" and "observed" distributions and does not involve calculation of posterior probability.

In practice, the divergence difference condition cannot be satisfied exactly and the rigorous condition results in low recall. In our experiment, we assume there exists certain amount of noise in the input data. Thus, another empirical parameter TH_N (called the noise factor) is introduced into the second inequity to balance the effect of the noise, resulting in the equation $D_{KL}(P \| Q) - D_{KL}(Q \| P) < TH_N$. The introduction of the constant TH_N increases the recall, while the precision is only reduced slightly (The recall, precision, and F1 measures of the experimental results are illustrated in Section "Evaluation").

ONTOLOGY LEARNING ALGORITHM

The "related" function defined in the SKOS model is rather ambiguous and in this paper it is interpreted as follows: if similarity between two concepts satisfies the similarity condition while not the divergence difference condition, the two concepts are said to be related. The intuition is that even though a "broader" relation cannot be established between them, they are very similar to each other. Together with the principle for establishing "broader" relationship defined in the previous section, the next step is to automatically organising concepts into hierarchies and then terminological ontologies. An additional constraint on the concept hierarchy to be learned is that a node can only have one parent.

We have developed a recursive algorithm which is named as Global Similarity Hierarchy Learning (GSHL). In another work, we also developed an algorithm called Local Similarity Hierarchy Learning (LSHL) which is only able to learn concept hierarchies. Comparison of the two algorithms can be found in (Wang et al., 2009). To learn "broader" relations, the algorithm recursively searches for the most similar concepts of the current "root" concept (the root node is specified by users) and eliminates those do not fulfill the divergence difference condition. The criteria for termination is either pre-defined number of iterations is reached or all concepts have been organised into an ontology. There are some parameters defined in the algorithms whose values can be modified to generate different ontology structures. Effect of these parameter values on precision of learned ontologies are discussed in Section "Evaluation". The parameters defined in the algorithm are listed as follows:

1. N_c — The number of topics or classes used to learn parameters in LDA model.
2. M_c — The maximum number of designated sub-nodes for a particular node.
3. TH_S and TH_D — The thresholds for similarity and divergence measures.
4. TH_N — The noise factor, which is the threshold for the difference between two KL divergence measures $D_{KL}(P \| Q)$ and $D_{KL}(Q \| P)$.
5. I — Maximum number of iterations.

The constant parameters TH_S, TH_D, TH_N can be modified to generate different results and they have direct effect on recall, precision and F1 measures. The parameter N_c defines the dimension of the semantic space and is used to identify appropriate number of latent classes in LDA learning. The parameter M_c is defined to assess the optimum number of sub-nodes of a particular node. In our experiment the number is assumed to be between 5 to 10. The result shows that the constant has no effect on those concepts which have less than 5 sub concepts (concepts which have more than 10 sub concepts are rare in our

sample dataset). In addition, three pair-wise similarity and divergence matrices (denoted using M) are pre-calculated to improve performance of the algorithms.

Global Similarity Hierarchy Learning

The ontology learning algorithm first specifies the root concept and adds it into the Processing Vector, V. The vector V_{temp} stores most similar concepts of the current "root" node using either Cosine similarity measure or JS divergence measure. Then the algorithm eliminates those concepts following a two-step procedure: first, those concepts whose KL divergence values with the current "root" do not satisfy the divergence difference condition are removed from V_{temp}. Then, for each concept left in the V_{temp}, only if the similarity value between the concept and the current "root" is greater than similarity value between the concept and any of the siblings of the current "root", a "broader" relation statement is asserted. Otherwise, a "related" relation statement is asserted. The pseudo-code is given in Figure 1. Algorithm 1: where the function $Sim(a,b)$ returns similarity (i.e., Cosine similarity) or divergence (JS divergence) values between concepts a and b. The function $Sibling(root)$ returns the siblings of the current "node". To establish "broader" relation between two concepts, the algorithm searches for the most similar concepts "globally" because of which we name it as Global Similarity Hierarchy Learning algorithm. After testing the divergence difference condition for a topic and the current root topic, the algorithm will conduct another search for the most similar topics among siblings of the current root. The time complexity of GSHL algorithm is $O(m^2 \cdot n^2)$, where $m = M_c$, $n = N$, and $n \gg M_c$. In (Wang et al., 2009), we also analysed the time complexity of another ontology learning approach ($O(n^3)$) (Zavitsanos et al., 2007) and reported that our algorithm is more

Figure 1.

Algorithm 1 $GSHL(root)$

Require: Initialise V, M_s, I, TH_s, TH_d, TH_n, and M_c.
Ensure: A terminological ontology with "broader" and "related" relations.
1: Initialise V, M_s, I, TH_s, TH_d, TH_n, and M_c;
2: **while** $(i < I$ and V is not empty$)$ **do**
3:     Add current root into V;
4:     Select most similar M_c nodes of root from M_s;
5:     Add similar nodes into V_{temp};
6:     Remove nodes in V_{temp} against Definition 2;
7:     **for** (all nodes n_i in V_{temp}) **do**
8:         **if** $(\text{Sim}(n_i, \text{root}) > \text{Sim}(n_i, \text{Sibling(root)}))$ **then**
9:             Assert broader relations between root and topic n_i;
10:         **else**
11:             Assert related relation between root and topic n_i;
12:         **end if**
13:         Move topic n_i from V_{temp} to V;
14:         Increment i by 1;
15:     **end for**
16:     Remove current root from V;
17: **end while**

---

efficient. In our experiment, the best precision is achieved using GSHL with 40 classes for LDA training (see Section "Evaluation" for evaluation details). The best precision for statements of "broader" relation is about 86% and for "related" relation is up to 90%.

EXPERIMENT

The experiment of using the GSHL algorithm to learn terminological ontologies with LDA models consists of the following four steps:

1. Dataset preparation and concepts extraction,
2. Learning LDA models with different number of classes,
3. Folding-in documents of concepts to learned LDA models,
4. Running GSHL algorithms to learn terminological ontologies.

Each of the steps is elaborated in the subsequent sections.

DATASET PREPARATION AND CONCEPT EXTRACTION

Around 5,000 Web pages containing abstracts of published work (conference paper, journal articles, and book chapters) in the Semantic Web research area are collected from the ACM digital library[12]. A Web page scraper is developed using the NekoHTML[13] HTML parser to extract relevant information, such as abstract, category annotation using terms from the ACM classification tree, user specified keywords, and related bibliographic information. Annotations of an article in a Web page normally consists of three types of terms: terms from the ACM classification tree, general terms (such as "Algorithm" and "Experiment"), and user supplied keywords. The ACM classification tree is maintained manually and seems a bit outdated for some research areas, for example, the term

"Semantic Web" does not exist in the tree. By using the user specified keywords the classification tree can be extended to deeper levels and expanded to broader range. The concept extraction process is done using a simple statistics on these keywords, that is, keywords appeared more than ten times in the whole corpus are regarded as stable concepts to be organised in the ontology. The approach for extracting concepts is similar to the one used in (Diederich & Balke, 2007). To increase recall of concepts extraction, a simple syntactical method is used to identify synonyms and plural form of some keywords, for example, ontology and ontologies. In total 80 concepts are extracted.

The corpus is further processed using some shallow natural language processing techniques. The standard English stopwords as well as a list of customised stopwords (which consists of words such as "1977" and "1st") are removed. The Stanford Log-linear Part-Of-Speech Tagger[14] is used to POS-tag all documents in the corpus and only nouns, verbs, and adjectives are preserved for training LDA models. All words are also stemmed using the Porter's stemmer[15] packaged in the Apache's Lucene Java[16], resulting in approximately 7000 unique words in total.

The extracted concepts are represented using documents which are annotated by the concepts. There are two main reasons for doing this. First, LDA is an efficient dimension reduction technique for documents, and it is able to capture the semantic relations between words, topics, and documents. A new document can be conveniently folded-in to the LDA model and represented using topic distributions. Second, as discussed earlier, a document represents a concrete context in which a concept is mentioned and explained.

LEARNING LDA MODELS

We use the Gibbs sampling algorithm provided by LingPipe[17] to learn LDA models (LingPipe is a Java library for linguistic analysis). In the experiment, seven LDA models are trained using different number of classes (i.e., from 30 to 90) in order to find out reasonable number of classes that can achieve better precision measures. The values of parameters for training LDA models are set as follows:

$$\alpha = 0.1,$$

$$\beta = 0.01,$$

$$number of Gibbs samples = 1000,$$

$$burn - in epochs = 1000,$$

$$Sample Lag = 1.$$

The values of α and β are selected according to the experiment presented in (Steyvers & Griffiths, 2005) which shows satisfying results. The Gibbs sampling algorithm starts with random assignment of a topic to every word token in the corpus, every subsequent assignment of topic is determined by keeping previous assignments fixed (a complete Gibbs sample consists of topic assignment to every word token in the corpus). The algorithm is then run for specified number of times (2000 in our experiment). The first 1000 Gibbs samples are discarded due to poor estimates of the target distribution. After the "burn-in" period (assume after the first 1000 Gibbs samples), the subsequent Gibbs samples start to approach the target distribution. Another 1000 Gibbs samples are saved at regular intervals to prevent correlations between samples (T. Griffiths, 2002, T. L. Griffiths & Steyvers, 2004, Steyvers & Griffiths, 2005). The probability values of $p(w \mid z)$, and $p(z \mid d)$ are saved for purpose of folding in new documents, i.e., the documents which represent concepts.

Figure 2 shows the LDA model learned using 30 topics. Only the top-10 words with highest topic-word probability values are shown. The first column is the index of word in the corpus, the second column is the stemmed word, and the third column is the topic-word probability. Four topics (topic 2, 5, 10, and 25) are excerpted from all the topic-word distributions and shown here. Topic 2 can be interpreted as "Agent" and Topic 5 is about "Ontology". However, it is difficult to associate concepts or literal labels to the Topic 10 and 25. Figure 3 shows the LDA model learned using 90 topics. Topic 0 is related to "Information Retrieval", or more precisely "Ranking". Topic 2 is about "Web Service". As the topics learned using 30 classes, it is confusing to associate meaningful labels or extracted concepts to the Topics 12 and 87.

Similar to the examples, among all topic models learned, there are always some topics that can be interpreted using the extracted concepts or labels easily, while others are difficult to be interpreted in the Semantic Web research area. By representing concepts as documents, our method does not suffer from such a problem. Through folding-in these concept documents and using the "Information Theory Principle for Concept Relationship", concepts can be organised into hierarchies or ontologies in an unsupervised manner.

FOLDING-IN DOCUMENTS OF CONCEPTS

The concept of document "folding-in" is first introduced in the original LSA papers (Deerwester et al., 1990, Berry, Dumais, & O'Brien, 1995) in order to represent previously unseen documents (also referred to as "pseudo-documents" or query) in the reduced latent semantic space. In conventional information retrieval models, a document is represented using a vector of all indexed words (i.e., the vector space model) (Baeza-Yates & Ribeiro-Neto, 1999), while in LSA, a document is approximated by a vector which can be viewed as coordinates in the reduced latent dimension space (Deerwester et al., 1990, Berry et al., 1995). The similarity between documents can then be calculated using their low dimension vector representations. While the vectors of words are often sparse, the vectors in the low dimension space are dense (i.e., without zero values). Thus, to a great extent the problem of data sparseness or "zero-frequency" can be resolved. As such, LSA is often regarded as an effective technique to deal with the synonym and polysemy problems in information retrieval (Manning, Raghavan, & Schôtze, 2008).

In probabilistic topic models (i.e., LDA) (Steyvers & Griffiths, 2005), the document "folding-in" process follows a similar idea, which is, to calculate a lower dimension representation of previously unseen documents. In pLSA, a new document is folded in by a similar procedure as in the model learning phase using the EM algorithm. The difference is that in the folding-in phase, the EM algorithm is conditioned on the parameter $p(w \mid z)$ (i.e., keeping $p(w \mid z)$ fixed).

Similarly, the "fold-in" process in LDA is performed using the Gibbs sampling algorithm as in the learning phase[18]. A new document is folded into a learned LDA model by running the Gibbs sampling in which the topic-word distribution are kept constant and assigning topics to every word token in the new document.

The documents which represent the extracted concepts are treated as new documents[19]. We wrote a program using the Gibbs sampling to calculate document-topic distributions conditioned on the learned topic-word distributions for all new documents. Parameters settings are same as those used during LDA training. Document-topic distributions for all new documents are then used to compute pair-wise similarity (Cosine similarity) and divergence values (JS and KL divergence) before running the ontology learning algorithms.

Figure 2. Topic-word distributions learned using 30 classes

TOPIC 10 SYMBOL	WORD	PROB
6886	document	0.102
3098	structur	0.041
4207	multimedia	0.041
4572	content	0.031
2093	link	0.031
601	adapt	0.026
410	hypermedia	0.025
948	hypertext	0.025
3452	media	0.023
2787	author	0.020

(a) Topic 2

TOPIC 25 SYMBOL	WORD	PROB
987	research	0.046
6078	comput	0.027
5454	commun	0.023
4613	develop	0.020
6441	technolog	0.019
1020	issu	0.017
2933	challeng	0.015
5844	scienc	0.014
4223	discuss	0.013
5643	futur	0.011

(c) Topic 10

TOPIC 2 SYMBOL	WORD	PROB
737	agent	0.221
5055	system	0.081
5862	multi	0.043
1953	base	0.033
2643	intellig	0.033
5454	commun	0.021
3100	softwar	0.020
618	interact	0.013
1569	distribut	0.012
3723	architectur	0.012

(b) Topic 5

TOPIC 5 SYMBOL	WORD	PROB
3893	ontolog	0.308
5079	semant	0.035
1683	domain	0.031
4581	map	0.028
6805	concept	0.028
1953	base	0.025
2254	approach	0.016
68	web	0.014
1644	construct	0.014
2387	relat	0.013

(d) Topic 25

Figure 3. Topic-word distributions learned using 90 classes

TOPIC 0 SYMBOL	WORD	PROB
1873	search	0.269
2831	rank	0.046
1953	base	0.043
534	engin	0.037
1103	keyword	0.036
1767	result	0.034
1669	index	0.031
3093	user	0.031
5292	queri	0.031
2168	relev	0.025

(a) Topic 0

TOPIC 2 SYMBOL	WORD	PROB
6397	servic	0.280
3923	composit	0.160
68	web	0.126
4471	compos	0.034
5393	autom	0.026
5523	automat	0.023
2254	approach	0.016
1180	describ	0.013
5146	techniqu	0.012
5361	net	0.012

(c) Topic 12

TOPIC 12 SYMBOL	WORD	PROB
2971	medic	0.077
3551	biomed	0.039
1410	clinic	0.031
624	health	0.027
6230	patient	0.027
5500	guidelin	0.026
987	research	0.024
5639	terminolog	0.024
5315	care	0.023
6642	us	0.022

(b) Topic 2

TOPIC 87 SYMBOL	WORD	PROB
5454	commun	0.230
6170	wiki	0.051
1613	share	0.031
4697	paper	0.027
6400	directori	0.026
3901	practic	0.024
4223	discuss	0.024
1180	describ	0.023
5814	extens	0.022
2836	collabor	0.021

(d) Topic 87

LEARNING TERMINOLOGICAL ONTOLOGIES

Ontology learning using GSHL is straightforward once the LDA models are learned and concept documents are folded-in. The algorithm is executed using different parameter values (for example, the number of classes used for training LDA, similarity and divergence threshold values and maximum number of sub-nodes) to find optimum parameter combinations. According to our experiment, satisfying results are achieved by setting the range of similarity threshold $TH_S \subset [0.5, 0.75]$, the divergence threshold $TH_D \subset [0.25, 0.45]$, and the noise factor $TH_N \subset [0.3, 0.5]$. The best result in terms of precision is achieved when Cosine similarity measure and 40 classes (for training LDA) are used. In (Wang et al., 2009), we reported that in terms of "broader" relation learning, the GSHL algorithm performs slightly better than LSHL in almost all cases. Another finding is that in most cases, the GSHL algorithm performs better when Cosine similarity measure is used, while the LSHL algorithm performs better with JS divergence measure. In a different experiment, we used the GSHL algorithm to learn a number of ontologies based on another topic model, pLSA, using same number of classes. The results show that overall precision of the ontological statements learned using LDA model is higher than those learned using pLSA.

We have re-implemented the concept hierarchy construction algorithms proposed in (Sanderson & Croft, 1999, Zavitsanos et al., 2007). The algorithms were then applied to the same dataset with similar parameter settings. The results produced using the algorithms (COO is the algorithm used in (Sanderson & Croft, 1999) and CIT is the algorithm used in (Zavitsanos et al., 2007)) are compared to ours, i.e., GSHL combined with the LDA. The precision curves are shown in Figure 3. As can be seen, our method performs notably better than the other two in terms of recall, precision, and F1 measures.

An example of a learned ontology is provided in the following with parameter settings: GSHL algorithm, Cosine similarity measure, LDA model with 40 classes, and the maximum number of sub-nodes equal to 8. The top level concept "Semantic Web" is predicted by the algorithm being broader than the following seven concepts: "Ontology", "RDF", "OWL", "Semantic Annotation", "Semantic Web Services", "Web", "Reasoning". All of the sub-concepts are correctly predicted except "Web", the reason is that there are few documents whose topics are directly related to "Web" in the corpus. Therefore, a problem of the method is that it is unable to exclude a concept which is not subsumed by the top concept. Although it can be eliminated during the concept extraction phase, for example, manually exclusion of such concepts, we aim to solve the problem using an automated approach in the future work.

Figure 5 shows a snippet of the automatically generated ontology[20] centering on the concept "Semantic Web" with "broader" relations only. The concept "Ontology" is one of the sub-concepts of "Semantic Web". In this particular case, the GSHL algorithm predicts that "Ontology" is a broader concept of "Ontology Evolution", "Information Integration", "Ontology Mapping", "Semantic Interoperability", and "Knowledge Acquisition". The diagrams (Figure 5 and 6) are generated using Protege[21] with "OntoViz" plugin.

Figure 6 shows a snippet of the ontology centering on the concept "Reasoning" with both "broader" and "related" relations. The GSHL algorithms predicts that "Reasoning" is related to "Ontology Mapping", "Knowledge Acquisition", "Ontology Evolution", and "Knowledge Representation".

Figure 4. Precision measures between COO, CIT, GSHL+LDA, and GSHL+pLSA

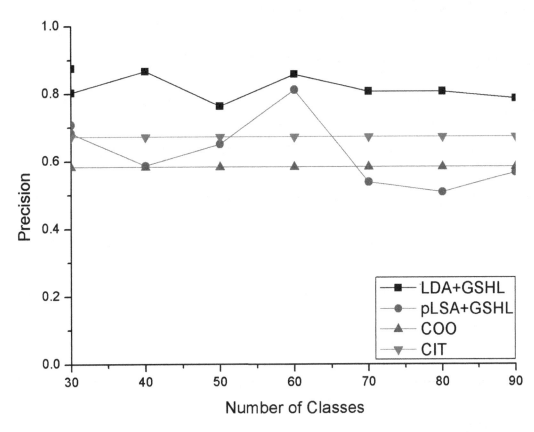

Figure 5. A snippet of the learned ontology centering on the concept "Semantic Web" with "broader than" relations

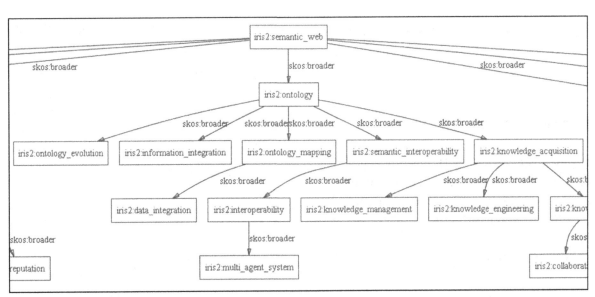

Figure 6. A snippet of the ontology centering on the concept "Reasoning" which is a sub-concept of "Semantic Web" with "broader" and "related" relations

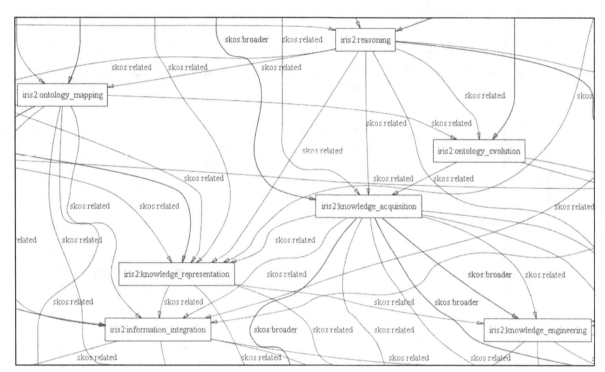

EVALUATION

The learned ontologies are transformed into the RDF format with respect to the SKOS model and evaluated by domain experts. The following sections report the evaluation results and also discuss the effect of different parameter values on the results.

EVALUATION METHODS

We use recall, precision and F1 measures (Manning et al., 2008) to assess the correctness of learned ontology statements. These metrics are popular measures of search performance for text retrieval. For our evaluation purpose, these metrics are defined as follows:

$$R = \frac{n_{tc}}{N_{cs}}$$

where n_{tc} is the number of correct learned statements given by the algorithms, N_{cs} is the total number of correct statements. We assume that a concept can only have one broader concept, thus the value of Ncs is equal to Nc-1, where Nc is the total number of topics.

Precision is defined as:

$$P = \frac{n_{tc}}{N_{ls}}$$

where n_{tc} is the number of correct learned statements, N_{ls} is the total number of learned state-

Table 1. Precision of ontology statements generated using different parameter values

Algorithm Settings\LDA classes			30	40	50	60	70	80	90	Average
5	LSHL	COS	0.684	0.694	0.645	0.737	0.685	0.743	0.815	0.715
		JS	0.813	0.653	0.657	0.788	0.667	0.721	0.661	0.709
	GSHL	COS	0.697	0.791	0.693	0.73	0.806	0.767	0.734	0.745
		JS	0.787	0.746	0.746	0.828	0.769	0.738	0.729	0.763
6	LSHL	COS	0.697	0.764	0.724	0.724	0.671	0.716	0.815	0.73
		JS	0.828	0.625	0.589	0.833	0.689	0.662	0.621	0.692
	GSHL	COS	0.684	**0.866**	0.763	0.743	0.778	0.681	0.781	0.757
		JS	0.787	0.803	0.697	0.81	0.761	0.738	0.767	0.766
7	LSHL	COS	0.724	0.75	0.724	0.803	0.685	0.743	0.723	0.736
		JS	0.844	0.712	0.644	0.773	0.608	0.647	0.593	0.689
	GSHL	COS	0.684	0.851	0.684	0.733	0.792	0.694	0.703	0.734
		JS	0.803	0.789	0.703	0.857	0.746	0.742	0.783	0.775
8	LSHL	COS	0.724	0.778	0.684	0.816	0.685	0.73	0.769	0.741
		JS	**0.875**	0.685	0.644	0.776	0.649	0.706	**0.576**	0.702
	GSHL	COS	0.71	**0.866**	0.737	0.787	0.792	0.681	0.683	0.751
		JS	0.816	0.764	0.697	0.833	0.731	0.723	0.767	0.762
9	LSHL	COS	0.724	0.736	0.671	0.789	0.685	0.73	0.776	0.73
		JS	0.859	0.712	0.603	0.806	0.608	0.691	**0.55**	0.69
	GSHL	COS	0.71	**0.866**	0.763	0.829	0.792	0.792	0.646	0.771
		JS	0.803	0.736	0.697	0.848	0.716	0.723	0.783	0.758
10	LSHL	COS	0.724	0.75	0.697	0.803	0.658	0.73	0.761	0.732
		JS	0.828	0.698	0.616	0.806	**0.568**	0.643	**0.55**	0.673
	GSHL	COS	0.789	0.836	0.75	0.803	0.75	0.806	0.785	0.788
		JS	0.803	0.722	0.716	0.848	0.735	0.754	0.78	0.765
Averge			0.767	0.758	0.689	0.796	0.709	0.721	0.715	-

ments by the algorithms. The results are marked as true, only if all domain experts give positive confirmation of the result, otherwise the statement is regarded as false. The difference with the precision measure used in Information Retrieval is that ranking of results does not need to be taken into account. For this reason, ad-hoc measures such as precision at n and average precision which are widely used to measure the ranking of relevant results are not used.

The F1 measure is defined as a harmonic mean of recall and precision to balance effects of both, same as the one used in information retrieval.

$$F1 = \frac{2 * R * P}{R + P}$$

EVALUATION OF RESULTS FOR "BROADER" RELATIONS

Seven LDA models are trained using different number of latent classes (i.e., 30, 40, 50, 60, 70, 80, and 90). For each model, ontologies are learned using different maximum number of sub-nodes (i.e., from 5 to 10). The two algorithms LSHL and GSHL are tested with Cosine similarity and JS divergence measures respectively (details of the LSHL algorithm can be found in (Wang et al., 2009)). The precision values for all ontological statements learned are shown in Table 1.

In our previous work, ontologies learned based on the pLSA and LDA models have been compared in terms of recall, precision, and F1 (Wang et al., 2009). The results show that the highest precision measure of pLSA is 81.1% for the "broader" relation, and the lowest precision is about 31.5%. Precision with LDA has the highest value (87.5%) when 30 clasess are used in training, the lowest precision is about 55% when 90 classes are used in training. Overall precision measure of ontologies learned using the LDA model is higher than those learned using the pLSA model. Another finding is that structure and precision measure of the ontologies learned using LDA are not affected as significantly as using pLSA when number of training classes are changed.

The performance difference between the two probabilistic topic models probably attributes to the difference of their capability of generalising to new documents. In a sense, the pLSA is incomplete because it does not provide probabilistic modelling at the document level. New documents are assumed to have similar semantic structures as the training documents, which is not always true in many situations, resulting in poor topic modelling for those new documents. In contrast, LDA is a well defined probabilistic model and generalises easily to previously unseen documents.

EVALUATION OF RESULTS FOR "RELATED" RELATIONS

The establishment of "broader" relations among concepts forms a concept hierarchy, which can be seen as the "back bone" of a terminological ontology. The presence of "related" relation interconnect concepts on same or different levels, forming a graph structure. In fact, research (especially in computer science) in one area (i.e., Semantic Web) often utilises techniques from others, such as artificial neural network borrows ideas from biological science, and computational linguistics emerges from joint research of computer science and natural language processing. Intuitively, concepts are also interconnected with and often dependent on each other. A terminological ontology is able to reflect the interaction and model the hierarchical information in a more complete manner than a typical concept or topic hierarchy.

The "related" relation defined in the SKOS model is an ambiguous term which is not formally defined. In our method, we interpreted the "related" relation as being hold between two concepts if the similarity condition in Definition holds while the divergence difference condition does not. The idea is that related concepts tend to have certain amount of similarity (for example, two concepts are mentioned in a similar context), even if the "subsumption" relation can not be established between them.

Statements of "related" relation between concepts are only generated by the GSHL algorithm because the LSHL algorithm does not perform a "global" similarity search. In the GSHL algorithm, if a concept is more similar to its current parent node's sibling, the "subsumption" relation between the concept and its parent is substituted with a "related" relation. The evaluation of "related" relation is similar to the evaluation of the "broader" relation. As expected, the GSHL algorithm combined with Cosine measure performs better in most of the cases and the highest precision is about 90%.

EFFECT OF NUMBER OF SUB-NODES

Another important parameter in ontology learning algorithms is the maximum number of sub-nodes, which is used to predict the possible number of concepts that a concept subsumes (in our experiment, we set the parameter values from 5 to 10).

In particular, we would like to assess the effect of the parameter on the precision of statements as well as the number of same statements across ontologies. The evaluation shows that precision measure with the LDA model is not sensitive to variation of this parameter (as shown in the Table 1 the precision difference is less than 5%). Further, the ontological statements generated using different maximum number of sub-nodes vary slightly. In the learned ontologies, there are many cases where one concept is only more general than exactly one other concept. This overcomes the problem in (Zavitsanos et al., 2007) in which one concept has to subsums at least two other concepts, if there are any.

DISCUSSION AND FUTURE WORK

Learning of concept hierarchy or terminological ontology is in fact a process of automated knowledge acquisition in which the main task is to extract concepts and then connect concepts using specified relations. The current work provides an alternative method for learning two ontology relations, "broader" and "related" as specified in the SKOS ontology model. It is based on a well defined probabilistic model for analysing and exploring intrinsic relations between words and documents.

The first step in learning relations is to provide a reasonable measure that specifies conditions based on which a relation can be established. We propose such an assumption inspired by the information theory, calling it "Information Theory Principle for Concept Relationship". The principle stipulates that two conditions, the similarity condition and divergence difference condition, must be satisfied in order to establish a "broader" relation between any two concepts. The principle borrows ideas from the information theory and specifies a quantitative measure in terms of Kullback-Leibler divergence. Another feature that distinguishes our work from existing work is that our method is able to learn a terminological ontology instead of traditional concept hierarchies.

The extracted concepts are represented using documents which are then folded into the learned LDA models using the Gibbs sampling algorithm. Based on the concept relationship principle and the trained LDA models, the ontology learning algorithm is then used to connect concepts with "broader" and "related" relations. An extensive evaluation using recall, precision, and F1 measures has been performed by domain experts. The results show that overall accuracy of the learned ontology statements is above 70%. In the best situations, the precision is around 85%. The learned ontology statements in terms of "broader" and "related" relations are stable when parameter values are changed, such as the maximum number of sub-nodes of a concept.

The proposed approach is not dependent on any specific domains since the underlying LDA model is also domain-independent. The evaluation shows that it has achieved encouraging results with a dataset constructed from documents related to the Semantic Web research area. The future work will involve applying the method into other domains such as medical research, where terminological ontologies also have important applications. The current implementation of the method utilises a simple approach for extracting concepts from user annotated keywords in the corpus. Other methods such as information extraction (Cunningham, 2005) or machine learning based methods for identifying key phrases proposed in (Frank, Paynter, Witten, Gutwin, & Nevill-Manning, 1999) can be used to improve concept extraction from full text. This will not only increases the number of concepts that can be extracted, but also will help producing better concept representation.

REFERENCES

Andrieu, C., de Freitas, N., Doucet, A., & Jordan, M. I. (2003). An introduction to mcmc for machine learning. *Machine Learning, 50*(1-2), 5–43. doi:10.1023/A:1020281327116

Baeza-Yates, R. A., & Ribeiro-Neto, B. A. (1999). *Modern information retrieval*. ACM Press / Addison-Wesley.

Berners-Lee, T., Hendler, J., & Lassila, O. (2001). The Semantic Web. *Scientific American, 284*(5). doi:10.1038/scientificamerican0501-34

Berry, M. W., Dumais, S. T., & O'Brien, G. W. (1995). Using linear algebra for intelligent information retrieval. *SIAM Review, 37*, 573–595. doi:10.1137/1037127

Biemann, C. (2005). Ontology learning from text: A survey of methods. *LDV Forum, 20*(2), 75–93.

Blei, D. M., Ng, A. Y., & Jordan, M. I. (2003). Latent dirichlet allocation. *Journal of Machine Learning Research, 3*, 993–1022. doi:10.1162/jmlr.2003.3.4-5.993

Brin, S., & Page, L. (1998). The anatomy of a large-scale hypertextual Web search engine. *Computer Networks and ISDN Systems, 30*(1–7), 107–117.

Cimiano, P. (2006). *Ontology learning and population from text: Algorithms, evaluation and applications*. Secaucus, NJ: Springer-Verlag New York, Inc.

Cimiano, P., Pivk, A., Schmidt-Thieme, L., & Staab, S. (2005). Learning taxonomic relations from heterogeneous sources of evidence. In *Ontology learning from text: Methods, evaluation and applications* (pp. 59–73). IOS Press.

Cimiano, P., & Staab, S. (2004). Learning by Googling. *SIGKDD Explorations, 6*(2), 24–33. doi:10.1145/1046456.1046460

Cimiano, P., & Völker, J. (2005). Text2onto. In *Natural language processing and information systems* (pp. 227-238).

Cunningham, H. (2005). *Information extraction, automatic* (2nd ed.). Encyclopedia of Language and Linguistics.

D'Agostini, G. (2003). Bayesian inference in processing experimental data: Principles and basic applications. *Reports on Progress in Physics, 66*(9), 1383–1419. doi:10.1088/0034-4885/66/9/201

Deerwester, S. C., Dumais, S. T., Landauer, T. K., Furnas, G. W., & Harshman, R. A. (1990). Indexing by latent semantic analysis. *JASIS, 41*(6), 391–407. doi:10.1002/(SICI)1097-4571(199009)41:6<391::AID-ASI1>3.0.CO;2-9

Diederich, J., & Balke, W. T. (2007). The semantic growbag algorithm: Automatically deriving categorization systems. In *European Conference on research and advanced technology for digital libraries* (pp. 1-13).

Frank, E., Paynter, G. W., Witten, I. H., Gutwin, C., & Nevill-Manning, C. G. (1999). Domain-specific keyphrase extraction. In *IJCAI* (p. 668-673). Morgan Kaufmann.

Griffiths, T. (2002). *Gibbs sampling in the generative model of latent dirichlet allocation. (Tech. Rep.)*. Stanford University.

Griffiths, T., & Steyvers, M. (2002). A probabilistic approach to semantic representation. In *Proceedings of the 24th annual Conference of the cognitive science society.*

Griffiths, T. L., & Steyvers, M. (2004, April). Finding scientific topics. *Proceedings of the National Academy of Sciences of the United States of America, 101*(1), 5228–5235. doi:10.1073/pnas.0307752101

Gruber, T. R. (2003). A translation approach to portable ontology specifications. *Knowledge Acquisition, 5*(2), 199–220. doi:10.1006/knac.1993.1008

Harris, Z. (1968). *Mathematical structures of language*. Wiley.

Hearst, M. A. (1992). *Automatic acquisition of hyponyms from large text corpora*. In International Conference on computational linguistics (pp. 539-545).

Hofmann, T. (1999a). Probabilistic latent semantic analysis. In *Proceedings of uncertainity in artificial intelligence* (pp. 289-296).

Hofmann, T. (1999b). Probabilistic latent semantic indexing. In *Annual ACM SIGIR Conference* (pp. 50-57).

Hofmann, T. (2001). Unsupervised learning by probabilistic latent semantic analysis. *Machine Learning, 42*(1/2), 177–196. doi:10.1023/A:1007617005950

Itti, L., & Baldi, P. (2006). Bayesian surprise attracts human attention. [Cambridge, MA: MIT Press.]. *Advances in Neural Information Processing Systems, 19*, 547–554.

Kiryakov, A., Popov, B., Terziev, I., Manov, D., & Ognyanoff, D. (2004). Semantic annotation, indexing, and retrieval. *Journal of Web Semantics, 2*(1), 49–79. doi:10.1016/j.websem.2004.07.005

Lemaire, B., & Denhière, G. (2006). Effects of high-order co-occurrences on word semantic similarities. *Current Psychology Letters, 18*(1).

MacKay, D. J. (2003). *Information theory, inference, and learning algorithms*. Cambridge University Press.

Maedche, A., Pekar, V., & Staab, S. (2002). Ontology learning part one - on discovering taxonomic relations from the Web. *Web Intelligence*, 301–322.

Manning, C. D., Raghavan, P., & Schôtze, H. (2008). *Introduction to information retrieval*. Cambridge University Press.

Sanderson, M., & Croft, W. B. (1999). *Deriving concept hierarchies from text* (pp. 206–213). In SIGIR.

Steyvers, M., & Griffiths, T. (2005). Probabilistic topic models. In T. Landauer, D. Mcnamara, S. Dennis, & W. Kintsch (Eds.), *Latent semantic analysis: A road to meaning*. Laurence Erlbaum.

Wang, W., Barnaghi, P., & Bargiela, A. (2009). Probabilistic topic models for learning terminological ontologies. *IEEE Transactions on Knowledge and Data Engineering*, 99.

Zavitsanos, E., Paliouras, G., Vouros, G. A., & Petridis, S. (2007). Discovering subsumption hierarchies of ontology concepts from text corpora. In *Wi '07: Proceedings of the IEEE/WIC/ACM International Conference on Web intelligence* (pp. 402–408). Washington, DC: IEEE Computer Society.

KEY TERMS AND DEFINITIONS

Ontology Learning: is the task to build ontologies from scratch, enriching adapting an existing ontology in (semi)automatic fashion using information from different sources.

Terminological Ontologies: is an ontology whose categories need not be fully specified by axioms and definitions.

SKOS: is an area of work developing specifications and standards to support the use of knowledge organization systems such as thesauri, classification schemes, subject heading lists and taxonomies within the framework of the Semantic Web.

Semantic Web: describes methods and technologies to allow machines to interpret meaning or "semantics" of data on the World Wide Web. According to Tim Berners-Lee (Berners-Lee et al., 2001), the Semantic Web is not a separate Web but an extension of the current one, in which information is given well-defined meaning, better enabling computers and people to work in cooperation.

Probabilistic Topic Model: are models based on Bayesian inference for various applications, in particular, document modelling.

Latent Dirichlet Allocation: is a statistical generative model for analysing latent topics in documents.

Information Theory Principle for Concept Relationship: is a principle for establishing relations, in particular, SKOS relations, for the purpose of learning terminological ontologies.

Gibbs Sampling: is an algorithm to generate a sequence of samples from the joint probability distribution of two or more random variables.

ENDNOTES

[1] http://www.w3.org/TR/skos-primer/

[2] http://www.jfsowa.com/ontology/gloss.htm

[3] In Semantic Web terminology "broader" and "narrower" relations are said to be inverse properties with each other.

[4] http://www.acm.org/class/1998/

[5] http://www.nlm.nih.gov/mesh/

[6] In Cimiano's publication (Cimiano, 2006), the word "concept" is used to denote "class", where "term" denotes instance. In a traditional concept hierarchy, no explicit distinctiveness has been made between "class" and "instance".

[7] High-order co-occurrence is often used to analyse strong associations between words even though they do not co-occur in the same documents (Lemaire & Denhière, 2006).

[8] http://dblp.l3s.de/

[9] These parameters are derived from the parameters specified in the generative process using the Bayes' rule. Derivation of equations on parameter estimation in pLSA can be found in (Hofmann, 2001).

[10] In Gibbs samplers, it is difficult to determine when the chain approaches stationarity. In practice, one often discards an initial set of samples (e.g., 1000) to avoid starting biases (Andrieu et al., 2003).

[11] A document constructed from words in the vicinity of the concept is a better representation for that concept. In a sense, the document is able to explain the concept and can be viewed as a collection of context in which the concept is mentioned. This in fact coincides with Harris' "distributional hypothesis" assumption.

[12] http://portal.acm.org

[13] http://sourceforge.net/projects/nekohtml

[14] http://nlp.stanford.edu/software/tagger.shtml

[15] http://tartarus.org/:$\sim$:>>martin/Porter-Stemmer/

[16] http://lucene.apache.org/

[17] http://alias-i.com/lingpipe/

[18] If the LDA model learning uses variational inference algorithms as proposed in the original LDA paper (Blei et al., 2003), one can condition on the distributions over words for the topics and run the variational algorithm to infer the distribution over topics for the query.

[19] The documents representing the concepts are not the original documents used in the LDA training; thus they are treated as new documents and folded-in to the trained LDA models.

[20] Due to the large number of concepts and concept relations, it is not possible to provide visualisation of the whole ontology.

[21] http://protege.stanford.edu/

Section 2
Applications of Ontologies and Knowledge Bases

Chapter 8
Incorporating Correlations among Gene Ontology Terms into Predicting Protein Functions

Pingzhao Hu
York University & University of Toronto, Canada

Hui Jiang
York University, Canada

Andrew Emili
University of Toronto, Canada

ABSTRACT

One of the key issues in the post-genomic era is to assign functions to uncharacterized proteins. Since proteins seldom act alone, but rather interact with other biomolecular units to execute their functions, the functions of unknown proteins may be discovered through studying their associations with proteins having known functions.

In this chapter, the authors discuss possible approaches to exploit protein interaction networks for automated prediction of protein functions. The major focus is on discussing the utilities and limitations of current algorithms and computational techniques for accurate computational function prediction. The chapter highlights the challenges faced in this task and explores how similarity information among different gene ontology (GO) annotation terms can be taken into account to enhance function prediction.

The authors describe a new strategy that has better prediction performance than previous methods, which gives additional insights about the importance of the dependence between functional terms when inferring protein function.

DOI: 10.4018/978-1-60960-625-1.ch008

INTRODUCTION

Currently the sequencing of many genomes has brought to light the discovery of thousands of putative open reading frames which are all potentially transcribed and translated into protein products. For many of these proteins, little is known beyond their primary sequences, and for the typical proteome, between one-third and one-half of all proteins remains functionally uncharacterized. For example, despite being the most highly studied model bacterium, a comprehensive community annotation effort indicated that only half (~54%) of the protein-coding gene products of *E. coli* currently have experimental evidence indicative of a biological role (Riley, 2006). The remaining genes have either only generic (homology-derived) functional attributes (e.g. 'predicted DNA-binding') or no discernable physiological role. Some of these functional 'orphans' may have eluded characterization because they lack obvious mutant phenotypes, are expressed at low or undetectable levels, or have no obvious homology to annotated proteins. Moreover, since proteins often perform different roles in alternate biological contexts, due to the complexity of biological systems, many functions of these alternate functions may not have yet been discovered. As a result, a major challenge in modern biology is to develop efficient methods for determining protein function at the genomic scale (Eisenberg, 2000; Brun, 2003; Barabasi, 2004; Chen 2006; Hu, 2009a).

Given the slow, laborious and expensive nature of experimenttation, computational procedures to systematically predict the functions of uncharacterized proteins from their molecular relationships are increasingly seen to be useful (Vazquez, 2003; Zhou, 2005; Zhao, 2007 and 2008; Hu, 2009a). The most handy and well-known computational method for function prediction is based on the detection of significant sequence similarity to gene products of known function, using such basic bioinformatic software tools as BLAST (Basic Local Alignment Search Tool) (Altschul, 1997).

The assumption is that proteins that are similar in sequence likely have similar biological properties. A major caveat with this simplistic approach is that only those functions are obviously and directly tied to sequence, such as enzymatic activity, can be predicted accurately.

However, proteins seldom act alone, but rather interact with other biomolecular units to execute their biological functions. For example, physical interactions operate at almost every level of cellular functions (Chien, 1991; Jansen, 2003; Wodak, 2004). Thus, implications about function can often be made via the study of such molecular interactions. These inferences are based on the premise that the function(s) of unknown proteins may be gleaned from their interaction partners having a known function. In fact, it has been postulated that protein function and the higher-level organization of proteins into biological pathways can be reliably deduced by studying protein interaction networks generated via proteomic, genomic and bioinformatic approaches, providing insights into the molecular mechanisms underlying biological processes (Huynen, 2000; Gavin, 2002 and 2006; Jansen, 2003; Asthana, 2004; Altaf-Ul-Amin, 2006; Chua, 2007; Hu, 2009a). Systematic functional predictions based on computational integration of high-throughput interaction datasets have gained popularity among computational biologists for investigating gene action in model organisms such as yeast (Chen, 2004) and prokaryote such as *E. coli* (Hu, 2009a). For example, a recent integrative analysis of large-scale phenotypic, phylogenetic and physical interaction data in bacteria revealed an evolutionarily conserved set of novel motility-related proteins (Rajagopala, 2007).

In this chapter, we introduce some state-of-the-art computational procedures that allow for the automated prediction of protein functions based on the analysis of the patterns of functional associations of both known and unannotated proteins in the context of interaction networks. We discuss the potential and caveats of existing algorithms for accurate function prediction and describe new approaches incorporating the correlations among gene ontology annotation terms to improve the performance of function prediction procedures. We also highlight outstanding challenges that must be overcome to increase the impact of such predictions.

BACKGROUND

Generation of Protein Interaction Networks and Their Integration

It has been a long practice to determine protein interaction networks (PINs) using experimental and computational tools in biological systems (Jansen, 2003; Gavin, 2002 and 2006; Krogan, 2006; Chen, 2008; Hu, 2009a). From an experimental view, traditionally, protein interactions (PIs) have typically been examined by intensive small-scale experiments on a small set of proteins of interest. Recently, it has become more and more popular to generate PIs using high-throughput techniques such as the yeast two-hybrid (Y2H) assay (Ito, 2001) and tandem affinity purification-tagging (TAP) (Krogan, 2006; Hu, 2009a). These strategies have been applied in many genome-wide studies. For example, genome-wide Y2H studies have been conducted in S. cerevisiae (Ito, 2001) and flies (Giot, 2003), while TAP coupled with mass spectrometry has also been used in S. cerevisiae (Gavin, 2002 and 2006). However, coverage of protein interaction data made by the experiments is still quite limited. Moreover, large data sets generated from by high-throughput studies, are not completely reliable, and data quality varies greatly from one data set to another (Bader, 2004).

High confidence PIs generated using experimental methods currently cover only a fraction of the complete PINs (Han, 2005). For example, although it has been estimated that the complete set of interactions in the yeast S. cerevisiae varies from 37,800 to 75,500 interactions, where a protein has on average 5 to 10 interacting

partners (Hart, 2006). Currently, the number of experimentally detected interacting components found in stable protein complexes is about 14,300 despite recent exhaustive experiments (Krogan, 2006; Yu, 2008) suggesting current maps are far from complete. Therefore, computational methods for the prediction of PIs have become popular (Wodak, 2004; Myers, 2007; Hu, 2009). For example, PIs were predicted based on genomic sequence comparisons by analyzing amino acid sequences between known interacting proteins (Bock, 2001; Chou 2006; Shen, 2007) and their phylogenetic profiles by accounting for patterns of presence or absence of a given protein in a set of genomes (Hu, 2009a). The prediction of functional relationships between two proteins according to the order and adjacency in the chromosomal location of the corresponding genes is widely used in bacteria (Hu, 2009a). Another major source of functional information is potentially buried in the thousands of genome-scale mRNA profiles in the Gene Expression Omnibus (GEO). Tissue and organelle protein expression profiles are potentially useful for functional inference (Kislinger, 2006). It has been shown that gene products that have similar expression patterns often participate in the same biological process (Segal, 2004) and that the corresponding proteins have a higher likelihood of physically associated (Jansen, 2003). Co-expression is not sufficient, however, for reliable function prediction since many genes involved in multiple cellular processes may be expressed at the same time, but is still informative, especially when combined with other data types, like molecular interaction networks. Table 1 lists publicly accessible resources useful for inferring functional associations, which serve as the basis for the systematic predictions using computational procedures.

Therefore, in order to improve accuracy and coverage of molecular interaction networks, it is necessary to combine information from multiple data sources, which can help uncover proteins that are represented with different types of inter-

Table 1. Publicly available data sources to examine gene product function

Name	Data Type	URL	Source / Reference
GO (Gene Ontology)	Gold-standard	www.geneontology.org	Ashburner, 2000
MIPS (Munich Information Center for Protein Sequence)	Gold-standard & Interaction	http://mips.gsf.de	Mewes, 2002
Gene Map Annotator and Pathway Profiler (GenMAPP)	Gold-standard & Interaction	www.genmapp.org	Dahlquist, 2002
Kyoto Encyclopedia of Genes and Genomes(KEGG)	Gold-standard & Interaction	www.genome.jp/kegg	Kanehisa, 2004
BioCarta	Gold-standard & Interaction	www.biocarta.com	---
SwissProt	Gold-standard & Interaction	www.expasy.org/uniprot/	Boeckmann, 2003
BIND	Interaction	www.bind.ca/Action	Bader, 2003
IntAct	Interaction	www.ebi.ac.uk/intact/site/	Hermjakob, 2004
HPRD	Interaction	www.hprd.org/	Peri, 2003
DIP	Interaction	http://dip.doe-mbi.ucla.edu/	Xenarios, 2002
MINT	Interaction	http://mint.bio.uniroma2.it/mint/	Zanzoni, 2002
Stanford Microarray Database (SMD)	Gene Expression Profiling	http://genome-www5.stanford.edu	Stanford University
Gene Expression Omnibus (GEO)	Gene Expression Profiling	www.ncbi.nlm.nih.gov/geo	National Center for Biotechnology Information, NIH

actions thereby providing a more comprehensive view on their cellular relationships. For example, Han (2004) demonstrated that interacting gene pairs predicted from multiple data sources are more likely to share the same GO functional categories, indicating improved predictive power through data integration. Jansen (2003) and Hu (2009a) showed that integration of the physical interactions and functional interactions generated by genomic context methods can likewise improve protein function predictions.

It has been a long practice to develop different approaches to incorporate various genomic data sources for improving protein interaction network prediction (Tanay, 2004). For example, Troyanskaya (2003) developed Bayesian network based method to incorporate knowledge from multiple data sources by taking into account their relative likelihood to predict if two proteins are function-

ally interacted. They estimated the posterior probability that each pair of proteins u and v has a functional relationship, given different genome-wide data sources. The approach outputs a functional association network in which reliability score (probability) is assigned to each edge between two proteins representing their functional similarity. von Mering (2003) assumed the reliabilities of the functional associations generated by different experimental and computational sources are independent. Therefore, an integrated weight score w_{uv} for a functional association between protein u and protein v can be defined as

$$w_{uv} = 1 - \prod_{r=1}^{t} \left(1 - w_{uv}^r\right) \tag{1}$$

where w_{uv}^r ($0 \leq w_{uv} \leq 1$) is the estimated weight score of the interaction between protein u and protein v in data source r, and t is the number of data sources the interaction was found. The method treats each w_{uv} as a probability. Similar methods have been used by other groups to integrate different functional association evidences (Nabieva, 2005; Chua, 2006 and 2007; Hu, 2009a).

Ben-Hur (2005) reported kernel based methods to integrate different data sources. They represented each data source using a kernel matrix, which essentially measures similarity between pairs of proteins. Different kernel functions have been designed for different data sources. Once specific kernel functions are constructed for different genomic data sources, there are different ways to integrate the kernel matrixes generated from different kernel functions. The simplest approach is to use the sum of the different kernels, which is equivalent to take the average kernel. However, not all data have equal quality. Some weighted sum approaches have been used to combine all the kernel matrices in a linear form (Lanchriet, 2004), in which the coefficients are estimated using a semidefinite program (SDP) approach. Tsuda (2005) developed a similar kernel method to integrate different PINs where the coefficients are estimated using convex optimization.

Gene Ontology as a Unifying Functional Annotation Schema

Biological functions must be clearly defined in order to set the stage for computational prediction (Hu, 2007). Yet protein function has many facets, reflecting the diversity of cellular activities and biochemical properties, ranging from the basic attributes of a protein product (such as an enzyme, like a protein kinase), to the nature of physical and regulatory interactions (such as protein-protein interactions), to membership in a given pathway (such as a signaling cascade). Explicitly defining these functions in a concise manner is difficult, as the functional terms must reflect the complex multi-faceted networks of proteins that often interact dynamically across a wide range of spatial and temporal scales, ranging from subcellular compartments to entire tissues systems or a whole organism. Therefore, when speaking of a protein function, one must always specify the relevant aspect (s) of the functional description under scrutiny. When setting out to use a function prediction tool, let alone to develop a new one, one must keep in mind which functional aspect(s) one is trying to predict, and use the appropriate vocabulary.

Many annotation schemas for the representation of gene product function have been devised, of which several prominent examples are listed in Table 1 (labeled as "Gold-standard"). The most widely adopted system is the gene ontology (GO) database (Ashburner, 2000), which uses a clearly defined, and computationally friendly, vocabulary for representing the cellular, biochemical and physiological roles of gene products in a systematic manner. From the perspective of functional computation, GO provides a standardized way to assess whether a set of proteins have similar functions, which has led to its increasing popularity for the many function prediction procedures used in model organism settings (Jansen, 2004). GO terms are organized in a tree-like structure, starting from most general (e.g. biological process) at the root to the most specific at the leaves (e.g. regulation of DNA recombination) distributed across three major semantic domains – molecular function, biological process, and cellular location. Since terms may have more than one parent, they are technically structured as a network called a directed acyclic graph (Figure 1). For instance, "Translation (GO: 0006412)" represents a sub-type of both the term "Cellular Biopolymer Biosynthetic Process (GO: 0034961)" and "Cellular Protein Metabolic Process (GO: 0044267)". Hence, functional classes are not necessarily independent of one another, and the dependencies are explicitly defined. Additionally, GO allows for a single gene product to be associated with more than one functional term during the curation process rather than being restricted to a single functional class. As discussed below, though, this flexibility for allowing multiple-label classifications has not yet been fully exploited by computational prediction methods.

In general, GO provides for a computationally accessible, organism-independent means for examining and reporting gene function (Ashburner, 2000). While expert curators manually assign terms based on published experimental evidence, most terms are electronically inferred based on sequence similarity to other well-studied gene products or other criteria. Each term is assigned an evidence code (www.geneontology.org/GO.evidence.shtml) (not shown in the diagram in Figure 1) stating how the annotation is supported, which allows one to assess the annotation reliability. If the annotation is based on experimental evidence traceable to an author or publication, it is presumably more reliable than if it was simply inferred through sequence similarity. The

GO has over ten such evidence codes, which are not part of the core ontology.

A shortcoming of the natural language-based representations, like the GO, is that complex biological functions and relationships, such as regulatory relationships like signaling cascades, cannot be finely tuned to reflect their true biological complexity. Many of the existing GO annotations for gene products have been made using very high-level (i.e. general) terms, which limit their usefulness.

Measure Semantic Similarity of Function Terms in Gene Ontology

Different methods have been developed to determine the similarity of two GO terms based on their distances to the closest common ancestor term and/or the annotation statistics of their common ancestor terms (Resnik, 1999; Lord, 2003; Lin, 2008). These measures evaluate the similarity

Figure 1. Example of GO hierarchy representing as a directed acyclic graph

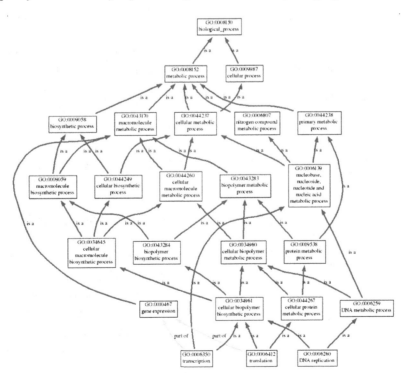

of two GO terms in terms of their proximity in the ontology, as well as their content. There are some drawbacks in these GO semantic similarity measurement methods. For example, Resnik method only considers information content of a functional term derived from the corpus statistics while the location of a GO term in GO graph is usually ignored. Wang (2008) recently proposed a novel method to encode a GO term's semantics (biological meanings) into a numeric value by aggregating the semantic contributions of their ancestor terms (including this specific term) in the GO graph (Figure 1). Here we detail the algorithm to measure the semantic similarity of GO terms as follows:

Assume that there are two GO terms: l_i and l_k, which are represented as two directed acyclic graphs (DAGs):

$$DAG_{l_i} = (l_i, Q_{l_i}, E_{l_i}) \text{ and } DAG_{l_k} = (l_k, Q_{l_k}, E_{l_k}),$$

respectively, where Q_{l_i} (Q_{l_k}) is the set of GO terms in DAG_{l_i} (DAG_{l_k}), including term l_i (l_k) and all of its ancestor terms in the GO graphs, and E_{l_i} (E_{l_k}) is the set of edges (semantic relations) connecting the GO terms in DAG_{l_i} (DAG_{l_k}). The semantic similarity between GO terms l_i and l_k is defined as

$$C(l_i, l_k) = \frac{\sum_{q \in Q_{l_i} \cap Q_{l_k}} (S_{l_i}(q) + S_{l_k}(q))}{SV(l_i) + SV(l_k)} \quad (2)$$

where $SV(l_i) = \sum_{q \in Q_{l_i}} S_{l_i}(q)$ and $S_{l_i}(q)$ is the similarity score of GO functional term q associated to term l_i. Here $S_{l_i}(q)$ is defined as:

$$\begin{cases} S_{l_i}(l_i) = 1 \\ S_{l_i}(q) = \max\{r_e * S_{l_i}(q') \mid q' \in childrenof(q)\} \text{ if } q \neq l_i \end{cases} \quad (3)$$

where $0 < r_e < 1$ measures the contribution of edge $e \in E_{l_i}$ linking term q with its child term q'. $SV(l_k)$ and $S_{l_k}(q)$ are defined in the same ways as $SV(l_i)$ and $S_{l_i}(q)$, respectively.

CHALLENGES IN NETWORK-BASED PROTEIN FUNCTION PREDICTION

Despite the utility of existing GO and PIN databases, several troublesome issues make it difficult to apply computational methods to annotate proteins in a practical, effective and comprehensive manner. Two, in particular, stand out and are described below.

The first one is related to the choice of gold-standards. The suitability of a high quality reference protein set for stringently assessing functional predictions is determined by two factors: (i) the projected coverage or overlap relative to the target proteins under consideration, which should ideally be large enough to offer a statistically reliable evaluation using the available interaction data; (ii) the resolution or specificity of the annotations, which must be consistent with the functional categories or resolution that one wishes to draw. For example, the fact that two proteins co-localize to the inner mitochondrial membrane supports the possibility of a functional interaction, but the association is too general to draw a detailed functional inference.

Currently, there is an obvious functional bias in the current GO database (Myers, 2006). Some biological processes have been studied in greater depth experimentally than others, thus generating more data. Proteins associated with these processes are far more likely to be correctly detected by computational prediction.

The second one is a computational issue that is related to the fact that individual genes may perform multiple functions (that is, are pleiotropic) during the various stages of biological processes

(Mateos, 2002; Ravasz, 2002; Palla, 2005). This property poses a challenge by re-setting functional prediction into a multi-class classification problem, wherein the classes (i.e. functions) are mutually-exclusive by definition; that is, each case (i.e. gene product) can be assigned to only one of two or more alternate classes at a given time. Gene products with multiple functions cause the actual functional classes to overlap by definition, yielding multiple labels as well as multiple classes, even for the reference gold standard annotations. To compound matters, it is unlikely that all of the relevant functions and pleiotropic overlap have been equally well explored by experimentalists.

Previous studies predicting gene function on a genome-wide basis (Letovsky, 2003; Deng, 2003; Nabieva, 2005; Murali, 2006; Massjouni, 2006) did not directly consider this multi-label predicament, and their networks only supported one functional assignment at a time. This strategy fails to capture the correlation structure linking functional classes into the prediction process. In other words, the biological functions are treated independently. For example, in 'supervised' prediction approaches, each function is learned, separately.

It has been pointed out that biological functions represented in most functional annotation schemas (e.g GO) are correlated each other and the incorporation of correlations among function categories can significantly improve the performance of function prediction (Barutcuoglu, 2006; Lee, 2006; Tao, 2007). Therefore, it would be interesting to explore more general constraint functional association networks in which the relationship between functional terms and network representation of functional association can be considered directly.

NETWORK-BASED PROTEIN FUNCTION PREDICTION

Once the functional terms used as labels are described by a system like the GO, the protein function prediction problem then becomes the task of assigning labels to all vertices in a functional association network (Figure 2). This labeled graph representation makes the function prediction problem amenable to the wealth of techniques developed in the graph theory and network analysis communities. For example, the idea of guilt-by-association, which is widely used by most approaches (Schwikowski, 2000; Vazquez, 2003; McDermott, 2005; Chua, 2006; Massjouni, 2006), turns the problem of function prediction into the problem of identifying (possibly overlapping) regions in the network that participate in the same biological process (i.e., should be assigned the same vertex label) (Rives, 2003; Hart, 2007). Broadly speaking, most of the methods used for the network-based functional annotation utilize and extend well-understood concepts from graph theory and graphical models.

In classical supervised learning methods, the prediction of protein function is usually treated as a classification problem, in which each protein is first represented by a set of features, and then learning algorithms are applied to infer the functional association relationship between the features and the biological functions. Here we relax the definition and refer supervised prediction methods to those that use functional label information in the prediction procedure. Many computational methods have been devised to automatically assign functional labels, such as GO terms, to the uncharacterized proteins in an interaction network in the 'supervised' manner according to the annotations of the broader neighborhood of interacting gene products (Schwikowski, 2000; Vazquez, 2003; Nabieva, 2005; Massjouni, 2006; Chua, 2006; Hu, 2009a; Hu, 2010). These approaches often exploit both the local and global properties of network graphs. Based on the possibility to incorporate correlations among GO terms into function prediction procedure, we classify the methods into two categories: one treats GO terms to be independent once they are selected as labels in function prediction procedure while another

Figure 2. Systematic flow of network-based function prediction

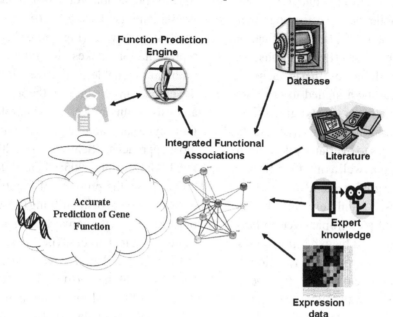

does take the correlations among hierarchically organized GO terms into account.

FUNCTION PREDICTION WITH HIERARCHICALLY INDEPENDENT GENE ONTOLOGY TERMS

Local Neighborhood Based Methods

The most straightforward method for annotating a protein v is to investigate the functions of its immediate partners in the PIN. The hypothesis is that nearest neighbors in the interaction network tend to share the same functions.

Schwikowski (2000) considered all labeled proteins in the first-neighbors n_v of a functional unknown protein v and count the number of times $(n_v(l_i))$ function l_i occurs for the protein. Functional unknown protein is annotated with the most commonly occurring functions of its interaction partners. For a weighted interaction network, the function score $F(v, l_i)$ of a given protein v with function l_i can be computed as

$$F(v, l_i) = \frac{\sum_{u \in n_v} w_{uv} *, (u, l_i)}{\sum_{u \in n_v} w_{uv}} \qquad (4)$$

where $, (u, l_i)$ is equal to 1 if protein u has functional annotation l_i, otherwise 0. w_{uv} is the weight between proteins u and v. The functional unknown protein v is then annotated with the function with the largest function score $F(v, l_i)$. A similar idea was developed by McDemott (2005), although they used a slightly different way to define denominator of the above formula as a source factor for adjusting the contribution of predicted interactions derived from public databases. In the literature, the unweighted approach is usually called the majority rule method while the weighted method is called as weighted majority rule method. These methods only use the first order neighbors of the unannotated proteins and do not take the whole topology of the network into account. Hence, it becomes problematic when the immediate neighbors of the unannotated proteins have no or only few annotations.

Hishigaki (2001) computed a chi-square statistic for function l_i in the neighbors of a functional unknown protein v as

$$F^k(v, l_i) = \frac{(n_v(l_i) - e_v(l_i))^2}{e_v(l_i)} \qquad (5)$$

where $n_v(l_i)$ is the number of times function l_i occurs for protein v in the k order neighbor (k is the network distance between two given proteins) and $e_v(l_i)$ is the expected number of times function l_i occurs for protein v in the k order neighbor. They considered both the first and second order neighbors ($k=2$). The top ranking functions $F^k(v, l_i)$ are assigned to the functional unknown protein. This approach alleviates the constraints of the (weighted) majority rule methods to some extent by taking the direct and indirect neighbors into account. However, the method treats proteins at different network distance (neighbors) to the unknown protein have the same weight and to some sense it ignores the network topology with local neighborhoods. Recent studies (Nabieva, 2005; Hu, 2009a) show the performance is even worse than that of (weighted) majority rule methods.

Letovsky (2003) developed a Markov random field (MRF) model for protein function prediction subject to a conditional independence assumption that the number of neighbors of a protein that are annotated with a given function is binomially distributed and this probability distribution for any protein (vertex) is conditionally independent of all other proteins given its neighbors. Therefore, the algorithm assigns functions to an unannotated protein only based on the functional annotations of its direct interaction parterres and the functions are considered to be independent. The algorithm starts with initializing the label (function) probabilities for unannotated proteins (vertices) to the frequency of the label and propagates frequencies iteratively. In the second iteration unlabeled proteins adjust the probabilities based on their neighbors using Bayes' rule. The algorithm stops after the second iteration to avoid self-reinforcement, and classifies the unlabeled proteins whose probability exceeds a threshold by assigning them the current label.

Chua (2006) explored the relationship between functional similarity and network distance from first and second-order neighbors to unannotated proteins, respectively. They found besides the strong functional relationship between first-order neighbors and the unannotated proteins, this functional relationship is also observable between second-order neighbors. Therefore, they developed a method to measure the functional similarity by taking both the first and second –order neighbors of the protein pairs into account. The likelihood of each function assigned to a given protein is scored based on the weighted frequency to the proteins in the first and second-order neighbors according to the local topology of the interaction network. Comparing with other methods (Schwikowski, 2000; Hishigaki, 2001; Nabieva, 2005), they showed their method has better prediction performance. Our group (Hu, 2009a) further developed the above approaches. They first defined functional profiles for each function based on the first and second-order neighbors of functional unknown proteins, respectively; then they modeled the functional profiles using a probability-based method with a step-wise procedure applied to select correlated functional profiles. A probability is assigned to un-annotated proteins for a given function in the network for predicting their functions. These approaches take function similarity of protein pairs into account, but they do not directly use the correlation among GO terms of the protein pairs into function prediction procedure.

Global Optimization Approaches

The major shortcoming in the neighborhood-based methods is that they do not take the global topology of the whole interaction network into account. Moreover, in very sparse PINs, it can be expected that the neighborhood methods will not work well since the neighbors (either first or second neighbors) of the unannotated proteins usually have no or only few annotations.

To tackle these problems, Vazquez (2003) determined globally optimal functional assignments to all uncharacterized proteins in the network so that the number of the same annotations associating with its neighbors is maximized.

Deng (2003) further explored the idea of Letovsky (2003) by considering the frequency of proteins having the function of interest with less weight placed on far away neighbors in the network than on the close neighbors. Their approach considers each function separately and globally takes into account the annotations of all proteins in the interaction network. They estimated the parameters in the MRF model based on the proteins whose functions are known using a quasi-likelihood approach. Conditioned on the functional annotation of each annotated protein in the network, the posterior probability for each uncharacterized protein to have a particular functional annotation is estimated using Gibbs sampling. This approach is theoretically elegant and better performance was achieved than those neighborhood based methods.

The functional flow algorithm described by Nabieva (2005) treated each protein of known functional annotation as a source of functional flow, which is then propagated to unannotated proteins (vertices) using the weighted edges in the interaction graph. The effect of each annotated protein on any other unannotated protein decreases with an increase in distance between them. Simulating the flow for a few iterations lets the function to travel into all uncharacterized proteins (vertices). The scores correspond to the amount of flow for the function the protein has received over the course of the simulation. In contrast to the majority vote algorithm (Schwikowski, 2000), functional flow considers functional annotations from proteins that are not immediate neighbors, and thus can annotate proteins that have no neighbors with known annotations. They demonstrated that the method has better performance than neighborhood based approaches (such as Schwikowski, 2000; Letovsky, 2003)

Lee (2006) developed a kernel logistic regression (KLR) method by incorporating diffusion kernels into Deng's method (Deng, 2003). The diffusion kernel measures the similarity distance between any two proteins in the network. The authors indirectly incorporated the correlation among biological functions into their model by identifying a set of functions that are highly correlated with the function of interest using χ^2 test. The prediction accuracy is comparable to another protein function classifier based on the support vector machine (SVM) with a diffusion kernel, but the KLR has been shown to outperform the basic MFR method.

Function Prediction with Hierarchically Dependent Gene Ontology Terms

As discussed before, although function terms taken from GO are hierarchically dependent, most network-based computational procedures for function prediction only support one function assignment per uncharacterized protein at a time. Therefore, these function terms are treated to be independent. Here we explore more general computational approaches in which the relationships among function terms defined by the hierarchical structure of GO and interaction networks can be considered directly in a function prediction procedure. We focus this on two approaches we developed recently.

The first approach (Hu, 2009b) is a variant of the local neighborhood-based method defined in formula (4). We measure the inter-relationship between the function terms in GO using the method defined in formula (2), which is then incorporated in our new functional prediction framework to assign functions to uncharacterized proteins as follows:

$$F(v,l_i) = \frac{\sum_{u \in n_v} w_{uv} * C(l_i,l_j)}{\sum_{u \in n_v} w_{uv}} \qquad (6)$$

where $0 \leq C(l_i,l_j) \leq 1$. It is obvious that $C(l_i,l_j) = 1$ if the function l_i being considered for protein v and function l_j of protein u are the same. Therefore, the functional prediction framework defined in formula (4) is a special case of the functional prediction framework defined in formula (6). Under suitable transformations, the correlation measure $C(l_i,l_j)$ can be also incorporated in other local neighborhood approaches (Hishigaki, 2001; Chua, 2006, Hu, 2009a), but we will not discuss this in detail here.

The second approach (Hu, 2010) is a network relaxation labeling method to take the correlations among GO terms globally. The method can be summarized as follows: In an interaction network, let us assume that L is the set $\{l_1,...,l_m\}$ of m possible function labels (GO terms). Let $P_v(l_i)$ be the probability that the label l_i is the correct label for protein v and each probability satisfies $0 \leq P_v(l_i) \leq 1$ where $P_v(l_i) = 0$ implies that label l_i is impossible for protein v and $P_v(l_i) = 1$ implies that this labelling is certain.

The relaxation labeling process includes three steps: (1) Initialize the probability $P_v(l_i)$ of protein v for function l_i. This can be done by assigning an initial and perhaps arbitrary probability for each label and uncharacterized protein. Here, we consider all labeled proteins in the direct neighbors of a given uncharacterized protein v, and calculate the initial probability $P_v(l_i)^{(0)}$ of protein v for function l_i given by:

$$P_v(l_i)^{(o)} = \frac{\sum_{u \in n_v} w_{uv} * ,(u,l_i)}{\sum_{u \in n_v} w_{uv}} \qquad (7)$$

If protein v has no neighbors with function l_i, we estimate $P_v(l_i)^{(0)}$ based on the function's prior in GO gold standard we construct. (2) Update the probability $P_v(l_i)$ of protein v for function l_i. This is done by considering the probabilities of labels for neighboring proteins. Let us assume that we have changed all probabilities up to some step, T, and we now seek an updated probability for the next step $T+1$. We can estimate the change in confidence of $P_v(l_i)$ by:

$$\Delta P_v(l_i) = \sum_{u \in n_v} \sum_{l_j \in L} C(l_i,l_j) P_u(l_j)^{(T)} \qquad (8)$$

where $C(l_i,l_j)$ is the correlation between protein function labels defined as the conditional probability that protein v has a label l_i given that protein u has a label l_j, i.e. $C(l_i,l_j) = P(l_i|l_j)$. We estimate $C(l_i,l_j)$ based on semantic similarity between function terms in GO discussed in formula (2). The new probability $P_v(l_i)$ for label l_i in generation $T+1$ can be computed from the values from generation T using

$$P_v(l_i)^{(T+1)} = \frac{P_v(l_i)^{(T)}\left[1 + \Delta P_v(l_i)\right]}{\sum_l P_v(l_l)^{(T)}\left[1 + \Delta P_v(l_l)\right]} \qquad (9)$$

Table 2. A summary of protein function prediction approaches

Algorithms	Dependence of GO Terms	Advantages	Disadvantage	Examples
Neighborhood based	GO terms treated as independent functions	1) Simple and effective	1) Full network topology is ignored 2) Each function is predicted independently 3) Hard to assign functions if neighbor proteins have no or few annotations	Schwikowski, 2000; Chua, 2006; Hu, 2009a
	GO terms treated as dependent functions	1) Simple and effective 2) Multiple functions can be predicted simultaneously	1) Full network topology is ignored 2) Hard to assign functions if neighbor proteins have no or few annotations	Jiang, 2008; Hu, 2009b
Global based	GO terms treated as independent functions	1) Full network topology is considered 2) More suitable for poorly annotated genomes	1) Each function is predicted independently 2) Computation is more expensive	Vazquez, 2003; Nabieva, 2005; Lee, 2006
	GO terms treated as dependent functions	1) Full network topology is considered 2) More suitable for poorly annotated genomes 3) Multiple functions can be predicted simultaneously	1) Computation is more expensive	Mostafavi, 2009; Hu, 2010

(3) The process of step (2) is repeated until the labelling method converges or stabilises. This occurs when there is little or no change between successive sets of probability values.

Recommendation for Selecting Function Prediction Approaches

Table 2 summarizes the advantages and disadvantages of the major function prediction algorithms discussed in this chapter. The focus is on neighborhood and global based approaches. Overall, if a protein is interacting with many proteins with known annotation, local neighborhood-based methods usually perform well. However, when a protein is known to interact with few annotated or only unannotated proteins, local neighborhood-based methods cannot make any predictions, whereas the global based methods may work well. In this sense, the neighborhood based approaches are more suitable for predicting protein functions for well-annotated genomes while global based approaches can be used for predicting protein

functions for poorly-characterized genomes since the methods can take the full network topology into account. It is also generally recommended that methods using GO relationships be used in inferring protein functions since they showed good performance than those ignoring GO correlations.

CONCLUSION AND FUTURE DIRECTIONS

In this chapter, we discussed generation of interaction networks and protein function prediction via analyzing interaction network. The basic idea of the computational procedure is to assign function terms to previously uncharacterized proteins based on the categorical properties of their annotated interaction partners. The underlying assumption is that the closer the two proteins are in the network, the more similar their function annotations are. We discussed two widely used approaches: local and global prediction methods. They differ mainly in the way they represent and exploit this relationship. Furthermore, since function terms are often interrelated (e.g. the GO hierarchies), the correlation structure of the respective function terms can be exploited. We showed the strategies to incorporate this relationship into both local- and global- based prediction methods.

Overall, function prediction via the evaluation of interaction network is still a relatively new area. With the increasing of PINs and other types of molecular interaction networks generated by both experimental and computational techniques, these advancements promise to give network-based methods a prominence position in automatic function prediction. Therefore, some promising directions are warranted for further research in this field.

First, it has been widely known that topology-sharing proteins have similar functions or co-exist in a pathway (Barabasi, 2004; Pˇrzulj, 2004; Zhang, 2005; Han, 2005; Chua, 2006; Lubovac, 2006). This implies that relaxation labeling approaches as outlined here may benefit from integrating this information in the function prediction framework. As shown before, our relaxation labeling method includes two major steps: first, initial label assignment is made by a local classifier; second, the dependencies among GO labels are taken into accounted and propagated using an iterative relaxation procedure. The potential trade-off implies that additional error or uncertainty may have occasionally been introduced by assuming function similarity among more loosely connected proteins. Therefore, better performance may be obtained by propagating the functions of the proteins sharing similar topology structure.

Second, many approaches have been developed to measure the similarity between function terms (e.g. GO). It has been known that there is a significant function bias in the current GO database since certain biological processes have been studied in far greater depth experimentally than others. Genes associated with these processes are much more likely to be correctly detected by computational prediction procedures (Barutcuo-

glu, 2006). Therefore, it is necessary to evaluate which similarity measures between GO terms are more easily affected by this issue in our function prediction frameworks.

Finally, it would be a useful exploration to extend the function prediction frameworks described herein to other prediction contexts. For example, a basic assumption is that genes causing similar diseases should be neighbors to each other. Therefore, when attempting a network-based disease gene prediction, it is possible to more efficiently prioritize disease genes present in interaction networks by taking into account the similarity of their disease associations defined by a public disease ontology (Du, 2009; Osborne, 2009).

REFERENCES

Altaf-Ul-Amin, M., Shinbo, Y., Mihara, K., Kurokawa, K., & Kanaya, S. (2006). Development and implementation of an algorithm for detection of protein complexes in large interaction networks. *BMC Bioinformatics*, 7, 207. doi:10.1186/1471-2105-7-207

Altschul, S. F., Madden, T. L., Schäffer, A. A., Zhang, J., Zhang, Z., Miller, W., & Lipman, D. J. (1997). Gapped BLAST and PSI-BLAST: A new generation of protein database search programs. *Nucleic Acids Research*, 25(17), 3389–3402. doi:10.1093/nar/25.17.3389

Ashburner, M., Ball, C. A., Blake, J. A., Botstein, D., Butler, H., Cherry, J. M., & Davis, A. P. (2000). Gene ontology: Tool for the unification of biology. The gene ontology consortium. *Nature Genetics*, 25(1), 25–29. doi:10.1038/75556

Asthana, S., King, O. D., & Gibbons, F. D. (2004). Predicting protein complex membership using probabilistic network reliability. *Genome Research*, 14(6), 1170–1175. doi:10.1101/gr.2203804

Bader, G. D., Betel, D., & Hogue, C. W. (2003). BIND: The biomolecular interaction network database. *Nucleic Acids Research, 31*(1), 248–250. doi:10.1093/nar/gkg056

Bader, J. S., Chaudhuri, A., Rothberg, J. M., & Chant, J. (2004). Gaining confidence in high throughput protein interaction networks. *Nature Biotechnology, 22*(1), 78–85. doi:10.1038/nbt924

Barabasi, A. L., & Oltvai, Z. N. (2004). Network biology: Understanding the cell's functional organization. *Nature Reviews. Genetics, 5*(2), 101–113. doi:10.1038/nrg1272

Barutcuoglu, Z., Schapire, R. E., & Troyanskaya, O. G. (2006). Hierarchical multi-label prediction of gene function. *Bioinformatics (Oxford, England), 22*(7), 830–836. doi:10.1093/bioinformatics/btk048

Ben-Hur, A., & Noble, W. S. (2005). Kernel methods for predicting protein-protein interactions. *Bioinformatics (Oxford, England), 21*(1), i38–i46. doi:10.1093/bioinformatics/bti1016

Bock, J. R., & Gough, D. A. (2001). Predicting protein - protein interactions from primary structure. *Bioinformatics (Oxford, England), 17*(5), 455–460. doi:10.1093/bioinformatics/17.5.455

Boeckmann, B., & Bairoch, A. (2003). The SWISS-PROT protein knowledgebase and its supplement TrEMBL in 2003. *Nucleic Acids Research, 31*(1), 365–370. doi:10.1093/nar/gkg095

Brun, C., Chevenet, F., Martin, D., Wojcik, J., Guenoche, A., & Jacq, B. (2003). Functional classification of proteins for the prediction of cellular function from a protein–protein interaction network. *Genome Biology, 5*(1), R6. doi:10.1186/gb-2003-5-1-r6

Chen, J. C., & Yuan, B. (2006). Detecting functional modules in the yeast protein–protein interaction network. *Bioinformatics (Oxford, England), 22*(18), 2283–2290. doi:10.1093/bioinformatics/btl370

Chen, P. (2008). Predicting and validating protein interactions using network structure. *PLoS Computational Biology, 4*(7), e1000118. doi:10.1371/journal.pcbi.1000118

Chen, Y., & Xu, D. (2004). Global protein function annotation through mining genome-scale data in yeast Saccharomyces cerevisiae. *Nucleic Acids Research, 32*(21), 6414–6424. doi:10.1093/nar/gkh978

Chien, C., Bartel, P., Sternglanz, R., & Fields, S. (1991). The two-hybrid system: A method to identify and clone genes for proteins that interact with a protein of interest. *Proceedings of the National Academy of Sciences of the United States of America, 88*(21), 9578–9582. doi:10.1073/pnas.88.21.9578

Chou, K. C., & Cai, Y. D. (2006). Predicting protein–protein interactions from sequences in a hybridization space. *Journal of Proteome Research, 5*(2), 316–322. doi:10.1021/pr050331g

Chua, H. N., Sung, W. K., & Wong, L. (2006). Exploiting indirect neighbours and topological weight to predict protein function from protein–protein interactions. *Bioinformatics (Oxford, England), 22*(13), 1623–1630. doi:10.1093/bioinformatics/btl145

Chua, H. N., Sung, W. K., & Wong, L. (2007). An efficient strategy for extensive integration of diverse biological data for protein function prediction. *Bioinformatics (Oxford, England), 23*(24), 3364–3373. doi:10.1093/bioinformatics/btm520

Dahlquist, K. D., Salomonis, N., Vranizan, K., Lawlor, S. C., & Conklin, B. R. (2002). GenMAPP, a new tool for viewing and analyzing microarray data on biological pathways. *Nature Genetics*, *31*(1), 19–20. doi:10.1038/ng0502-19

Deng, M., Zhang, K., Mehta, S., Chen, T., & Sun, F. (2003). Prediction of protein function using protein–protein interaction data. *Journal of Computational Biology*, *10*(6), 947–960. doi:10.1089/106652703322756168

Du, P., Feng, G., Flatow, J., Song, J., Holko, M., Kibbe, W. A., & Lin, S. M. (2009). From disease ontology to disease-ontology lite: Statistical methods to adapt a general-purpose ontology for the test of gene-ontology associations. *Bioinformatics (Oxford, England)*, *25*(12), i63–i68. doi:10.1093/bioinformatics/btp193

Eisenberg, D., Marcotte, E. M., Xenarios, I., & Yeates, T. O. (2000). Protein function in the postgenomic era. *Nature*, *405*(6788), 823–826. doi:10.1038/35015694

Gavin, A. C., Aloy, P., Grandi, P., Krause, R., Boesche, M., Marzioch, M., & Rau, C. (2006). Proteome survey reveals modularity of the yeast cell machinery. *Nature*, *440*(7084), 631–636. doi:10.1038/nature04532

Gavin, A. C., Bösche, M., Krause, R., Grandi, P., Marzioch, M., Bauer, A., & Schultz, J. (2002). Functional organization of the yeast proteome by systematic analysis of protein complexes. *Nature*, *415*(6868), 141–147. doi:10.1038/415141a

Giot, L., Bader, J. S., Brouwer, C., Chaudhuri, A., Kuang, B., Li, Y., & Hao, Y. L. (2003). A protein interaction map of Drosophila melanogaster. *Science*, *302*(5651), 1727–1736. doi:10.1126/science.1090289

Han, J. D., & Bertin, N. (2004). Evidence for dynamically organized modularity in the yeast protein-protein interaction network. *Nature*, *430*(6995), 88–93. doi:10.1038/nature02555

Han, J. D., Dupuy, D., Bertin, N., Cusick, M. E., & Vidal, M. (2005). Effect of sampling on topology predictions of protein-protein interaction networks. *Nature Biotechnology*, *23*(7), 839–844. doi:10.1038/nbt1116

Hart, G. T., Lee, I., & Marcotte, E. R. (2007). A high-accuracy consensus map of yeast protein complexes reveals modular nature of gene essentiality. *BMC Bioinformatics*, *8*, 236. doi:10.1186/1471-2105-8-236

Hart, G. T., Ramani, A. K., & Marcotte, E. M. (2006). How complete are current yeast and human protein-interaction networks? *Genome Biology*, *7*(11), 120. doi:10.1186/gb-2006-7-11-120

Hermjakob, H., & Monetcchi-Palazzi, L. (2004). IntAct: An open source molecular interaction database. *Nucleic Acids Research*, *32*, D452–D455. doi:10.1093/nar/gkh052

Hishigaki, H., Nakai, K., Ono, T., Tanigami, A., & Takagi, T. (2001). Assessment of prediction accuracy of protein function from protein–protein interaction data. *Yeast (Chichester, England)*, *18*(6), 523–531. doi:10.1002/yea.706

Hu, P., Bader, G., Wigle, D. A., & Emili, A. (2007). Computational prediction of cancer gene function. *Nature Reviews. Cancer*, *7*(1), 23–34. doi:10.1038/nrc2036

Hu, P., & Janga, S. C. (2009a). Global functional atlas of Escherichia coli encompassing previously uncharacterized proteins. *PLoS Biology*, *7*(4), e96. doi:10.1371/journal.pbio.1000096

Hu, P., Jiang, H., & Emili, A. (2009b). A topology-sharing based method for protein function prediction via analysis of protein functional association networks. *Proceedings of 2009 IEEE International Conference on Bioinformatics and Biomedicine (BIBM'09) Workshops*, (pp. 243-248). Washington D.C., USA, November, 2009.

Hu, P., Jiang, H., & Emili, A. (2010). Predicting protein functions by relaxation labelling protein interaction network. *BMC Bioinformatics, 11*(1), S64. doi:10.1186/1471-2105-11-S1-S64

Huynen, M., Snel, B., Lathe, W. III, & Bork, P. (2000). Predicting protein function by genomic context: Quantitative evaluation and qualitative inferences. *Genome Research, 10*(8), 1204–1210. doi:10.1101/gr.10.8.1204

Ito, T., Chiba, T., Ozawa, R., Yoshida, M., Hattori, M., & Sakaki, Y. (2001). A comprehensive two hybrid analysis to explore the yeast protein interactome. *Proceedings of the National Academy of Sciences of the United States of America, 98*(8), 4569–4574. doi:10.1073/pnas.061034498

Jansen, R., & Gerstein, M. (2004). Analyzing protein function on a genomic scale: The importance of gold-standard positives and negatives for network prediction. *Current Opinion in Microbiology, 7*(5), 535–545. doi:10.1016/j.mib.2004.08.012

Jansen, R., Yu, H., Greenbaum, D., Kluger, Y., Krogan, N. J., & Chung, S. (2003). A Bayesian networks approach for predicting protein–protein interactions from genomic data. *Science, 302*(5644), 449–453. doi:10.1126/science.1087361

Jiang, X., Nariai, N., Steffen, M., Kasif, S., & Kolaczyk, E. D. (2008). Integration of relational and hierarchical network information for protein function prediction. *BMC Bioinformatics, 9*, 350. doi:10.1186/1471-2105-9-350

Kanehisa, M., Goto, S., Kawashima, S., Okuno, Y., & Hattori, M. (2004). The KEGG resource for deciphering the genome. *Nucleic Acids Research, 32*, D277–D280. doi:10.1093/nar/gkh063

Kislinger, T., Cox, T. B., Kannan, A., Chung, C., Hu, P., & Ignatchenko, A. (2006). Global survey of organ and organelle protein expression in mouse: Combined proteomic and transcriptomic profiling. *Cell, 125*(1), 173–186. doi:10.1016/j.cell.2006.01.044

Krogan, N. J., & Cagney, G. (2006). Global landscape of protein complexes in the yeast Saccharomyces cerevisiae. *Nature, 440*(7084), 637–643. doi:10.1038/nature04670

Lanckriet, G. R., De Bie, T., Cristianini, N., Jordan, M. I., & Nobel, W. S. (2004). A statistical framework for genomic data fusion. *Bioinformatics (Oxford, England), 20*(16), 2626–2635. doi:10.1093/bioinformatics/bth294

Lee, H., Tu, Z., Deng, M., Sun, F., & Chen, T. (2006). Diffusion kernel-based logistic regression models for protein function prediction. *OMICS: J Integr Biol, 10*(1), 40–55. doi:10.1089/omi.2006.10.40

Letovsky, S., & Kasif, S. (2003). Predicting protein function from protein-protein interaction data: a probabilistic approach. *Bioinformatics (Oxford, England), 19*(1), i197–i204. doi:10.1093/bioinformatics/btg1026

Lin, D. (2008). *An information-theoretic definition of similarity, semantic similarity based on corpus statistics and lexical taxonomy.* Fifteenth International Conference on Machine Learning. (pp. 296–304).

Lord, P. W., Stevens, R. D., Brass, A., & Goble, C. A. (2003). Investigating semantic similarity measures across the gene ontology: The relationship between sequence and annotation. *Bioinformation, 19*(10), 1275–1283. doi:10.1093/bioinformatics/btg153

Lubovac, Z., Gamalielsson, J., & Olsson, B. (2006). Combining functional and topological properties to identify core modules in protein interaction networks. *Proteins, 64*(4), 948–959. doi:10.1002/prot.21071

Massjouni, N., Rivera, C. G., & Murali, T. M. (2006). VIRGO: Computational prediction of gene functions. *Nucleic Acids Research, 34*, W340–4. doi:10.1093/nar/gkl225

Mateos, A., Dopazo, J., Jansen, R., Tu, Y., Gerstein, M., & Stolovitzky, G. (2002). Systematic learning of gene functional classes from DNA array expression data by using multilayer perceptrons. *Genome Research, 12*(11), 1703–1715. doi:10.1101/gr.192502

McDermott, J., Bumgarner, R., & Samudrala, R. (2005). Functional annotation from predicted protein interaction networks. *Bioinformatics (Oxford, England), 21*(15), 3217–3226. doi:10.1093/bioinformatics/bti514

Mewes, H. W. (2002). MIPS: A database for genomes and protein sequences. *Nucleic Acids Research, 30*(1), 31–34. doi:10.1093/nar/30.1.31

Mostafavi, S., & Morris, Q. (2009). Using the gene ontology hierarchy when predicting gene function. In *Proceedings of the Twenty-Fifth Conference on Uncertainty in Artificial Intelligence (UAI-09)* (pp. 419-427). Oregon: AUAI Press.

Murali, T. M., Wu, C. J., & Kasif, S. (2006). The art of gene function prediction. *Nature Biotechnology, 24*(12), 1474–1475. doi:10.1038/nbt1206-1474

Myers, C. L., & Troyanskaya, O. G. (2007). Context-sensitive data integration and prediction of biological networks. *Bioinformatics (Oxford, England), 23*(17), 2322–2330. doi:10.1093/bioinformatics/btm332

Nabieva, E., Jim, K., Agarwal, A., Chazelle, B., & Singh, M. (2005). Whole proteome prediction of protein function via graph-theoretic analysis of interaction maps. *Bioinformatics (Oxford, England), 21*(1), i302–i310. doi:10.1093/bioinformatics/bti1054

Osborne, J. D., & Flatow, J. (2009). Annotating the human genome with disease ontology. *BMC Genomics, 10*(1), S6. doi:10.1186/1471-2164-10-S1-S6

Palla, G., Der'enyi, I., Farkas, I. J., & Vicsek, T. (2005). Uncovering the overlapping modular structure of protein interaction networks. *Nature, 435*(7043), 814–818. doi:10.1038/nature03607

Peri, S., & Navarro, J. D. (2003). Development of human protein reference database as an initial platform for approaching systems biology in humans. *Genome Research, 13*(10), 2363–2371. doi:10.1101/gr.1680803

Pˇrzulj, N., Wigle, D., & Jurisica, I. (2004). Functional topology in a network of protein interactions. *Bioinformatics (Oxford, England), 20*(3), 340–348. doi:10.1093/bioinformatics/btg415

Rajagopala, S. V., & Titz, B. (2007). The protein network of bacterial motility. *Molecular Systems Biology, 3*, 128. doi:10.1038/msb4100166

Ravasz, E., Somera, A. L., Mongru, D. A., Oltvai, Z. N., & Barabási, A. L. (2002). Hierarchical organization of modularity in metabolic networks. *Science, 297*(5586), 1551–1555. doi:10.1126/science.1073374

Resnik, P. (1999). Semantic similarity in a taxonomy: An information-based measure and its application to problems of ambiguity in natural language. *Journal of Artificial Intelligence Research, 11*(2), 95–130.

Riley, M., & Abe, T. (2006). Escherichia coli K-12: A cooperatively developed annotation snapshot–2005. *Nucleic Acids Research, 34*(1), 1–9. doi:10.1093/nar/gkj405

Rives, A. W., & Galitski, T. (2003). Modular organization of cellular networks. *Proceedings of the National Academy of Sciences of the United States of America, 100*(3), 1128–1133. doi:10.1073/pnas.0237338100

Schwikowski, B., Uetz, P., & Fields, S. (2000). A network of protein–protein interactions in yeast. *Nature Biotechnology, 18*(12), 1257–1261. doi:10.1038/82360

Segal, E., Yelensky, R., & Koller, D. (2003). Genome-wide discovery of transcriptional modules from DNA sequence and gene expression. *Bioinformatics (Oxford, England), 19*(1), 1273–1282. doi:10.1093/bioinformatics/btg1038

Shen, J., Zhang, J., Luo, X., Zhu, W., Yu, K., & Chen, K. … Jiang, H. (2007). Predicting protein-protein interactions based only on sequences information. *Proceedings of the National Academy of Sciences USA, 104*(11), 4337–41.

Tanay, A., Sharan, R., Kupiec, M., & Shamir, R. (2004). Revealing modularity and organization in the yeast molecular network by integrated analysis of highly heterogeneous genomewide data. *Proceedings of the National Academy of Sciences of the United States of America, 101*(9), 2981–2986. doi:10.1073/pnas.0308661100

Tao, Y., Sam, L., Li, J., Friedman, C., & Lussier, Y. A. (2007). Information theory applied to the sparse gene ontology annotation network to predict novel gene function. *Bioinformatics (Oxford, England), 23*(13), i529–i538. doi:10.1093/bioinformatics/btm195

Troyanskaya, O. G., Dolinski, K., Owen, A. B., Altman, R. B., & Botstein, D. (2003). A Bayesian framework for combining heterogeneous data sources for gene function prediction in Saccharomyces cerevisiae. *Proceedings of the National Academy of Sciences of the United States of America, 100*(14), 8348–8353. doi:10.1073/pnas.0832373100

Tsuda, K., Shin, H., & Schölkopf, B. (2005). Fast protein classification with multiple networks. *Bioinformatics (Oxford, England), 21*(2), ii59–ii65. doi:10.1093/bioinformatics/bti1110

Vazquez, A., Flammini, A., Maritan, A., & Vespignani, A. (2003). Global protein function prediction from protein–protein interaction networks. *Nature Biotechnology, 21*(6), 697–700. doi:10.1038/nbt825

Von Mering, C., Huynen, M., Jaeggi, D., Schmidt, S., Bork, P., & Snel, B. (2003). STRING: A database of predicted functional associations between proteins. *Nucleic Acids Research, 31*(1), 258–261. doi:10.1093/nar/gkg034

Wang, J. Z., Du, Z., Payattakool, R., Yu, P. S., & Chen, C. F. (2007). A new method to measure the semantic similarity of GO terms. *Bioinformatics (Oxford, England), 23*(10), 1274–1281. doi:10.1093/bioinformatics/btm087

Wodak, S. J., & Mendez, R. (2004). Prediction of protein-protein interactions: The CAPRI experiment, its evaluation and implications. *Current Opinion in Structural Biology, 14*(2), 242–249. doi:10.1016/j.sbi.2004.02.003

Xenarios, I., Salwinski, L., Duan, X. J., Higney, P., Kim, S. M., & Eisenberg, D. (2002). DIP, the database of interacting proteins: A research tool for studying cellular networks of protein interactions. *Nucleic Acids Research, 30*(1), 303–305. doi:10.1093/nar/30.1.303

Yu, H., Braun, P., Yildirim, M. A., Lemmens, I., Venkatesan, K., & Sahalie, J. (2008). High-quality binary protein interaction map of the yeast interactome network. *Science, 322*(5898), 104–110. doi:10.1126/science.1158684

Zanzoni, A., Montecchi-Palazzi, L., Quondam, M., Ausiello, G., Helmer-Citterich, M., & Cesareni, G. (2002). MINT: a Molecular INTeraction database. *FEBS Letters, 513*(1), 135–140. doi:10.1016/S0014-5793(01)03293-8

Zhang, B., & Horvath, S. (2005). A general framework for weighted gene co-expression network analysis. *Statistical Applications in Genetics and Molecular Biology, 4*, 17. doi:10.2202/1544-6115.1128

Zhao, X. M., Chen, L. N., & Aihara, K. (2007). Gene function prediction with the shortest path in functional linkage graph. *Lect Notes Oper Res, 7*, 68–74.

Zhao, X. M., Wang, Y., Chen, L. N., & Aihara, K. (2008). Gene function prediction using labeled and unlabeled data. *BMC Bioinformatics*, *9*, 57. doi:10.1186/1471-2105-9-57

Zhou, X. J., Kao, M. C., Huang, H., Wong, A., Nunez-Iglesias, J., & Primig, M. (2005). Functional annotation and network reconstruction through cross-platform integration of microarray data. *Nature Biotechnology*, *23*(2), 238–243. doi:10.1038/nbt1058

KEY TERMS AND DEFINITIONS

Interaction Networks: A graphical description of a large ensemble of molecular associations, whose nodes correspond to gene products and whose edges reflect direct links or connections between the gene products.

GO Correlation Structure: A statistical measure of the relationships observed between all pair-wise functional classes examined.

Directed Acyclic Graph: A network data structure used to represent gene function classification system in the Gene Ontology, having ordered relationships between nodes (e.g. parent and child terms, wherein the graph direction indicates which term is subsumed by the other), and no cycles (no path returns to the same node twice). Terms can have multiple parents.

GO Gold Standard: A reference gene set used for labeling protein functions, both for building prediction models and for creating test data to evaluate classifier performance.

Multi-Function Prediction: A computational procedure wherein a gene product is assigned to at least two or more functional classes.

Supervised Learning: A computational procedure to identify sets of gene products that are similar to a reference set of manually-defined examples using a principled prediction rule or criteria. Any genes of unknown function that are grouped with the set of pre-defined genes are deemed similar in function.

Majority Voting: The annotated functions of all direct neighbors (interacting partners) of a given gene/protein in a network are ordered in a list, from the most-to-least frequent. The function of an associated uncharacterized gene product(s) is then predicted to be the top k (a value defined by the user) or fewer functions in this list. This method is simple and fast, but takes only limited advantage of the overall network topology or any relationship among annotations.

Chapter 9
GO–Based Term Semantic Similarity

Marco A. Alvarez
Utah State University, USA

Xiaojun Qi
Utah State University, USA

Changhui Yan
North Dakota State University, USA

ABSTRACT

As the Gene Ontology (GO) plays more and more important roles in bioinformatics research, there has been great interest in developing objective and accurate methods for calculating semantic similarity between GO terms. In this chapter, the authors first introduce the basic concepts related to the GO and then briefly review the current advances and challenges in the development of methods for calculating semantic similarity between GO terms. Then, the authors introduce a semantic similarity method that does not rely on external data sources. Using this method as an example, the authors show how different properties of the GO can be explored to calculate semantic similarities between pairs of GO terms. The authors conclude the chapter by presenting some thoughts on the directions for future research in this field.

GENE ONTOLOGY AND GENE ONTOLOGY ANNOTATION

The most successful effort for systematically describing current biological knowledge is the GO project (Ashburner et al., 2000), which maintains a dynamic, structured, precisely defined, and controlled vocabulary of terms for expressing the roles of genes and gene products. The GO is dynamic in the sense that its structure changes as more information is available. The GO consists of three different ontologies describing: 1) biological processes (BP), where a process often involves a chemical or physical transformation (e.g. cell growth); 2) molecular functions (MF), where functions are defined as the biochemical activity of gene products (e.g. enzyme); and 3) cellular components (CC), which refers to places in the cell where gene products are active (e.g. nuclear membrane). Each ontology contains nodes (GO

DOI: 10.4018/978-1-60960-625-1.ch009

terms) linked to each other through *"is-a"* or *"part-of"* relationships forming a directed acyclic graph. Such organization enables the retrieval and visualization of biological knowledge at different levels.

The Gene Ontology Annotation (GOA) project (Barrell et al., 2009) at the European Bioinformatics Institute (EBI) is a project that aims to provide high-quality electronic and manual associations (annotations) between GO terms and UniProt KnowledgeBase (UniProtKB) entries (Consortium, 2009). Crucial to this project is the integration of different databases, a problem that has been addressed by the GO project. The GO maintains a common vocabulary of terms that can be applied to all organisms enabling the annotation across species and databases. The GOA project associates GO terms to UniProtKB entries using strictly controlled manual and electronic methods where every association is supported by a distinct evidence source. A protein can be annotated to multiple GO terms from any of the three ontologies in GO. Functional annotations of UniProtKB proteins currently consists of over 32 million annotations to more than 4 million proteins (Barrell et al., 2009).

SEMANTIC SIMILARITY BETWEEN GENE ONTOLOGY TERMS

The calculation of semantic similarity between pairs of ontology terms aims to capture the relatedness between the semantic content of the terms. Researchers have made great efforts to develop objective and accurate methods to calculate term semantic similarity. For example, semantic similarity between concepts has been a central topic in natural language processing where several robust methods have been proposed based on the WordNet ontology (Budanitsky & Hirst, 2006). In recent years, ontologies have grown to be a popular topic in the biomedical research community creating a demand for computational methods that can

exploit their hierarchical structure, in particular, methods for calculating semantic similarity between terms in the GO. Such methods are designed to reflect the closeness or distance between the semantic content of the terms, in other words, their biological relationships.

Additionally, semantic similarity methods can easily be extended to infer higher level semantic relationships. For example, at the protein level, scores for a given protein pair can be calculated by combining the pairwise semantic similarities for the GO terms associated with the proteins. These scores can be used in a broad range of applications such as clustering of genes in pathways (Wang, Du, Payattakool, Yu, & Chen, 2007, Sheehan, Quigley, Gaudin, & Dobson, 2008, Nagar & Al-Mubaid, 2008, Du, Li, Chen, Yu, & Wang, 2009), protein-protein interaction (Xu, Du, & Zhou, 2008), expression profiles of gene products (Sevilla et al., 2005), protein sequence similarity (Pesquita et al., 2008, Mistry & Pavlidis, 2008, Lord, Stevens, Brass, & Goble, 2003), protein function prediction (Fontana, Cestaro, Velasco, Formentin, & Toppo, 2009), and protein family similarity (Couto, Silva, & Coutinho, 2007). An armada of semantic similarity measures using the GO are available in the biomedical literature. A representative collection of available methods have been reviewed and categorized by (Pesquita, Faria, Falcão, Lord, & Couto, 2009).

SEMANTIC SIMILARITY BETWEEN GENE PRODUCTS

In the research related to biological ontologies, great interest has been seen in exploiting ontological annotations to estimate the relationship between gene products, particularly proteins. The use of ontological annotations to measure the similarities between gene products was first introduced in (Lord et al., 2003), where three different methods (Jiang & Conrath, 1997, Lin, 1998, Resnik, 1995) originally designed for the

WordNet ontology were evaluated under the biological context.

Bearing in mind that each gene product is annotated by multiple GO terms, we focus our attention on pairwise approaches that measure semantic similarities between gene products by combining the pairwise semantic similarities between their terms. Three methods have been widely used for this purpose: average (Lord et al., 2003), maximum (Sevilla et al., 2005), and the best match average (Couto et al., 2007, Schlicker, Domingues, Rahnenfuhrer, & Lengauer, 2006, Wang et al., 2007). Such methods can be explained using the following example.

Let P_k be a protein, and $A(P_k) = \{t_{k1}, t_{k2}, \ldots\}$ be the set of non-redundant GO terms that annotate P_k. Then, given two input proteins P_i and P_j with annotation sets $A(P_i) = \{t_{i1}, t_{i2}, \ldots, t_{im}\}$ and $A(P_j) = \{t_{j1}, t_{j2}, \ldots, t_{jn}\}$, we obtain the similarity matrix $M_{m \times n}$ where every $M(a, b)$ is the semantic similarity between GO terms t_{ia} and t_{jb}. The similarity matrix $M_{m \times n}$ is not necessarily square or symmetric since proteins may be annotated by any number of GO terms. Let's assume that $SSA(t_1, t_2)$ denotes the semantic similarity between GO terms t_1 and t_2 calculated by our method.

In the maximum method, the semantic similarity between proteins P_i and P_j is the largest term similarity found in the similarity matrix $M_{m \times n}$. This approach can be expressed as:

$$P_{max}(P_i, P_j) = \max_{1 \le a \le m, 1 \le b \le n} SSA(t_{ia}, t_{jb})$$

Similarly, the average method defines the semantic similarity between proteins P_i and P_j as the average over all term similarities in the matrix. This approach can be expressed as:

$$P_{avg}(P_i, P_j) = \frac{\sum_{a=1}^{m} \sum_{b=1}^{n} SSA(t_{ia}, t_{jb})}{m + n}$$

The best match average method is based on the different meanings of rows and columns in the similarity matrix $M_{m \times n}$. Note that the values in row a represent the similarities between term t_{ia} and all the terms in $A(P_j)$, while column b contains the similarities between term t_{jb} and all the terms in $A(P_i)$. Let's define the row maxima of a row of matrix $M_{m \times n}$ as the maximum value in that row and column maxima of a column of $M_{m \times n}$ as the maximum value in that column. Then, the vector consisting of all row maxima represents the best hits when comparing one protein with the other, and the vector consisting of all column maxima represents the best hits when comparisons are made in the other direction. The best match average method calculates the averages of both vectors and then takes the average of them. This method is summarized below:

$$row_{max}(P_i, P_j) = \frac{1}{m} \cdot \sum_{a=1}^{m} \max_{1 \le b \le n} SSA(t_{ia}, t_{jb})$$

$$col_{max}(P_i, P_j) = \frac{1}{n} \cdot \sum_{b=1}^{n} \max_{1 \le a \le m} SSA(t_{ia}, t_{jb})$$

$$P_{bma}(P_i, P_j) = \frac{row_{max}(P_i, P_j) + col_{max}(P_i, P_j)}{2}$$

According to (Pesquita et al., 2008), from a biological point of view there are limitations to the average and maximum approaches. Imagine two functionally identical proteins with more than one annotation. The average method will yield a similarity below 1.0 because the average is calculated over all the pairwise combinations. On the other hand, the maximum approach can yield similarities of 1.0 even when the proteins are not functionally identical, because it ignores unrelated terms. In (Pesquita et al., 2008) the authors claimed that the best match average approach does not suffer from the above limitations, and accounts for both similar and dissimilar terms as expected biologically. In our experiments, we tested these three methods with our proposed semantic similarity algorithm. The results confirm that the best match average is a better way to combine GO term similarities to obtain semantic similarities between proteins.

EVALUATION OF METHODS FOR COMPUTING SEMANTIC SIMILARITY BETWEEN GO TERMS

Although there exist a few methods for calculating the semantic similarity between GO terms, the fair evaluation and comparison of these methods has proven very difficult. The main challenge is that there is no gold standard to compare with, more specifically, there is no well-accepted quantitative definition for semantic similarities between GO terms. An approach used in several studies is to calculate semantic similarities for a set of proteins and correlate the resulting semantic similarities with sequence similarity (Lord et al., 2003), Pfam similarity (Couto et al., 2007), protein interactions (Guo, Liu, Shriver, Hu, & Liebman, 2006), among others. In general, correlations are determined by the Pearson Correlation Coefficient, which is in the range of $[-1, 1]$. Then the correlation is used as a measure to evaluate the performance of the proposed method. Better methods are expected to achieve higher correlation. Two different types of functional similarities have been used in our study for this purpose. In the first type, sequence similarity between proteins is used to estimate functional similarity. The foundation of this approach is that similar sequence leads to

similar function. The second type of function similarity is based on the Pfam (Finn et al., 2008) annotations of proteins. Let families $F(P_i) = \{f_{i1}, f_{i2}, \ldots, f_{im}\}$ and $F(P_j) = \{f_{j1}, f_{j2}, \ldots, f_{jn}\}$ be the Pfam families that protein P_i and P_j are associated with respectively. Then the functional similarity between the two proteins is calculated similarly to (Couto et al., 2007), where the Jaccard coefficient between the two sets is defined as shown below:

$$P_{pfam}(P_i, P_j) = \frac{|F(P_i) \cap F(P_j)|}{|F(P_i) \cup F(P_j)|}$$

PREVIOUS METHODS FOR COMPUTING SEMANTIC SIMILARITY BETWEEN GO TERMS

Given two input terms, a semantic similarity algorithm returns a numerical score that quantifies the relatedness of the input terms. Based primarily on the structure of the GO and GOA annotations, several algorithms for estimating the semantic similarity of GO terms have been proposed in the biomedical literature. In one dimension, they can be roughly classified as node-based methods (Couto et al., 2007, Lord et al., 2003, Schlicker et al., 2006), edge-based methods (Cheng et al., 2004, Wu, Zhu, Guo, Zhang, & Lin, 2006), and hybrid methods (Wang et al., 2007, Othman, Deris, & Illias, 2008). In edge-based methods, the semantic similarity varies according to the shortest distance connecting the input terms, while in node-based methods the similarity is evaluated by comparing specific properties of the input terms, and optionally their ancestors. In a second dimension, they can be classified as intrinsic methods that only rely on the ontologies and external methods that depend on additional information from external data sources. For example, annotation databases

Table 1. Statistics for the Gene Ontology. For each of the ontologies we show respectively the number of GO terms, the number of "is-a" links, the number of "part-of" links, and the maximum depth.

Ontology	Terms	*"is-a"* **links**	*"part-of"* **links**	*max-depth*
Biological Process	16,819	27,532	3,446	14
Molecular Function	8,628	10,079	3	14
Cellular Location	2,416	3,670	941	10

like GOA can be used to calculate the frequency of annotation and/or information content scores for any node. Several existing semantic similarity algorithms include in their calculations information content measures determined from an external corpus. For instance, algorithms reported in (Pesquita et al., 2009) use, direct or indirectly, information content calculations proposed by (Resnik, 1995, Jiang & Conrath, 1997, Lin, 1998).

A limitation of methods that rely on external data sources is their sensitivity to changes in the involved corpus. If the lexical corpus is changed, the semantic similarity values will also change. In our context, GOA annotations are commonly used as a corpus. As the GOA is updated, the semantic similarity between the same pair of GO terms will also change. However, an ideal semantic similarity method should only rely on the ontologies and should not be affected by the change of the external corpus. In this regard, semantic similarity methods that are intrinsic to the ontologies should be the target of future research. In the following section, we will use an example to show how to develop a semantic similarity method that only relies on the ontologies.

A SEMANTIC SIMILARITY METHOD THAT DOES NOT RELY ON EXTERNAL DATA SOURCES

Dataset

For our experiments we downloaded the revision 1.723 of the GO. Table 1 shows the number of

terms, *"is-a"* links, *"part-of"* links, and maximum depth of the three ontologies in such version of the GO.

Evaluation

For the purpose of evaluating our method, we downloaded the release 15.6 of the UniProtKB database, which is the most comprehensive and highly annotated publicly accessible protein sequence database, having recorded more than 6.6 million proteins through a combination of manual and electronic techniques. Then the annotations of the proteins in UniProtKB were extracted from the release 74.0 of GOA-UniProt, which provides the mapping of GO terms to UniProtKB entries. The mapping is done in the GOA project using both manual and electronic methods, both of which are strictly controlled to produce high-quality GO annotation and both require the involvement of biologists and software engineers (Barrell et al., 2009). Bear in mind that our semantic similarity method does not use the information in GOA-UniProt to calculate the semantic similarity. From the UniProtKB protein database, we selected the top 500 proteins with the highest number of annotations. We ensure that all the selected proteins have at least one annotation in GOA-UniProt for each of the three GO ontologies. In Figure 1 we can observe the density function for the number of annotations existing in our selected dataset of the top 500 most annotated proteins. In total we count 16,248 unique annotations for Biological Process, 5,029 for Molecular Function, and 4,298 for Cellular Component ontologies.

Figure 1. Histogram for the number of BP annotations considering the dataset of the top

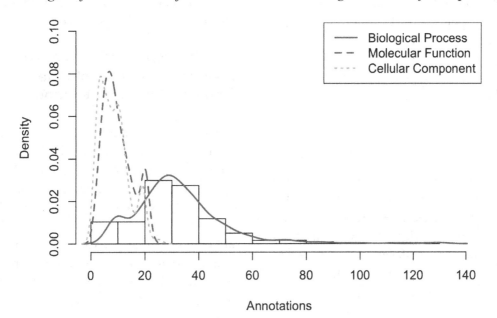

500 most annotated proteins. The figure also shows the probability density estimate for the number of annotations in the BP, MF, and CC ontologies in the same dataset. Note how the proteins have considerably fewer MF and CC annotations than BP ones.

To evaluate our method, we calculated the pairwise semantic similarities between the top 500 proteins. For every pair of proteins we used our method to calculate pairwise semantic similarities between the GO terms annotating them and combined those similarities using the best match average method. Then, the resulting semantic similarities between the top 500 proteins were compared with the functional similarities between these proteins using the Pearson Correlation Coefficient (PCC). Higher PCC values imply a better semantic similarity method. The pairwise functional similarities between proteins were calculated based on the Pfam annotations associated with the proteins. For this purpose, when we selected the top 500 proteins, we also guaranteed that the selected proteins have at least one Pfam-A annotation by checking the online service available at http://pfam.sanger.ac.uk/ protein/ provided by the Pfam database. According to recommendations found in (Yon Rhee, Wood, Dolinski, & Draghici, 2008), we excluded all annotations containing the *not*, *contributes_to*, and *colocalizes_with* qualifiers.

Semantic Similarity Method that only Considers the Shortest Path Between GO Terms on the Ontology

The first information that we explored to calculate semantic similarity between two GO terms was the shortest path that connects them on the ontology following either *"is-a"* and *"part-of"* links. We used the length of the path as a measure for the relatedness of the terms. The hypothesis is that if two GO terms are semantically similar, they should be close to each other in the ontology. The edges at different depths of the GO imply different distances in the biological setting, with the edges closer to the root implying longer distances than edges farther from the root. Thus, we assigned weights to edges based on the depths of their endpoints in the ontology. For example an edge with endpoints t_1 and t_2 is given a weight as follows:

$$weight(t_i, t_j) = 1 - \frac{depth(t_i) + depth(t_j)}{2 \cdot max}$$

where $depth(t_i)$ and $depth(t_j)$ are their corresponding depths in the graph, and max is the maximum depth in the respective ontology. Due to multiple inheritance there are special cases where a given node can have different paths from the root with different lengths. We choose to consider the maximum depth possible which indicates the higher degree of specialization of the node.

The length of the path between two GO terms is defined as the sum of edge weights on the path. The shortest path is then the path with the smallest length. We transform the length of the path into a similarity measure using the following quadratic function so that shorter distances imply higher similarities:

$$spsim(t_i, t_j) = \left(\frac{sp(t_i, t_j)}{max} - 1 \right)^2$$

where $sp(t_i, t_j)$ is the length of the shortest path between node t_i and node t_j, and max is the maximum depth in the ontology. It can be easily proven that the similarity values are in the range of $[0,1]$. We use this function to express a similarity score between two GO terms as follows:

$$SSA(t_1, t_2) = spsim(t_1, t_2)$$

When this method was used to calculate semantic similarity between GO terms, the correlation between semantic similarities and functional similarities for the top 500 proteins was

0.668, 0.600 and 0.444 respectively when BP, MF and CC ontologies were considered.

Add the Depth of the Nearest Common Ancestor into the Semantic Similarity Method

The second property that we explored to calculate semantic similarity between two GO terms was the depth of the nearest common ancestor (NCA) for a pair of nodes in the ontologies. The hypothesis for this is that two semantically similar GO terms should share a long common path from the root and only branch at a place close to the bottom of the ontology. Based on this assumption, the deeper the NCA, the more similar the terms are. We used the following function to convert the depth of NCA into a similarity score:

$$nca(t_i, t_j) = \frac{dnca(t_i, t_j)}{max}$$

where $dnca(t_i, t_j)$ simply returns the depth of the NCA between terms t_i and t_j, and max is the maximum depth of the ontology. The output of $nca(t_i, t_j)$ is also in the interval $[0,1]$. Then, we combined this function with the length of the shortest path to develop a similarity score between two GO terms as follows:

$$SSA(t_1, t_2) = \frac{spsim(t_1, t_2) + nca(t_1, t_2)}{2}$$

When this function was used to calculated semantic similarity between GO terms, the correlation between semantic similarities and functional similarities for the top 500 proteins was 0.787, 0.765 and 0.510 respectively when BP, MF and CC ontologies were considered. Compared these results with those in the previous section, we can see that adding depth of NCA into the semantic similarity method significantly improve

CONSIDER THE SIMILARITY BETWEEN THE DEFINITIONS OF GO TERMS

On the GO, each term is associated with a definition which is a textual description of the term. If two GO terms are similar in semantics, they are very likely to share some common words in their definitions. Thus, we also explored the definition of GO terms to calculate semantic similarity between GO terms. First we defined the long definition of a term as the union of the terms' name and definition. We refined every long definition by removing common words (e.g. of, a, the) and applied the Porter algorithm (Porter, 1980) for stemming. Then, we created long definition vectors in a n dimensional ontological space. The value of n is the total number of unique stemmed words found in all long definitions for the respective ontology, which is $10,130$ for the biological process ontology, $12,979$ for the molecular function ontology and $5,884$ for the cellular component ontology. Every value in the long definition vector represents the *tf-idf* weight (term frequency-inverse document frequency) for the corresponding word. This weight evaluates how important a word is to its long definition. A high *tf-idf* weight is reached by words with high frequency in the long definition and with low frequency in the corpus (i.e. the collection of all long definitions in the respective ontology), therefore *tf-idf* weights tend to filter out common words. The similarity score is the cosine similarity defined by:

$$ld(t_i, t_j) = \frac{\overrightarrow{ld_i} \cdot \overrightarrow{ld_j}}{\| \overrightarrow{ld_i} \| \cdot \| \overrightarrow{ld_j} \|}$$

where $\overrightarrow{ld_i}$ and $\overrightarrow{ld_j}$ are the long definition vectors for terms t_i and t_j respectively.

We then combined all the three functions to obtain a score for the semantic similarity between two GO terms:

$$SSA(t_1, t_2) = \frac{spsim(t_1, t_2) + nca(t_1, t_2) + ld(t_1, t_2)}{3}$$

When this function was used to calculate semantic similarity, the correlation between semantic similarities and functional similarities for the top 500 proteins was increased to 0.804, 0.780 and 0.544 respectively for BP, MF and CC ontologies.

DISCUSSION AND FUTURE DIRECTIONS

Till this point, we have shown how to use different properties of the ontologies to calculate semantic similarity between GO terms. Figure 2, shows how the performance of the method is improved gradually by including more properties from the GO.

We also compared our method with other semantic similarity methods using the CESSM Web server available at http://xldb.fc.ul.pt/biotools/cessm developed by the XLDB research group at the University of Lisbon. CESSM currently implements 11 semantic similarity measures, all of which rely on external data sources. CESSM allows users to evaluate their semantic similarity algorithms using sequence similarities, which are calculated by means of RRBS (Pesquita et al., 2008), a relative measure of sequence similarity based on BLAST bitscores. Instead of using PCC, CESSM provides a resolution score which represents how well semantic similarities match sequence similarities. According to CESSM, resolution is the relative intensity where variations in

Figure 2. The performance of the semantic similarity method improves gradually as more properties of the ontologies are included. BP: biological process ontology; MF: molecular function ontology; CC; cellular component ontology; sp : the length of the shortest path between GO terms; nca : the depth of the nearest common ancestor; and ld : the similarity between long definitions.

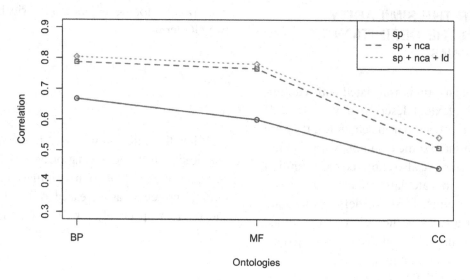

the sequence similarity scale are translated into the semantic similarity scale. Higher resolution values mean that the semantic similarity method has higher capability to distinguish between different levels of protein function.

In the comparison, we only use the MF ontology because BP and CC ontologies present poor correlation with sequence similarity, as stated in (Lord et al., 2003). In this context, the best result achieved by the 11 methods in CESSM is a resolution score of 0.967. In contrast, our method achieves a resolution score of 0.972. In addition to the high performance, the key advantage of our method is that it is intrinsic to the ontology, that is, it does not rely on the external data sources in the calculation of semantic similarity.

Future research can be performed in the following directions in the search of better semantic similarity algorithms.

Different Weightings for Terms

In the method we developed, when we combined different properties of the ontologies to obtain a similarity score, equal weights are given to the three different terms: sp, nca, and ld. But it is possible to obtain a better combination by assigning different weights to the three terms. As a simple exploration, we tried every combination of the weights in the range of $[0, 2]$ (with increments of 1) for the three terms. No combination can improve the performance consistently across the three ontologies. One possibility is that the relationships among the three terms are not linear. Thus, to find the optimal weighting, systematic research will be needed to explore the individual contribution of each term and the mutual dependency among these properties.

More Properties of the Ontology

Exploring other properties of the ontology may also help improve the performance in calculating semantic similarity. For example, there are two different types of links between GO terms: *"is-a"* and *"part-of"*. In different studies, these two types of links have been used indiscriminately and represented by the same kind of edges. But since these links characterize different relationships, modeling separate types of links using different types of edges in the graph may better explore the knowledge in the ontologies.

Weighting Edges in the Ontology

Our results have shown that the length of the shortest path between two GO terms is a good indication of the semantic similarity between them. We assign weights to the edges based on the depth of their endpoints. Other strategies may be explored to assign biological weights to the edges of the ontologies. For example, weights corresponding to evolutionary distances may be considered. One simple way to do that is to assign weight to an edge by averaging the evolution distances between proteins associated with the two endpoints of the edge.

Evaluation Benchmarks

A very important but still unsolved problem in the development of semantic similarity measures is how to evaluate a semantic similarity method. Most researchers do this by comparing the semantic similarities between proteins given by a method with functional similarities between proteins. The functional similarities between proteins may be estimated using sequence similarity or annotations of the proteins in some functional databases. However, for a protein, there are many aspects that biologists are interested in. For example, the amino acid sequence, the 3D structure, and the evolutionary history of the protein. The semantic similarities between proteins given by a method should reflect all these aspects of a protein. Thus, an ideal evaluation should also compare the semantic similarity with the structural similarity,

evolutionary distance, and other biological aspects between proteins. In addition to that, the correlation between semantic similarity and functional similarity (or other aspects) may not be linear. So Pearson Correlation Coefficient may not be the best way to compare them. Other methods should also be explored. For example, one can compare the rankings of all pairwise similarities based on semantic similarity with that based on functional similarity.

ACKNOWLEDGMENT

The authors would like to thank the XLDB Research Team of the University of Lisbon for providing an online tool for the evaluation of GO-based semantic similarity measures. In particular, we thank Catia Pesquita for all the kind support given for using their tool.

REFERENCES

Ashburner, M., Ball, C. A., Blake, J. A., Botstein, D., Butler, H., & Cherry, J. M. (2000). Gene ontology: Tool for the unification of biology. *Nature Genetics, 25*(1), 25–29. doi:10.1038/75556

Barrell, D., Dimmer, E., Huntley, R. P., Binns, D., O'Donovan, C., & Apweiler, R. (2009). The GOA database in 2009–an integrated gene ontology annotation resource. *Nucleic Acids Research, 37*(1), D396–D403. doi:10.1093/nar/gkn803

Budanitsky, A., & Hirst, G. (2006). Evaluating wordnet-based measures of lexical semantic relatedness. *Computational Linguistics, 32*(1), 13–47. doi:10.1162/coli.2006.32.1.13

Cheng, J., Cline, M., Martin, J., Finkelstein, D., Awad, T., & Kulp, D. (2004). A knowledge-based clustering algorithm driven by gene ontology. *Journal of Biopharmaceutical Statistics, 14*(3), 687–700. doi:10.1081/BIP-200025659

Consortium, T. U. (2009). The universal protein resource (uniprot) 2009. *Nucleic Acids Research*, *37*(1), D169–D174. doi:10.1093/nar/gkn664

Couto, F. M., Silva, M. J., & Coutinho, P. M. (2007). Measuring semantic similarity between gene ontology terms. *Data & Knowledge Engineering*, *61*(1), 137–152. doi:10.1016/j. datak.2006.05.003

Du, Z., Li, L., Chen, C. F., Yu, P. S., & Wang, J. Z. (2009). G-sesame: Web tools for go-term-based gene similarity analysis and knowledge discovery. *Nucleic Acids Research*, *37*(2), W345–349.

Finn, R. D., Tate, J., Mistry, J., Coggill, P. C., Sammut, S. J., & Hotz, H. R. (2008). The pfam protein families database. *Nucleic Acids Research*, *36*(1), D281–D288.

Fontana, P., Cestaro, A., Velasco, R., Formentin, E., & Toppo, S. (2009). Rapid annotation of anonymous sequences from genome projects using semantic similarities and a weighting scheme in gene ontology. *PLoS ONE*, *4*(2), e4619. doi:10.1371/journal.pone.0004619

Guo, X., Liu, R., Shriver, C. D., Hu, H., & Liebman, M. N. (2006). Assessing semantic similarity measures for the characterization of human regulatory pathways. *Bioinformatics (Oxford, England)*, *22*(8), 967–973. doi:10.1093/bioinformatics/btl042

Jiang, J. J., & Conrath, D. W. (1997). *Semantic similarity based on corpus statistics and lexical taxonomy*. In International Conference Research on Computational Linguistics.

Lin, D. (1998). *An information-theoretic definition of similarity*. In International Conference on Machine Learning (pp. 296–304).

Lord, P. W., Stevens, R. D., Brass, A., & Goble, C. A. (2003). Investigating semantic similarity measures across the gene ontology: The relationship between sequence and annotation. *Bioinformatics (Oxford, England)*, *19*(10), 1275–1283. doi:10.1093/bioinformatics/btg153

Mistry, M., & Pavlidis, P. (2008). Gene ontology term overlap as a measure of gene functional similarity. *BMC Bioinformatics*, *9*(1), 327. doi:10.1186/1471-2105-9-327

Nagar, A., & Al-Mubaid, H. (2008). *A new path length measure based on GO for gene similarity with evaluation using sgd pathways*. In IEEE International Symposium on Computer-Based Medical Systems (pp. 590–595).

Othman, R., Deris, S., & Illias, R. (2008). A genetic similarity algorithm for searching the gene ontology terms and annotating anonymous protein sequences. *Journal of Biomedical Informatics*, *41*(1), 65–81. doi:10.1016/j.jbi.2007.05.010

Pesquita, C., Faria, D., Bastos, H., Ferreira, A. E., Falcão, A. O., & Couto, F. M. (2008). Metrics for GO based protein semantic similarity: A systematic evaluation. *BMC Bioinformatics*, *9*(5). doi:10.1186/1471-2105-9-S5-S4

Pesquita, C., Faria, D., Falcão, A. O., Lord, P., & Couto, F. M. (2009). Semantic similarity in biomedical ontologies. *PLoS Computational Biology*, *5*(7), e1000443. doi:10.1371/journal. pcbi.1000443

Porter, M. F. (1980). An algorithm for suffix stripping. *Program*, *14*(3), 130–137.

Resnik, P. (1995). *Using information content to evaluate semantic similarity in a taxonomy*. In International Joint Conference on Artificial Intelligence (vol. 1, pp. 448–453).

Schlicker, A., Domingues, F. S., Rahnenfuhrer, J., & Lengauer, T. (2006). A new measure for functional similarity of gene products based on gene ontology. *BMC Bioinformatics*, *7*, 302. doi:10.1186/1471-2105-7-302

Sevilla, J. L., Segura, V., Podhorski, A., Guruceaga, E., Mato, J. M., & Martinez-Cruz, L. A. (2005). Correlation between gene expression and GO semantic similarity. *IEEE/ACM Transactions on Computational Biology and Bioinformatics*, *2*(4), 330–338. doi:10.1109/TCBB.2005.50

Sheehan, B., Quigley, A., Gaudin, B., & Dobson, S. (2008). A relation based measure of semantic similarity for gene ontology annotations. *BMC Bioinformatics*, *9*(1), 468. doi:10.1186/1471-2105-9-468

Wang, J. Z., Du, Z., Payattakool, R., Yu, P. S., & Chen, C. F. (2007). A new method to measure the semantic similarity of GO terms. *Bioinformatics (Oxford, England)*, *23*(10), 1274–1281. doi:10.1093/bioinformatics/btm087

Wu, X., Zhu, L., Guo, J., Zhang, D. Y., & Lin, K. (2006). Prediction of yeast protein-protein interaction network: Insights from the gene ontology and annotations. *Nucleic Acids Research*, *34*(7), 2137–2150. doi:10.1093/nar/gkl219

Xu, T., Du, L., & Zhou, Y. (2008). Evaluation of go-based functional similarity measures using s. cerevisiae protein interaction and expression profile data. *BMC Bioinformatics*, *9*(1), 472. doi:10.1186/1471-2105-9-472

Yon Rhee, S., Wood, V., Dolinski, K., & Draghici, S. (2008). Use and misuse of the gene ontology annotations. *Nature Reviews. Genetics*, *9*(7), 509–515. doi:10.1038/nrg2363

KEY TERMS AND DEFINITIONS

Ontology.: The formal representation of knowledge for a given domain by a hierarchical organization of concepts and relationships between them.

Gene Ontology.: A project that provides a controlled vocabulary of terms describing gene product characteristics and relationships across all species.

Semantic Similarity.: A measure of how related two or more concepts are.

Gene Product.: Biochemical material, either RNA or protein, resulting from gene expression.

Chapter 10
Ontology Learning and the Humanities

Toby Burrows
The University of Western Australia, Australia

ABSTRACT

This chapter reviews the current state of play in the use of ontologies in the humanities, with best-practice examples from selected disciplines. It looks at the specific domain problems faced by the humanities, and examines the various approaches currently being employed to construct, maintain, and develop humanities ontologies. The application of ontology learning in the humanities is discussed by reviewing a range of research projects in different disciplines. The chapter concludes with an assessment of the future potential of ontology learning in the humanities, and an attempt to set out a research agenda for this field.

INTRODUCTION

The humanities are academic disciplines which study the nature of human life and experience. They are different from the natural and social sciences because they use methods which are mainly analytical, critical, or speculative. There are various different definitions of the scope of the humanities. According to the Australian Academy of the Humanities they cover the fol-

lowing disciplines: Archaeology; Asian Studies; Classical Studies; English; European Languages and Cultures; History; Linguistics; Philosophy, Religion and the History of Ideas; Cultural and Communication Studies; the Arts.[1]

Ontological frameworks are central to the work of humanities researchers. This is because most humanities research involves either the analysis and definition of concepts or the categorization of individual phenomena into broader classes. Philosophy is the pre-eminent academic discipline which focuses on concepts, while the focus

DOI: 10.4018/978-1-60960-625-1.ch010

of the disciplines of history and archaeology is largely on the categorization of specific instances (people, places, events, objects and so on). Other humanities disciplines rely on a mixture of these two approaches.

This paper reviews the current state of play in the use of ontologies in the humanities, with best-practice examples from selected disciplines. It looks at the specific domain problems faced by the humanities, and examines the various approaches currently being employed to construct, maintain and develop ontologies.

The application of ontology learning in the humanities is also examined, by reviewing a range of research projects in different disciplines. Areas discussed include the availability of text corpora and other sources of knowledge, and the use of text mining techniques and tools. The standards and tools used for expressing and developing ontologies are also covered.

The paper concludes with an assessment of the future potential of ontology learning in the humanities, and an attempt to set out a research agenda for this field. It also aims to identify areas where ontology learning is likely to prove most valuable and applicable.

Ontologies and the Humanities

The humanities are a particularly difficult area for the development and application of ontologies. The semantic context is complex and often ambiguous, and there are numerous existing vocabularies and taxonomies which often overlap. The multilingual nature of much humanities research has obvious implications for the use of ontologies. Not only are there different terms in different languages for the same concept; a term may be similar in appearance across different languages but have quite different meanings. Humanities research also often crosses different time periods, and the meanings of words and concepts tend to shift over time. Other worldviews and ways of categorizing the world – both current and past – also need to

be factored in. Indigenous knowledge (the Australian aborigines or the North American Indians, for example) has a radically different hierarchy of classes, in addition to the obvious linguistic differences. A further area of complexity is the enormous proliferation of instances, particularly of people and places.

Nagypál (2005, pp. 208-209) discusses four specific difficulties:

- Time dependence: almost every instance is time-dependent, e.g. Strasbourg is part of France today, but has been part of Germany at various times in the past. This means that the relationship between an instance and its class is likely to be different at different historical periods.

- Uncertainty: the documentation relating to instances is frequently missing or contradictory, especially about dates. There are at least two different recorded birth dates for Joseph Stalin, for instance: 21 December 1879 in the official Soviet records, and 6 December 1878 in the church records. In another typical example, the paintings of the Dutch artist Vermeer cannot be dated precisely. This kind of uncertainty may affect the relationship between an instance and its class.

- Subjectivity: "most complex historical notions are vaguely defined or open to multiple interpretations, and thus can be interpreted subjectively, making them difficult to model conceptually." Concepts like 'the Enlightenment' or 'the Middle Ages' do not have precise beginning and ending dates, for example, and it can be unclear whether a given temporal instance falls within the scope of a concept like this. Opinions and interpretations can differ considerably, even between experts.

- "Why" questions: historians tend to focus on this kind of question, and are interested in seeing facts in an explanatory context rather than on their own. Ontologies are much better at representing precise facts, and historical knowledge is particularly difficult to model in this way.

These difficulties have led some researchers to question the very applicability of ontologies in the humanities (Veltman 2004). Nevertheless, there has been a growing body of research in recent years which is aimed at the development and maintenance of such ontologies. There are also an increasing number of digital resources for the humanities which make use of ontologies, especially in the field of knowledge discovery for cultural heritage collections. Mark Greengrass (2007) has identified three basic approaches to the development of humanities ontologies:

- Top-down ontologies: generated from taxonomies accepted within a discipline;
- Middle-out ontologies: generated by intelligent iteration;
- Bottom-up ontologies: generated from a representative sample of canonical data.

Most of the work in the humanities to date has concentrated on the production of top-down and middle-out ontologies.

Two important examples of broad top-down ontologies relevant specifically to the humanities are VICODI and CIDOC-CRM. VICODI (Visual Contextualisation of Digital Content) was a European Union project which developed an ontology to serve as the basis for searching a European history portal. The VICODI ontology was developed using a middle-out iterative approach. A bottom-up approach was not thought to be possible because the project could not identify a suitable textual corpus to use for deriving such an ontology. The VICODI ontology consists of only seven basic concepts (or "flavours"), with a shallow hierarchy of two or three levels. This structure is designed to allow the population of the ontology with large numbers of instances and

relations. Over 15,000 instances were uploaded from Excel spreadsheets, though this work took about two years to carry out. The VICODI ontology instances referring to historical people and events have subsequently been translated into twelve European languages as part of the ENRICH project, which has been implementing a Web catalogue of medieval manuscripts.

The VICODI project encountered two major difficulties (Ciravegna, et al., 2008, p. 71). The first was that there is no accepted corpus of documents or texts from which a conceptual framework could be developed. There is also no organization with sufficient authority in the field of historical research to promulgate or sponsor the use of a particular scheme of knowledge classification. The second major difficulty was that there are major differences between the terminology used to write about history and the terminology used in the historical sources themselves. The project team concluded that "the VICODI ontology development process has shown that a complex humanities domain can be represented through a shallow ontology structure and a limited number of concepts and properties." But the project left open the question of whether "constructing an ontology for any humanities domain is too labour intensive and too costly" (Nagypál, Deswarte & Oosthoek, 2005, p. 346). It also led to the conclusion that "it is practically impossible to build a monolithic ontology for such a complex domain as history" (Nagypál 2005, p. 213).

The CIDOC Conceptual Reference Model (ISO 21127:2006) is a core high-level ontology for describing concepts and relationships used in cultural heritage documentation (Doerr, 2003; Gill, 2004). It was developed as a top-down ontology by Martin Doerr and his colleagues at the Foundation for Research and Technology (FORTH) in Heraklion, Greece. In its latest version, it defines 90 classes and 148 properties. It was designed to enable semantic interoperability between the disparate sources of information produced by libraries, archives, museums and galleries. The

CIDOC CRM has been used as "semantic glue" by a range of services and projects, mainly in the field of museum documentation. Among these is CLAROS (Classical Art Research Online Services), which combines more than two million database records for Greek and Roman art objects held in a variety of museums.

Because of its universal and high-level approach, the CIDOC-CRM is also being mapped to knowledge structures in closely related domains. The Text Encoding Initiative (TEI) is widely used as the accepted XML schema for text encoding in the humanities. A draft mapping of TEI elements to CIDOC-CRM was completed in 2007, and there is considerable current interest in modelling vocabularies within specific TEI elements using the CIDOC-CRM framework (Ore & Eyde, 2009). Another mapping is with FRBR (Functional Requirements for Bibliographic Records) – the internationally accepted XML schema for encoding bibliographic descriptions, which is being used to re-engineer the systems used by libraries to catalogue published materials. FRBR has been harmonized with CIDOC-CRM and transformed into an object-oriented version, FRBRoo (Riva, Doerr & Žumer, 2009).

In addition to high-level ontologies such as VICODI and CIDOC CRM, a wide range of more specific ontologies have been developed and used by humanities projects and services. One important example is the MuseumFinland project and its successor CultureSampo, which provide a range of different views of Finnish cultural heritage resources and collections (Hyvönen, et al., 2009). These services are built on various ontologies which make up the national FinnONTO infrastructure. This consists of a range of domain-specific ontologies mapped together to form a large national ontology called KOKO. Most of these ontologies were developed by transforming pre-existing thesauri into light-weight SKOS-based schemas, using semi-automatic processes. Among the components are an upper ontology YSO (20,600 concepts), a museum ontology MAO (6,800 concepts), an agriforestry ontology AFO (5,500 concepts), an applied art ontology TAO (2,600 concepts) and a photography ontology VALO (1,900 concepts). CultureSampo also makes use of a geographical registry of 800,000 places in Finland, an ontology of persons and organizations, and international vocabularies such as Iconclass and the Union List of Artists Names (ULAN).

Another important application of ontologies is in the prototype of the Europeana Digital Library, which uses them to underpin its semantic searching and browsing facilities. This applies the work originally done by the MultimediaN E-Culture project in the Netherlands, which built a sophisticated demonstrator system with more than 200,000 cultural heritage objects from six different cultural heritage collections (Schreiber, et al., 2008). No new ontologies were developed for this demonstrator. Four existing vocabularies were re-used instead: WordNet, and the three thesauri maintained by the Getty Research Institute – the Art & Architecture Thesaurus (AAT), the Union List of Artists Names (ULAN) and the Thesaurus of Geographic Names (TGN). These vocabularies were made interoperable through their conversion to the SKOS format and subsequent alignment using owl:sameAs and skos:exactMatch relations. The demonstrator has been limited to "simple syntactic alignments" aimed at boosting search results.

Other humanities research projects have developed and applied ontologies on a smaller scale. Mirzaee, Iverson and Hamidzadeh (2005) provide a useful example of an iterative middle-out approach to ontology-building, applied to a single book on the history of the Iranian constitution. They adopted the following steps:

1. Identifying the purpose, scope, and users
2. Domain analysis and knowledge acquisition
3. Building a conceptual (informal) ontology model
4. Formalization
5. Evaluation

They drew on various techniques: competency questions and scenarios, brainstorming, informal analysis of the text, other general ontologies and ontology libraries. After designing, building and formalizing their ontology, they populated it with more than 750 instances extracted from the history book. The same competency questions methodology was also used by the ONTO-H project to build a general humanities ontology for annotating texts, designed as a plugin to the Protégé software (Benjamins, et al., 2004).

Other humanities projects have reported using ontologies but have not described the methodology used to develop their ontology. The *Lands of the Normans* project, for example, applied a small-scale ontology to build a database of persons, places, source documents and relationships relevant to the land-holdings of the Norman aristocracy in twelfth-century England (Power, et al., 2007). But the methods used to build this ontology are not described in the project documentation. The report on the research by Gijs Geleijnse and Jan Korst (2007) aimed at populating an ontology on historical persons by using information extracted from the Web does not explain how the ontology itself was developed.

Ontology Learning and the Humanities

The complexity of the linguistic and conceptual environment for the humanities has made ontologies a difficult research field. It is hardly surprising, therefore, that the application of ontology learning techniques in this domain has been slow and infrequent. Four recent projects have broken important new ground, however, and shown considerable promise for the future. These projects are based on major textual corpora in different humanities disciplines: classical literature, 18th-century French writings, 13th-century Latin documents, and 18th-century accounts of trials.

Perseus Digital Library

The Perseus Digital Library is a major collection of literature and related resources in classical Greek and Latin, developed and maintained by a research team which has played a leading role in applying new semantic technologies to humanities data (Crane, Seales & Terras, 2009). One of its recent projects has been to investigate new approaches to the representation of fragmentary texts in the digital environment (Romanello, Berti, Boschetti, Babeu, & Crane, 2009). These fragments only survive as quotations or references embedded in the writings of later authors. They pose a particularly difficult challenge for scholars in identification, attribution, and dating, and hence in modelling and digital representation. This project involved designing an ontology to represent these fragmentary ancient texts and to make them available in RDF as linked data on the Web.

To design this ontology, an initial analysis of the knowledge domain was carried out using ontology learning techniques. A corpus of 170 research articles was assembled from journals on classical philology contained in the JSTOR archive. The selection of the articles was made by a philologist with particular expertise in the history of fragmentary texts. The articles were in English and covered a range of different genres. Three other specialist scholars worked with the project to assess and filter the results of the ontology learning process.

Initial pre-processing of the text corpus was done with the TreeTagger software, which tagged parts of speech and produced lemmatizations. The texts were then processed with Infomap, which was used to apply Latent Semantic Analysis. "Fragment" was chosen as the first seed term, and the Infomap associate tool was used to identify the terms mostly closely associated with it. Three categories of terms were then classified to form the second generation of seed terms:

- philological topics (e.g. "quotation");
- subjective evaluation and uncertainty (e.g. "supposition"); and,
- relationships – whole/part or spatial (e.g. "beginning" and "end").

From this, new seed terms were generated iteratively until no relevant new terms were provided. The semantic relationships were then reduced to two dimensions and clustered through the use of the k-means algorithm, enabling their representation in a two-dimensional graph.

The resulting ontology of concepts related to "fragment" was then linked into a broader ontological framework. A new class ("textual-interpretation") was created within the Philo-SURFical ontology of philosophical concepts, as a sub-class of the "interpretation" class. Authors (conjectural and certain) were modelled as part of the FOAF ontology (as instances of foaf:person), and also as part of the CIDOC-CRM ontology for cultural heritage objects (as instances of the "name" sub-class of the "appellation" class). The evidence for the fragment (i.e., the text and edition in which it was cited) was modelled through the BIBO ontology for bibliographical entities (as instances of the "book" class).

Using an ontology of this kind to represent fragments of classical texts was considered to be successful and valuable. The method used to build the ontology "demonstrated the importance of basing the ontology design on evidences that spontaneously emerge from a text corpus" (Romanello, et al., 2009, p.171).

Diderot's *Encyclopédie*

The *Encyclopédie ou Dictionnaire raisonné des sciences, des arts et des métiers* was published in Paris between 1751 and 1772, under the direction of Denis Diderot and Jean d'Alembert. It originally appeared in a total of 28 printed volumes, and contains more than 77,000 articles covering all areas of human knowledge. The articles appear in alphabetical order, but most of them are also assigned to categories and sub-categories in a scheme for the classification of knowledge. About 70% of the articles are classified in this way.

A project carried out by staff of the ARTFL Project at the University of Chicago used the *Encyclopédie* to experiment with supervised learning algorithms (Horton, Morrissey, Olsen, Roe, & Voyer 2009). There were three initial objectives:

- To train a classifier on the classified articles in the *Encyclopédie* and then apply it to classify the articles which were left unclassified in the original publication;
- To re-apply the classifier to the classified articles and compare the results to the original classifications; and,
- To apply the classification model to other French literary texts of the eighteenth century and to evaluate its applicability beyond the *Encyclopédie*.

Pre-processing of the data involved extracting the text of all the classified articles and removing the classification terms present at the beginning of these articles. TreeTagger was used to tokenize and lemmatize the texts, and frequencies for words and lemmas were computed. A Multinomial Native Bayesian classifier was then applied to the corpus. It was found to work most effectively when articles of 25 words or fewer were excluded, together with words which occurred in less than four articles. The classifier was then applied to the 22,000 unclassified articles from the original text. Manual analysis of a sample of results led to the assessment that the classifier had performed "reasonably well".

In the final stage of this project, the classifier was used to re-classify all the 54,289 originally classified articles. The classifier succeeded in assigning the "correct" classifications to 71.4% of the articles. This success rate could have been improved by some additional techniques, but it also reflects some anomalies in the original classifications. The "Grammar" class, for example, was used by the editors of the *Encyclopédie* to hide quite a few controversial and polemical entries on other subjects. A subsequent application of the classifier to 1,027 articles from an 18th-century French periodical, the *Journal de Trévoux*, led the researchers to an enhanced understanding of the meaning of several important concepts at that time. The concept of "Literature", for instance, had a much wider scope than its present-day meaning and referred to something like "universal erudition".

The next stages in this research programme will involve improving the performance of the classifiers, using such features as n-grams and information about parts of speech. Other machine learning techniques to be applied will include vector space analysis, latent semantic indexing, and other clustering models.

Henry III Fine Rolls Project

This project was carried out at the Centre for Computing in the Humanities at King's College London. It aimed to develop a range of print and digital editorial products relating to the "Fine Rolls" compiled in the reign of Henry III of England (Ciula, Spence & Vieira, 2008; Vieira & Ciula, 2007). These are parchment documents which record the amounts of money paid to the King in order to obtain various concessions and favours. The products included digital images of the original documents, English summaries and translations of the text, links between the images and the translations, indexes of people, places and subjects mentioned in the documents, and the ability to search across the whole corpus of texts. The translated summaries ("calendars") of the texts were encoded using the Text Encoding Initiative (TEI), which aimed to show the following characteristics:

- the physical structure of the rolls – they consist of several membranes sewn together;
- the structure of the English calendars; and,
- the semantic content of the roll: names of people, names of places, and key themes mentioned in the text.

The TEI only represents historical documents as a textual corpus which contains facts. It cannot give a full account of their significance and meaning as historical objects. In particular, only the immediate context given by the document is captured. An additional interpretative layer is required to capture more fully "the implicit associations between places, persons, and subjects in the documents" (Ciula, Spence & Vieira, 2008, p. 313). This layer should be connected to the encoding, but also independent of it.

The first step in developing an ontology for the Fine Rolls was to carry out a detailed analysis of what needed to be modeled. Various existing ontologies were then queried in order to identify predicates which could be reused. Among the ontologies used in this way were the CIDOC CRM, Geo, and the W3C Time ontology. The TEI-encoded documents themselves were used to populate the ontology through data extraction. This approach using a source-based model did produce a major issue: how to synchronize the data from the source documents with the ontology itself? If the text is edited and encoded first, and its information is then integrated into the ontology, what are the implications of new interpretations (e.g., of relationships between people) which are identified at the latter stage? How can these be reflected back into the encoding of the original documents?

Even allowing for this difficulty, the researchers concluded that "the use of an ontological approach, in conjunction with TEI XML mark-up for encoding the sources, represents a powerful technical framework for historical projects, which balances respect for the text as unique witness with the need to represent its historical context and interpretation" (Ciula, Spence & Vieira, 2008, p. 323). They were less convinced that the project had been able to develop an ontology which could be reused by other projects. The specific structure of the Fine Rolls was likely to limit its applicability beyond similar historical sources of the same general period.

Armadillo and Distributed Historical Sources

Armadillo is a software agent designed by the Natural Language Processing Group at the University of Sheffield. Its purpose is to provide machine readable content from large repositories for the Semantic Web, using automated methods. Doing this through manual or semi-automated annotation would be extremely costly and time-consuming. Techniques for information extraction are also unsuitable, because the documents have not already been annotated. Instead, Armadillo annotates texts automatically, with little or no manual intervention. It extracts information from a range of different sources and integrates this into a repository, from which it can be searched as well as linking back to (or annotating) the original source. These links ensure that the provenance and accuracy of the extracted information can be verified (Ciravegna, et al., 2008).

Armadillo relies primarily on redundancy – i.e., the fact that the sources contain multiple evidence for the same facts, in formats which are superficially different. Because a system knows the name of an author, for example, it can be used to identify other authors' names in digital resources, instead of relying on rule-based or statistical approaches, or manually constructed lists. By using this redundancy strategy, Armadillo can model the relevant domain, build an RDF ontology and a knowledge base, and connect findings across a corpus of distributed resources.

Armadillo was initially tested with technical documentation relating to jet engines and emer-

gency response. A project carried out between 2005 and 2007 then aimed to test its applicability to 18th-century historical sources. Its History demonstrator draws on five digital documentary collections: the Old Bailey Proceedings Online, fire insurance policies of the Sun and Royal Exchange, wills registered in the Prerogative Court of Canterbury wills, the Settlement Examinations for the parish of St Martin-In-the-Fields, and the Westminster Historical Database. The most important of these is the Old Bailey Proceedings Online, which contains the published accounts of more than 100,000 trials in the Old Bailey court in London between 1674 and 1834.

The first four of these sources are relational databases, each with their own defined set of tables. The Old Bailey Proceedings, on the other hand, are an XML encoded text repository, with more than forty tags and attributes. The problem faced by the project was how to integrate these different approaches into a single ontology. The first step was to generate RDF from each of the datasets, using XLST scripts to retain the underlying structures in the data. Rather than mapping these to a single pre-existing ontology like VICODI, however, the Armadillo project mapped the various fields into which the data had been divided, to form a relatively simple ontology for each dataset. Each of these was then linked to enable cross-searching.

Because of time constraints, several fields in the datasets were not mapped into the ontology – notably those relating to time and time-intervals. This was one of the major weaknesses of the demonstrator identified during a subsequent independent evaluation carried out by graduate students and data developers. While the Armadillo history demonstrator was acknowledged as being a very limited first step, it produced sufficient evidence to support the general value of using an ontological framework for linking distributed historical datasets.

FUTURE RESEARCH DIRECTIONS

Within this broad field, some more specific questions can be identified as constituting a future research agenda. The relationship between ontologies and text encoding is an interesting research area. Amélie Zöllner-Weber (2010) has reported on a project which takes TEI tags used for marking interpretations in a text and uses them to generate instances within an ontology which models literary characters according to their mental representations. This is a semi-automatic process which reduces the need for manual extraction and classification of data. There are numerous textual corpora which already use TEI encoding. Adding to their value through the use of ontology learning techniques will ensure that they remain a central component of the future Web of humanities data.

Zöllner-Weber's project also reflects another major area of research interest: the use of automated methods to identify instances and populate existing ontologies with them. Geleijnse and Korst (2007) describe a method of populating an ontology on historical people with information extracted from search engine query results. The first step on this process was to build a collection of snippets of text in response to Web queries. These snippets were analysed to identify names of people using a rule-based approach. An approach based on machine learning was not used, for three reasons:

- No representative training set was available. The corpus was fragmentary and multilingual.
- The corpus consisted of uncontrolled texts.
- The task of named entity recognition was simplified by the occurrence of patterns – primarily that a person's name preceded a pattern of dates (birth – death).

The results obtained from this rule-based approach compared very favourably with results obtained by using the Stanford Named Entity Recognizer.

Matching between different ontologies is another important area for future research, given the proliferation of vocabularies in the humanities and the work being done to convert them to ontology-like formats. Improving techniques for ontology matching, especially across different languages and different disciplines, has been the focus of several recent projects. Some work has already been done on using semi-automatic methods of identifying links between vocabularies, using art history texts (de Boer, van Someren & Wielinga, 2006). Two related Dutch projects also tested ontology matching techniques against cultural heritage vocabularies used by the Koninklijke Bibliotheek in the Netherlands and the Bibliothèque nationale de France (Isaac, et al., 2009; Angjeli, et al., 2009).

Designing ontologies to cope with concept shifting over time is another area of great relevance to the humanities. MuseumFinland is one of the few projects to date which has successfully addressed this problem. A spatiotemporal ontology of Finnish counties between 1865 and 2007 was developed as one of MuseumFinland's products. This was designed to enable information retrieval which takes into account more than 600 changes in the borders and names of local administrative areas in Finland during this period (Kauppinen & Hyvönen, 2007).

More large-scale textual resources are becoming available, accompanied by new search and analysis tools. There will be an increasing opportunity and incentive to apply data mining techniques to extract ontologies from these kinds of corpora. The recent "Digging into Data Challenge", sponsored jointly by the National Science Foundation (NSF), the National Endowment for the Humanities (NEH) and the Joint Information Systems Committee (JISC), is a sign of things to come. Eight projects are being funded to analyse large datasets in a variety of formats: texts, images, audio recordings, music, geographical and numerical. They include teams working with the Perseus Digital Library and the Old Bailey Proceedings (described above). The JISC-funded Connected Histories Project, being led by the University of Sheffield, is extending the work done by the Armadillo project (described above) to a total of fourteen structured and unstructured textual datasets.

A major potential impediment is the commercial ownership of important text corpora (like Early English Books Online) and existing vocabularies (like those produced by the Getty Research Institute). Geleijnse and Korst (2007, p. 156) start with the assumption that "when … all knowledge available on a domain can be found on the Web, this corpus can be used for ontology-driven information extraction." This is not the situation in many humanities fields, where key datasets and corpora are owned by commercial firms and are not freely available for ontology-related research and experimentation. This is likely to hinder future experimentation with ontology learning in the humanities.

CONCLUSION

There is a growing recognition that ontologies are vital for building next-generation Semantic Web services aimed at the humanities research community. This is despite the well-documented difficulties involved in applying ontologies to this knowledge domain. Some work has been done on developing general humanities ontologies using top-down and middle-out methodologies. VICODI and the CIDOC CRM are important examples of this process. But most research to date has gone into converting existing vocabularies and thesauri into ontology-like formats, particularly RDF and SKOS, as well as into identifying ways of matching related vocabularies.

As a result, ontology learning is still in its infancy in the humanities. Several recent projects have experimented with the application of data mining

techniques to textual corpora. For the most part, this work has emphasized using machine learning and data mining to identify instances to populate a limited range of classes, rather than building an entire ontology from scratch. The results have generally been quite encouraging. The ARTFL researchers working on the *Encyclopédie* project drew the conclusion that "traditional humanistic inquiry can be enhanced and broadened through the judicious application of machine learning and data mining techniques" (Horton, et al., 2009).

REFERENCES

Angjeli, A., Isaac, A., Cloarec, T., Martin, F., van der Meij, L., Matthezing, H., & Schlobach, S. (2009). Semantic Web and vocabulary interoperability: An experiment with illumination collections. *International Cataloguing and Bibliographic Control*, *38*(2), 25–29.

Benjamins, V. R., Contreras, J., Blázquez, M., Dodero, J. M., García, A., & Navas, E. … Wert, C. (2004). Cultural heritage and the Semantic Web. In C. Bussler, J. Davies, D. Fensel, & R. Studer (Eds.), *The Semantic Web: Research and applications: First European Semantic Web Symposium, ESWS 2004, Heraklion, Crete, Greece, May 10-12, 2004: Proceedings* (LNCS 3053), (pp.433–444). Berlin, Germany: Springer-Verlag.

Ciravegna, F., Greengrass, M., Hitchcock, T., Chapman, S., McLaughlin, J., & Bhagdev, R. (2008). Finding needles in haystacks: Data-mining in historical datasets. In Greengrass, M., & Hughes, L. (Eds.), *The virtual representation of the past* (pp. 65–79). Farnham, UK: Ashgate.

Ciula, A., Spence, P., & Vieira, J. M. (2008). Expressing complex associations in medieval historical documents: The Henry III Fine Rolls project. *Literary and Linguistic Computing*, *23*(3), 311–325. doi:10.1093/llc/fqn018

Crane, G., Seales, B., & Terras, M. (2009). Cyberinfrastructure for classical philology. *Digital Humanities Quarterly, 3*(1). Retrieved March 10, 2010, from http://www.digitalhumanities.org/dhq/vol/3/1/000023.html

de Boer, V., van Someren, M., & Wielinga, B. (2006). Extracting instances of relations from Web documents using redundancy. In Y. Sure & J. Domingue (Eds.), *The Semantic Web: Research and applications: 3rd European Semantic Web Conference, ESWC 2006 Budva, Montenegro, June 11-14, 2006, Proceedings* (LNCS 4011), (pp. 245-258). Berlin, Germany: Springer-Verlag.

Doerr, M. (2003). The CIDOC CRM: An ontological approach to semantic interoperability of metadata. *AI Magazine, 24*(3), 75–92.

Geleijnse, G., & Korst, J. (2007). Creating a dead poets society: Extracting a social network of historical persons from the Web. In K. Aberer, P. Cudré-Mauroux, K. Choi, N. Noy, D. Allemang, K. Lee, … G. Schreiber (Eds.), *Proceedings of the 6th International Semantic Web and 2nd Asian Conference on Asian Semantic Web Conference (Busan, Korea, November 11 - 15, 2007)* (LNCS 4825), (pp. 156-168). Berlin, Germany: Springer-Verlag.

Gill, T. (2004). Building semantic bridges between museums, libraries and archives: The CIDOC Conceptual Reference Model. *First Monday, 9*(5). Retrieved March 10, 2010, from http://firstmonday.org/htbin/cgiwrap/bin/ojs/index.php/fm/article/view/1145/1065

Greengrass, M. (2007). *Ontologies and semantic interoperability for humanities data.* Paper presented at Ontologies and Semantic Interoperability for Humanities Data workshop, Edinburgh. Retrieved March 10, 2010, from http://www.nesc.ac.uk/action/esi/download.cfm?index=3524

Horton, R., Morrissey, R., Olsen, M., Roe, G., & Voyer, R. (2009). Mining eighteenth century ontologies: Machine learning and knowledge classification in the Encyclopédie. *DHQ: Digital Humanities Quarterly, 3*(2). Retrieved March 10, 2010 from http://digitalhumanities.org/dhq/vol/3/2/000044.html

Hyvönen, E., Mäkelä, E., Kauppinen, T., Alm, O., Kurki, J., & Ruotsalo, T. … Nyberg, K. (2009). CultureSampo - a national publication system of cultural heritage on the Semantic Web 2.0. In L. Aroyo, P. Traverso, F. Ciravegna, P. Cimiano, T. Heath, E. Hyvönen, … E. Simperl (Eds.) *The Semantic Web: Research and applications: ESWC 2009 Heraklion, Crete, Greece, May 31–June 4, 2009 Proceedings* (LNCS 5554) (pp. 851-856). Berlin, Germany: Springer-Verlag.

Isaac, A., Wang, S., Zinn, C., Matthezing, H., van der Meij, L., & Schlobach, S. (2009). Evaluating thesaurus alignments for semantic interoperability in the library domain. *IEEE Intelligent Systems, 24*(2), 76–86. doi:10.1109/MIS.2009.26

Kauppinen, T., & Hyvönen, E. (2007). Modeling and reasoning about changes in ontology time series. In Kishore, R., Ramesh, R., & Sharman, R. (Eds.), *Ontologies: A handbook of principles, concepts and applications in Information Systems* (pp. 319–338). Berlin, Germany: Springer-Verlag.

Mirzaee, V., Iverson, L., & Hamidzadeh, B. (2005). Computational representation of semantics in historical documents. In *Humanities, Computers and Cultural Heritage: Proceedings of the XVI International Conference of the Association for History and Computing, 14-17 September 2005* (pp. 199-206). Amsterdam, The Netherlands: Royal Netherlands Academy of Arts and Sciences.

Nagypál, G. (2005). History ontology building: The technical view. In *Humanities, Computers and Cultural Heritage: Proceedings of the XVI International Conference of the Association for History and Computing, 14-17 September 2005* (pp. 207-214). Amsterdam, The Netherlands: Royal Netherlands Academy of Arts and Sciences.

Nagypál, G., Deswarte, R., & Oosthoek, J. (2005). Applying the Semantic Web: The VICODI experience in creating visual contextualization for history. *Literary and Linguistic Computing, 20*(3), 327–349. doi:10.1093/llc/fqi037

Ore, C., & Eide, Ø. (2009). TEI and cultural heritage ontologies: Exchange of information? *Literary and Linguistic Computing, 24*(2), 161–172. doi:10.1093/llc/fqp010

Power, D., et al. (2007). *The lands of the Normans in England (1204–1244): Technical background.* Retrieved August 6th, 2010, from http://www.hrionline.ac.uk/normans/technical.shtml

Riva, P., Doerr, M., & Žumer, M. (2009). FRBRoo: Enabling a common view of information from cultural heritage institutions. *International Cataloguing and Bibliographic Control, 38*(2), 30–34.

Romanello, M., Berti, M., Boschetti, F., Babeu, A., & Crane, G. (2009). Rethinking critical editions of fragmentary texts by ontologies. In S. Mornati & T. Hedlund (Eds.), *Rethinking Electronic Publishing: Innovation in Communication Paradigms and Technologies: Proceedings of 13th International Conference on Electronic Publishing* (pp. 155-174). Milan, Italy: CILEA.

Schreiber, G., Amin, A., Aroyo, L., van Assem, M., de Boer, V., & Hardman, L. (2008). Semantic annotation and search of cultural-heritage collections: The MultimediaN e-culture demonstrator. *Journal of Web Semantics, 6*(4), 243–249. doi:10.1016/j.websem.2008.08.001

Veltman, K. H. (2004). Towards a Semantic Web for culture. *JoDI: Journal of Digital Information, 4*(4). Retrieved March 10, 2010, from http://jodi.ecs.soton.ac.uk/Articles/v04/i04/Veltman/

Vieira, J. M., & Ciula, A. (2007). *Implementing an RDF/OWL ontology on Henry the III Fine Rolls.* Paper presented at OWLED 2007, Innsbruck, Austria. Retrieved March 10, 2010, from http://www.webont.org/owled/2007/PapersPDF/submission_6.pdf

Zhou, L. (2007). Ontology learning: State of the art and open issues. *Information Technology Management, 8*, 241–252. doi:10.1007/s10799-007-0019-5

Zöllner-Weber, A. (2010). *Text encoding and ontology – enlarging an ontology by semi-automatic generated instances.* Paper presented at Digital Humanities 2010. Retrieved August 5, 2010, from http://dh2010.cch.kcl.ac.uk/academic-programme/abstracts/papers/pdf/ab-643.pdf

ADDITIONAL READING

Antoniou, G., & van Harmelen, F. (2003). Web Ontology Language: OWL. In Staab, S., & Studer, R. (Eds.), *Handbook on Ontologies* (pp. 67–92). Berlin: Springer-Verlag.

Babeu, A., Bamman, D., Crane, G., Kummer, R., & Weaver, G. (2007). Named entity identification and cyberinfrastructure. In L. Kovács, N. Fuhr, & C. Meghini (Eds.) *Research and Advanced Technology for Digital Libraries: 11th European Conference, ECDL 2007, Budapest, Hungary, September 16-21, 2007: Proceedings* (Lecture Notes in Computer Science, 4675) (pp. 259-270). Berlin: Springer-Verlag.

Benjamins, V. R., Fensel, D., Decker, S., & Gómez Pérez, A. (1999). (KA)2: building ontologies for the Internet: a mid-term report. *International Journal of Human-Computer Studies, 51,* 687–712. doi:10.1006/ijhc.1999.0275

Berthold, M. (2003). Fuzzy logic. In Berthold, M., & Hand, D. J. (Eds.), *Intelligent Data Analysis* (pp. 321–350). Berlin: Springer-Verlag. doi:10.1007/978-3-540-48625-1_9

Breitman, K., Casanova, M. A., & Truszkowski, W. (2007). *Semantic Web: Concepts, Technologies and Applications.* London: Springer.

Cimiano, P., Völker, J., & Studer, R. (2006). Ontologies on demand? - A description of the state-of-the-art, applications, challenges and trends for ontology learning from text. *Information. Wissenschaft und Praxis, 57*(6-7), 315–320.

Cohen, D. J. (2006). From Babel to knowledge: data mining large digital collections. *D-Lib Magazine* 12 (3). Retrieved August 6 2010 from http://www.dlib.org/dlib/march06/cohen/03cohen.html

Delve, J. (2008). Humanities data warehousing. In Wang, J. (Ed.), *Encyclopedia of Data Warehousing and Mining* (2nd ed., pp. 987–992). Hershey: IGI Global. doi:10.4018/9781605660103.ch153

Delve, J., & Allen, M. (2006). Large-scale integrated historical projects – does data warehousing offer any scope for their creation and analysis? *History & Computing, 13*(3), 301–313. doi:10.3366/hac.2001.13.3.301

Delve, J., & Healey, R. (2005). Is there a role for data warehousing technology in historical research? In *Humanities, Computers and Cultural Heritage: Proceedings of the XVI International Conference of the Association for History and Computing, 14-17 September 2005* (pp. 106-111). Amsterdam: Royal Netherlands Academy of Arts and Sciences.

Deswarte, R., & Oostoek, J. (2005). Clio's ontology criteria: the theory and experience of building a history ontology. Paper presented at Humanities, Computers and Cultural Heritage: XVIth International Conference of the Association for History and Computing, Royal Netherlands Academy of Arts and Sciences, Amsterdam.

Farrar, S., Lewis, W. D., & Langendoen, D. T. (2002). An ontology for linguistic annotation. In *Semantic Web Meets Language Resources: Papers from the AAAI Workshop* (Technical Report WS-02-16) (pp. 11–19). Menlo Park, CA.

Halpern, J. Y. (2005). *Reasoning about uncertainty.* Cambridge, Mass: MIT Press.

Hudson, P. (2000). *History by Numbers: an Introduction to Quantitative Approaches.* London: Arnold.

Lüngen, H., & Storrer, A. (2007). Domain ontologies and wordnets in OWL: modelling options. *Zeitschrift für Computerlinguistik und Sprachtechnologie, 22*(2), 1–17.

McCarty, W. (2005). *Humanities Computing.* London: Palgrave Macmillan. doi:10.1057/9780230504219

Pasin, M., & Motta, E. (2009). Ontological requirements for annotation and navigation of philosophical resources. *Synthese* (Online First). Retrieved August 5, 2010, from http://www.springerlink.com/content/20275389857wj5v3/fulltext.pdf

Renear, A. H., Yunseon, C., Jin Ha, L., & Schmidt, S. (2006). Axiomatizing FRBR: An exercise in the formal ontology of cultural objects. In [Paris.]. *Proceedings of Digital Humanities, 2006,* 164–170.

Robertson, B. (2009). Exploring historical RDF with Heml. *DHQ: Digital Humanities Quarterly* 3 (1). Retrieved August 5, 2010, from http://www.digitalhumanities.org/dhq/vol/003/1/000026.html

Shirky, C. (2005). Ontology is overrated: categories, links, and tags. Retrieved August 5, 2010, from http://www.shirky.com/writings/ontology_overrated.html

Smith, D. C. P. (2008). Re-discovering Wittgenstein. In *Philosophy of the Information Society: Proceedings of 30th International Wittgenstein Symposium, vol. 2* (pp. 208-210). Heusenstamm: Ontos Verlag.

Tummarello, G., Morbidoni, C., Puliti, P., & Piazza, F. (2008). A proposal for textual encoding based on Semantic Web tools. *Online Information Review, 32*(4), 467–477. doi:10.1108/14684520810897340

Zöllner-Weber, A. (2007). Noctua literaria - A system for a formal description of literary characters. In Rehm, G., Witt, A., & Lemnitzer, L. (Eds.), *Data Structures for Linguistic Resources and Applications* (pp. 113–121). Tübingen: Günter Narr.

Zöllner-Weber, A., & Apollon, D. (2008). The challenge of modelling information and data in the humanities. In T. Hug (Ed.), *Proceedings of the International Conference on Explorations of New Spaces, Relations and Dynamics in Digital Media Ecologies*. Innsbrück: Innsbrück University Press.

Zöllner-Weber, A., & Pichler, A. (2008). Utilizing OWL for Wittgenstein's Tractatus. *In Philosophy of the Information Society: Proceedings of 30th International Wittgenstein Symposium, vol. 2* (pp. 248-250). Heusenstamm: Ontos Verlag.

Zöllner-Weber, A., & Witt, A. (2006). Ontology for a formal description of literary characters. In [Paris.]. *Proceedings of Digital Humanities, 2006,* 350–352.

KEY TERMS AND DEFINITIONS

Cultural Heritage: The artefacts and attributes of a society which are inherited from past generations.

Humanities: Academic disciplines which study the human condition.

Thesauri: A type of controlled vocabulary which shows the hierarchical relationships between terms.

Controlled Vocabulary: A list of words and phrases for use in information retrieval, showing authorized and preferred terms.

Bibliographical: Relating to the description and study of books and other publications.

Text Encoding: The representation of texts in digital form using a markup language.

Text Corpora: A large and structured collection of texts for linguistic analysis.

ENDNOTES

[1]   http://www.humanities.org.au/About/Overview.htm

Chapter 11
Ontology–Based Knowledge Capture and Sharing in Enterprise Organisations

Aba-Sah Dadzie
University of Sheffield, UK

Victoria Uren
University of Sheffield, UK

Fabio Ciravegna
University of Sheffield, UK

ABSTRACT

Despite years of effort in building organisational taxonomies, the potential of ontologies to support knowledge management in complex technical domains is under-exploited. The authors of this chapter present an approach to using rich domain ontologies to support sense-making tasks associated with resolving mechanical issues. Using Semantic Web technologies, the authors have built a framework and a suite of tools which support the whole semantic knowledge lifecycle. These are presented by describing the process of issue resolution for a simulated investigation concerning failure of bicycle brakes. Foci of the work have included ensuring that semantic tasks fit in with users' everyday tasks, to achieve user acceptability and support the flexibility required by communities of practice with differing local sub-domains, tasks, and terminology.

INTRODUCTION

Knowledge management (KM) in enterprise organisations involves the analysis of very large scale, distributed, multi- and cross-media data, in order to extract the information contained, and convert this to the knowledge required to support timely, effective decision-making. The X-Media project[1] (Ciravegna & Staab, 2005) aimed to enhance KM in such environments by harnessing the power of Semantic Web (SW) technology. In this chapter we describe the use of SW technology to support the KM lifecycle, from the retrieval of existing knowledge and the generation of new

DOI: 10.4018/978-1-60960-625-1.ch011

knowledge, through its capture and storage, to manipulation in use and the resulting enrichment of the knowledge, and finally to sharing and reusing the rich knowledge gained.

The issue investigation scenario used to guide the presentation of this chapter involves teams with varied expertise, working independently and collaboratively to identify the causes of mechanical issues. Findings during the course of an investigation and the lessons learnt when it is concluded are shared with interested parties. Flexible methods for each step of the knowledge lifecycle are therefore necessary to satisfy the variations in requirements of different user communities, to support the multiple perspectives each brings to their normal activities (Wenger, 2004).

Ontologies provide a useful tool for formalising, enriching and disseminating knowledge. KM and analysis structured around SW technology starts with the modelling of domain ontologies to provide formal definitions of users, their environments and the knowledge-intensive activities they engage in. We employ a modular ontology design, so as to allow a clear distinction between the sub-parts of each domain, and to allow reuse of relevant public ontologies (such as OWL-Time[2] to record event occurrence). Using the ontology, we formalise and capture the information end users interact with, and store it in shared semantic (knowledge) repositories. We also make use of ontology-based annotation to enrich knowledge capture. Further, we use the ontologies to guide exploratory knowledge discovery and analysis from the shared semantic knowledge repositories and other related sources of information (e.g., databases) and knowledge (e.g., as derived by human experts).

An evaluation of our approach with different groups of target end users in industrial settings confirmed the enhanced KM that results. Participants in the usability evaluations reported an increase in ability to retrieve information from distributed resources and collect this in a single workspace, allowing their analysis to be grounded in the

context of relevant evidence. The participants especially valued the increased "intelligence" of the knowledge framework evaluated – the interpretation of the domain knowledge captured to the ontologies used to support KM and the analytical activity. Overall, the participants noted increased confidence in decision-making based on the output of the semantic, context-driven KM and analysis.

This chapter is structured as follows: we summarise the limitations of the traditional approach to KM in large, complex organisations, and the potential claimed by SW technologies for enhancing KM. We then discuss the tools and functionality available to support SW-based KM and analysis. We introduce the Issue Resolution process and a test case developed during X-Media to demonstrate the research carried out. This leads to a review of the state of the art, with a focus on visual solutions. We continue to describe the ontology which serves as the spine around which we structure the interactive construction of knowledge workspaces that support intuitive information retrieval and analytics. This leads to a detailed description of the ontology-based knowledge creation, use and enrichment enabled, throughout the different phases of the knowledge lifecycle. A brief description of the final evaluation of the integrated knowledge framework developed is followed by an examination of the challenges faced in semantic KM, and our approach to resolving these. We conclude with a brief look at future research directions and a summary of our contribution to enhanced semantic KM.

BACKGROUND

Traditional approaches to KM, especially in large, hierarchical organisations, often assume centralised, pre-defined sources of information and knowledge that aim to cater to requirements across user groups and activities. In practice, this limits effective working practices (Hayes et al., 2005); the differences in tasks, individual users, organisational departments and the increasingly common Communities of Practice (CoPs) created to share knowledge and carry out specialised tasks (Wenger, 2004) mean that more flexible methods for knowledge generation, access and use must be established.

Golder and Huberman (2006), for instance, discuss the conflicts due to differing levels of granularity used to describe objects, and the variability in terminology used to verbalise the collective knowledge that contributes to sense-making. They highlight the difficulty this poses to information labelling and organisation and therefore, retrieval and reuse. It is important to ensure that the knowledge within an organisation can be shared across sub-groups and processes (within the restrictions of security) – this is the reasoning behind the creation of centralised data schemas and storage facilities. It is equally important that all users are able to interpret correctly this shared knowledge, to ensure effective (re)use that results also in the generation of new, richer knowledge (Wenger, 2004). We handle the inherent conflicts by adopting the formalism afforded by ontologies – from which commonly agreed terminology (with known, sometimes community-specific synonyms, acronyms, etc.) may be retrieved to describe or annotate information. This increases correctness in interpreting shared knowledge, leading ultimately to more confident and effective analysis and decision-making.

We take an approach to enhancing KM using SW technology, to cater to different CoPs interacting with each other and their collective knowledge spaces, each constructing their community- or task-specific perspective on shared organisational knowledge. We build on existing research (such as that of Bonifacio, Bouquet, & Cuel, 2002, Tempich, Pinto, & Staab, 2006), and model the users, dynamic CoPs, larger departments and the activities they carry out using a modular domain ontology. An important feature of our design is to support and enhance end users' regular activities without requiring significant changes to working practices. This is especially important in complex organisations where the high initial cost associated with significant changes to existing practice may impede the adoption of more effective tools and techniques.

Using a case study involving the analytical investigation carried out to determine the root causes of issues identified in complex domains, we will illustrate the solutions developed in X-Media to meet the requirements for semantic knowledge creation and management in such environments. To comply with data sensitivity issues we employ a simulated investigation that spans the complete knowledge lifecycle, derived by studying real users in large, complex enterprise organisations. The investigation concerns irregular mechanical brake failure in pedal cycles, a test case developed to illustrate all the key features of actual issue investigations.

The Issue Resolution (IR) process is triggered by the receipt of reports describing an issue discovered on a mechanical component or assembly. An issue owner is nominated and an Investigation Process Team (IPT) is formed to include a range of expertise and experience that brings multiple perspectives to the investigation. An initial search of legacy data is performed based on the issue description, to determine if information exists on the same or other closely related events. The IPT must analyse related information, most of which is found in legacy corpora, contextualise this information and convert it to knowledge, often relying on their collective experience and expertise. Figure 1 summarises the IR process.

IR routinely spans several weeks or months, during which time the IPT must identify the links between apparently disconnected pieces of evidence and build these into a set of arguments that lead to a verified and agreed conclusion. The IPT performs an exhaustive investigation of the evidence related to an issue, supported by the hierarchical breakdown and exploration of a set of hypotheses formulated for the root (and additional) causes of the issue. The members of the

Figure 1. Flow chart illustrating the Issue Resolution process

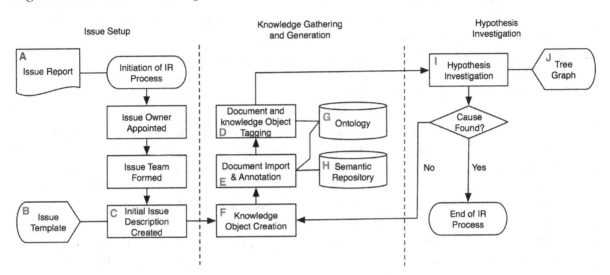

IPT work independently on various aspects of the investigation, consulting other (independent or external) experts as required. They meet regularly to share and collate their findings. The issue owner serves as the "knowledge gatekeeper", being responsible for validating knowledge generated as the investigation progresses. The investigation is concluded when the exit criteria set at the beginning of the process have been met, and a solution implemented, verified and validated. The lessons learnt should ideally be recorded such that the new knowledge acquired may be reused in subsequent investigations and other related activities. In X-Media we proposed the use of SW technology to support the knowledge-intensive activities carried out during issue investigation.

Proposing SW technology and in particular, ontologies, as a tool for managing work practices and knowledge is becoming increasingly popular. Early work includes that of (Ernst & Storey, 2003), who use the process of creating a wine ontology to illustrate the cycle between ontology engineering, knowledge creation and use. They begin by modeling the (wine) domain and knowledge in other closely related domains (in this case, meals corresponding to specific types of wine). After crafting the ontology they populate

it with instances; this requires the knowledge acquired by domain experts with experience. The knowledge base that results is then available to support activities in the domain. This leads in turn to further population and the recognition of the need to extend the original model, to include new knowledge or existing knowledge omitted at the original design stage, or to refine the original model in accordance with evolving requirements.

Each of these steps will be carried out by different users – domain experts as well as ontology engineers. It is necessary to support each of these end users (Ernst & Storey, 2003), to build and modify the knowledge base and to make use of the shared knowledge. Translating effective use of ontologies to different users and domains is however not a simple task. Significant amounts of effort are typically expended on building domain ontologies and/or adapting generalised ontologies to an environment; this effort is wasted if the subsequent evolution that naturally occurs, due to changes in working practices and knowledge, is not mapped to effective management and evolution of the ontologies. One of the better known ontology engineering tools is Protégé (Gennari et al., 2003). While Protégé is widely used in the knowledge engineering community, anecdotal evidence suggests that the domain experts who are often the owners of the ontologies in an organisation encounter difficulty using Protégé and other ontology engineering tools (see also Ernst & Storey, 2003). This is largely because these tools are built to support the knowledge engineering task, which is not core to the organisations that must manage KM activity structured around ontologies.

Among the solutions being developed to provide more effective support for browsing and editing ontologies is the use of visual interfaces. Ernst and Storey (2003), Mularz and Lyell (2004), among others, discuss the challenges inherent in the analysis of very large knowledge spaces, in order to extract relevant information and codify this in ways that support further knowledge discovery and analysis. Ernst and Storey (2003) consider the advantages information visualisation brings to data exploration and comprehension, and sharing its information content with others. Mularz and Lyell (2004) look at the use of SW technology with mind maps, and examine methods for conceptualising the entities within knowledge spaces; with an aim to create knowledge maps that support their exploration and obtain more effective decision-making.

Castro et al. (2006) use concept maps to support knowledge elicitation during the construction and maintenance of ontologies. They note the usefulness of the informal visual technique for capturing and sharing knowledge within distributed communities. Hayes et al. (2005) also make use of concept maps to provide user-centred elicitation, expression and communication of domain knowledge, such that it is easily formalised in ontologies. They found that the technique was successful predominantly because it supports flexible exploration, allowing end users to iteratively build meaningful knowledge structures. While for ontology-based KM the models are largely predetermined, visualisation can aid the understanding of shared ontologies and their extension for specialised tasks. Finally, (Katifori, Halatsis, Lepouras, Vassilakis, & Giannopoulou, 2007)

provide a detailed survey of ontology management tools, grouping functionality by characteristics such as visualisation type and the methods used to present the structure of ontologies.

To encourage successful uptake of novel solutions for KM they must be woven into users' regular activities. Working from the results of user studies in X-Media, and employing an iterative cycle of design and development, we built an integrated, interactive knowledge framework with a graphical user interface (UI) that allows access, from a single point, to a variety of tools for semantic KM and analysis. The *XMediaBox* provides a container in which to collect knowledge from multiple sources, creating a *knowledge space* that enables intuitive interaction with information, resulting in new knowledge generation and enrichment, and support for sharing this knowledge effectively with other interested parties. Dadzie, Iria, et al. (2009), Dadzie, Lanfranchi, and Petrelli (2009) detail the initial UI design and modules. This chapter describes the research carried out for the remainder of the project, based on a review of the outcomes of the initial stages.

Different options are made available, dependent on the user's task and the resources and artefacts they normally interact with. These include form-filling to capture the information that leads to ontology evolution – chiefly by creating new instances of existing concepts, and variation in terminology such as synonyms, acronyms and abbreviations. An example of such an information capture task is the recording of the metadata associated with a new task, to enable subsequent retrieval from shared semantic repositories (points B and C during *Issue Setup* in Figure 1).

As do, for e.g., Castro et al. (2006), Hayes et al. (2005), we provide visual support for working with the knowledge contained in ontologies. This allows the end user to focus on the task being performed, rather than on the (still necessary tasks) ontology management and evolution. The knowledge generated as a side effect of users' activities in this case is captured transparently. An example of a task where visual ontology management is performed is root cause analysis (see points I and J during *Hypothesis Investigation* in Figure 1).

We discuss next the use of ontologies and other relevant SW technology, via the X-Media knowledge framework, to enable more effective use, management and sharing of knowledge.

ONTOLOGY-BASED KNOWLEDGE MANAGEMENT

SW technology benefits complex scenario analysis, through the formalism provided by ontologies, used with semantic repositories, to support the retrieval of the knowledge contained within data, the enrichment and generation of new knowledge as end users interact with it, and finally the sharing and reuse of knowledge in related activities (Hayes et al., 2005). We introduce this section with a brief discussion of the design of the domain ontologies that serve as the spine on which we structure semantic KM. We then describe the flexible, customisable, SW-based solutions provided via the X-Media knowledge framework to support the variations in information and knowledge requirements of the different CoPs who must interact with each other and very large amounts of complex, distributed, heterogeneous data in order to obtain the knowledge required to carry out their normal working activities and critical decision-making. We illustrate this by mapping the distinct but overlapping phases in a typical issue investigation case to corresponding stages in the KM lifecycle.

A User-Centric, Modular Domain Ontology

We consider the construction of domain ontologies from the perspective of use – the goal being to support end users to more effectively and efficiently carry out knowledge intensive activities. We therefore look at ontologies as a source of

shared, formalised knowledge, a repository built by studying the types of users and CoPs in an organisation, the specific tasks each performs, and the artefacts users employ in their work.

The IR application described in this chapter addresses the diagnosis of issues arising in mechanical systems such as the pedal bicycle example we use. These issues may be of any kind affecting the in-service performance of mechanical systems. Therefore the ontology has to cover a broad spectrum of different kinds of information types for this case, concerning different bicycle models: the bicycle component parts and the materials they are made of, physical mechanisms that may cause issues, the locations, on the bicycle and geographically, where issues are reported, the different kinds of documents in which issues are described and so forth. As a consequence the ontology required has several distinct sub-domains. Figure 2 shows the sub-parts of the ontology relevant to the use case.

Other groups in the organisation can also benefit from the ontological information, however they don't necessarily need all the kinds of information used in IR: issue investigation has particularly complex requirements because it needs to be able to tackle all possible kinds of issues. For example, a group responsible for design would need all the knowledge about materials and components but would have lower interest in knowledge about specific in-service events.

After initial experiments with a monolithic ontology (one that was stored in a single OWL – Web Ontology Language – file), we changed to a modular design. Building modular ontologies is considered good practice for the same reasons that modular software is, i.e., they are "easier to understand, verify, debug, extend, reuse parts of, and thus facilitate collaborative development" (Grau, Parsia, Sirin, & Kalyanpur, 2006, pp. 198); (see also Gennari et al., 2003, Hayes et al., 2005). The X-Media developers found the modular ontology easier to use, because it was more apparent where each different kind of knowledge was located. It was also easier for the ontology

Figure 2. An extract from the domain ontology for the Bicycle Assembly, showing the sub-sections relevant to the test bed. On the left a simplified overview showing only inheritance properties. On the right, an extension of the general Mechanical System ontology created to provide a test case for root cause investigation is shown, with links from the top level ontology to selected concepts and information about other ontology relations (bottom, left and top, right)

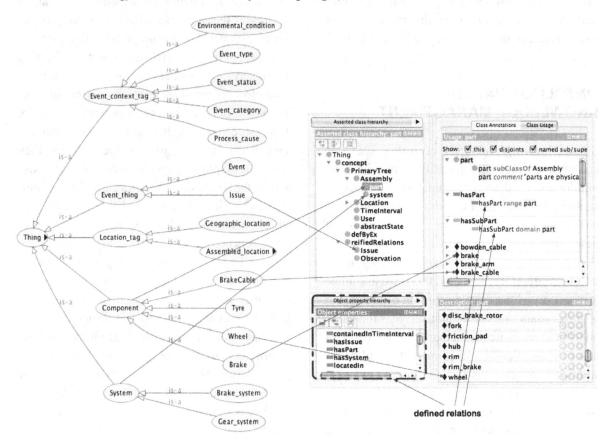

engineers to produce different versions of the ontology for different tasks, e.g., (sub-)ontologies were built for two different sub-domains in aerospace engineering, by extending and linking to relevant sub-parts of the Mechanical System ontology. These were Experimental Vibration, to support an engine testing group, and Issue Resolution, geared predominantly at service engineers.

The ontology modules that were incorporated into the ontology produced for IR comprised: Mechanisms, Bicycles, Systems, Components, Services, Locations, Events, Knowledge Sources (documents) and Agents (people and organisations). The example developed in the rest of this chapter will demonstrate how knowledge from these sub-domains is used in the IR process.

The Knowledge Management Lifecycle

We employ a bottom-up approach to semantic KM, and map the requirements of different CoPs to corresponding stages in the knowledge lifecycle and to the sub-parts of the domain ontologies that describe the tasks they perform. The support required for each stage of the knowledge lifecycle varies based on users' tasks, information requirements and the final end use of the knowledge gained.

Table 1. Mödritscher's lifecycle stages

X-Media knowledge lifecycle stage	Mödritscher (2009) stage
1. generation or retrieval	authoring, mining
2. capture and storage	modeling, authoring
3. interaction with knowledge, resulting in enrichment	modeling, application, evaluation
4. sharing	application
5. reuse (other users, in other tasks & scenarios)	application

However a single mechanism underlies our support for each – the ontologies that provide a formal description of the tasks that users must perform and the artefacts employed. We follow Bonifacio et al. (2002), Tempich et al. (2006), and maintain the autonomy of each sub-domain, independent tasks and activities and the different types of users and CoPs, by using the modular ontology design previously described. As do Bonifacio et al. (2002) we support co-ordination between different parts of the domain and the corresponding ontology by defining the relationships that cross sub-domains, allowing different units to map their context onto that of related units, much as is already done on an informal basis within knowledge networks and CoPs (Berners-Lee, Hendler, & Lassila, 2001). This highlights the links between communities, tasks and activities, resulting in more intuitive navigation through the larger knowledge space, and therefore, enhanced knowledge discovery and analysis. Each user or CoP is able to focus on the knowledge most pertinent to their environment and activities, within the context of the larger, complete, shared knowledge space, leading also to increased confidence in decision-making.

Mödritscher (2009) has proposed a lifecycle model specifically for semantic information systems. This has the stages modeling, application, authoring, mining and evaluation. The X-Media KM framework, although using a different design modeled based on the ontology, may be loosely mapped to the lifecycle stages defined by Mödritscher (2009) shown in Table 1.

Our lifecycle model is not dissimilar to other studies on the development of methodologies for building and maintaining ontologies for real-world use (e.g., Castro et al., 2006, Ernst & Storey, 2003, Tempich et al., 2006). In the XMediaBox, the applications built directly on the structure of the ontology are for knowledge retrieval and root cause analysis. Authoring occurs in several places in the XMediaBox, e.g., at the issue description stage and when the user annotates retrieved knowledge. Mining is not discussed in detail in this chapter; this however occurs during Information Extraction (IE), as a preliminary step to populating the knowledge base with automatically extracted annotation of legacy data. Evaluation in this model corresponds to evaluating and refining the semantic model of the knowledge end users interact with. This is demonstrated during root cause analysis, where the user examines evidence to determine its relevance to an investigation. Where necessary, users may formulate hypotheses for new root causes (which map to new concepts and instances in the domain ontology), and verify or validate these using knowledge derived from the evidence examined.

We present in the following sections the outcome of the research in X-Media into enhanced support for shared knowledge creation and interaction that results in an increasingly richer cycle of enrichment and further knowledge generation.

Knowledge Retrieval

The knowledge lifecycle starts with information retrieval, when evidence for the issue is collected, based on the information initially provided to the issue owner and the IPT (steps A-C in the *Issue Setup* in Figure 1). In the *Bike Brakes* case this will be the recorded statements of customers reporting the failure of their brakes and any repair reports generated for bikes taken into the workshop as a result. An ontology-backed form is used to record the initial description of each issue, from which a (domain-specific) terminology recogniser is used to extract key terms in the user's input, map these terms to corresponding ontology concepts and store the information as metadata for the issue in question. Form fields include product type, i.e., the bicycle model, and the component parts affected – valid values for each of these should be existing instances of the corresponding concepts in the domain ontology. However the (deterioration) mechanisms seen to contribute to the issue may match existing instances of the concept, e.g., commonly occurring *corrosion* or *wear*, or users may enter new terms corresponding to mechanisms not captured to the ontology – comprising new knowledge, or more commonly, variations in terminology and language local to specific CoPs. Such information will feed into ontology evolution, which we will discuss later. Values for the form fields are captured as metadata to the semantic repository; the formalised knowledge thus obtained is used to formulate and trigger ontology-based queries to retrieve information from legacy corpora related to the issue; the evidence retrieved is the base from which further user-driven information retrieval will occur (see Figures 3 and 4).

Hybrid querying (user-specified combinations of keyword- and ontology-based queries) of text documents is provided by a plug-in (Bhagdev, Chakravarthy, Chapman, Ciravegna, & Lanfranchi, 2008). This is used with content- and feature-based retrieval for image and cross-media docu-ments[3], work done as part of the X-Media project, to reduce users' cognitive load during information retrieval from the very large legacy databases that are the norm in today's knowledge-intensive society. However, retrieving relevant documents from the legacy data stores is only the first step in analysis. An important aim of X-Media was to move from the norm, interaction with data, to the more abstract but conceptual interaction with the knowledge contained within data (Ciravegna & Staab, 2005, Iria, 2009). The two main types of search available from the XMediaBox retrieve not just documents that satisfy queries, but also the knowledge contained within them. This is achieved by structuring the original knowledge capture (both user-controlled and automated IE) and continued enrichment around the domain ontologies (discussed next).

Knowledge Generation & Formalisation

A significant benefit of SW technology is the support for formalising and storing knowledge. Storing the context (of use) with information is key to ensuring the reusability of the knowledge thus derived; we therefore map the content and context of the data and information end users interact with to corresponding entities in ontologies, and capture the knowledge derived to shared semantic repositories. The ontologies that serve as the common, agreed domain knowledge therefore aid its interpretation, especially important for knowledge sharing and reuse, both within the domain itself and in other related areas.

Document annotation is an important contributor to semantic knowledge generation and retrieval (Brewster et al., 2007, Giovannetti, Marchi, Montemagni, & Bartolini, 2008), especially for IE from the very large amounts of distributed, heterogeneous data that is the norm in large, complex, enterprise organisations (step E under *Knowledge Gathering and Generation* in Figure 1, as a step to populating the *Ontology* (G) and *Semantic Repository* (H)). However, a significant lesson learnt during X-Media is the difficulty in obtaining sufficient amounts of high quality annotation across data and document types from domain experts (Iria, 2009). X-Media therefore explored automatic methods for annotating new corpora (Iria, 2009, provides an extensive discussion of the approach taken). Following this, as end users (domain experts) carry out their normal KM and analysis activities and interact with data and the knowledge extracted (as annotation), errors in the automatic IE are corrected and new annotation generated, using tools such as the ontology-based tagging accessed via the XMediaBox. The results are fed back to the automated IE, gradually increasing precision and recall in an iterative cycle of annotation and IE. Similar approaches to iterative refinement and enrichment of annotation are described in (Giovannetti et al., 2008, McShane, Nirenburg, Beale, & O'Hara, 2005).

Web sites such as *Flickr*[4] and *Del.icio.us*[5] allow users to (collaboratively) create key terms to tag content; this information is used to categorise data and aid retrieval, relying on consistency in tag labels for individuals and similarity in terminology between users (Golder & Huberman, 2006). We take a similar approach, allowing end users to label and categorise information imported into or created within the X-Media knowledge framework using descriptions meaningful to them (step D under *Knowledge Gathering and Generation* in Figure 1). Additionally, references to ontology-based search results, on import into the knowledge framework, are automatically stored with the values for the concept matches as metadata for each document. Documents referenced and other knowledge objects created within the XMediaBox, e.g., conversation threads or action lists (used to exchange and/or request information), may be tagged using the domain and other pre-selected ontologies, providing a simple method for whole-object annotation (steps D and F under *Knowledge Gathering and Generation* in Figure 1).

The user's input is formalised and transformed into enriched knowledge by linking the free text

tags to corresponding ontology concepts, capturing the context of use, improving information retrieval and supporting more correct and effective reuse. A tag will be one of: an ontology concept – the *subject*, or a relation between a *subject – predicate* pair of an RDF[6] statement. The value for the tag set by the user is the *object* – a *Literal*, which is used to complete the statement captured to the semantic repository. Figure 3 illustrates the formalisation of the tags attached to an image showing a component part of the *brake system* using the sub-ontology that describes issue reports. The image is tagged to record a brake_cable examined as part of the brake_failure investigation, on which the deterioration mechanism *wear* has been observed.

Automated Terminology Recognition (TR) provides additional annotation, by identifying key terms and concepts in free text input such as the comments users make (which serve as personal notes) as an investigation progresses. It may be necessary to verify the automatic extraction with human gatekeepers, at least till pre-set thresholds for accuracy, precision and recall are obtained. Once validated the terms are mapped to corresponding ontology concepts; attaching a comment to a document or other knowledge object therefore updates the metadata that describes the knowledge contained. Similarly, applying TR to the content of action lists and conversation threads generates additional metadata both for the knowledge objects themselves and the entire investigation. This simple method for verbalising and formalising the valuable implicit knowledge that domain experts bring to analysis promotes sharing and reuse; the content of the custom knowledge objects will be retrieved during subsequent ontology search.

Interaction with Knowledge

The knowledge lifecycle continues as the IPTs interact with the knowledge retrieved and generated in earlier steps. Increasingly refined queries are generated to retrieve specific information.

Figure 3. A sub-ontology (extract on left) is used to formalise the knowledge represented by the tags (centre) used to describe an image – a photograph showing brake cables, component parts whose deterioration may have contributed to the brake_failure event – from the perspective of the issue being investigated. The new knowledge is written to the shared semantic repository as RDF statements; this allows the image to be retrieved using ontology search, in addition to the default image similarity search

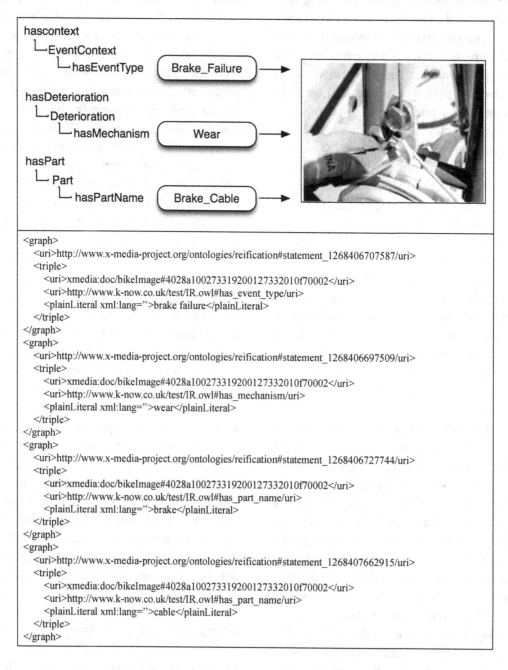

```
<graph>
   <uri>http://www.x-media-project.org/ontologies/reification#statement_1268406707587/uri>
   <triple>
      <uri>xmedia:doc/bikeImage#4028a100273319200127332010f70002</uri>
      <uri>http://www.k-now.co.uk/test/IR.owl#has_event_type/uri>
      <plainLiteral xml:lang=">brake failure</plainLiteral>
   </triple>
</graph>
<graph>
   <uri>http://www.x-media-project.org/ontologies/reification#statement_1268406697509/uri>
   <triple>
      <uri>xmedia:doc/bikeImage#4028a100273319200127332010f70002</uri>
      <uri>http://www.k-now.co.uk/test/IR.owl#has_mechanism/uri>
      <plainLiteral xml:lang=">wear</plainLiteral>
   </triple>
</graph>
<graph>
   <uri>http://www.x-media-project.org/ontologies/reification#statement_1268406727744/uri>
   <triple>
      <uri>xmedia:doc/bikeImage#4028a100273319200127332010f70002</uri>
      <uri>http://www.k-now.co.uk/test/IR.owl#has_part_name/uri>
      <plainLiteral xml:lang=">brake</plainLiteral>
   </triple>
</graph>
<graph>
   <uri>http://www.x-media-project.org/ontologies/reification#statement_1268407662915/uri>
   <triple>
      <uri>xmedia:doc/bikeImage#4028a100273319200127332010f70002</uri>
      <uri>http://www.k-now.co.uk/test/IR.owl#has_part_name/uri>
      <plainLiteral xml:lang=">cable</plainLiteral>
   </triple>
</graph>
```

The information collected on various aspects of an issue will include reports detailing the event(s) that triggered the investigation. For the case of mechanical systems such as the bicycle brake system, design documents, manuals and maintenance reports recording the history of components and systems are among the document types that may be retrieved.

Figure 4 illustrates a search to retrieve similar items to the image inspected in Figure 3. This starts with a region-based similarity search from the image. The tags attached to it, formalised and written to the shared semantic repository (refer Figure 3), are used to formulate an ontology search, by converting the tags into keyword-in-context queries. By propagating the search to different media and document types a simple form of integrated search is obtained across all the search modalities implemented using independent tools.

The information retrieved is processed to extract the knowledge contained, for use in subsequent analytical activity and decision-making. In our case study the varied information retrieved will point to alternative hypotheses for the root cause of the brake failure. It is therefore fed into the hypothesis investigation, the Root Cause Analysis (RCA), carried out to determine the root and other causes of the issue (the cycle started in step I under *Hypothesis Investigation* in Figure 1). Each potential cause must be assessed based on all the evidence that supports or contradicts the hypothesis that it is the root cause. Human cognitive limits however restrict the ability to exhaustively examine the very large amounts of distributed, heterogeneous data available (in the order of hundreds to thousands to tens of thousands and even larger amounts of potentially related documents), to determine what is relevant to the investigation of an issue and perform the analysis required to identify its root cause. Harnessing advanced human perception, we enhance users' sense-making and analytical capability through intuitive, visual, context-driven, hierarchical hypothesis breakdown and analysis.

A plug-in into the XMediaBox uses ontology-based, interactive tree graph construction to guide the hypothesis investigation. Starting from the most likely root cause of an issue a tree is built that explores the relationships between alternative, related or conflicting, hypotheses for the root cause, by selecting corresponding concepts from the domain ontology (step J, a component part of the *Hypothesis Investigation* in Figure 1). Recognising, however, that the ontology is neither exhaustive nor complete, the end user may define additional hypotheses to capture new knowledge discovered as their investigation progresses. The interactive visual representation of the user's analysis reveals the interlinking between hypotheses for the root cause and the evidence examined for each. Petrelli et al. (2009) describe the initial design for the visual RCA; the final prototype is shown in Figure 5.

In our scenario the user starts their RCA by defining the event that triggered the issue observed: Brake_Failure on a pedal bicycle. The analysis progresses along two branches: the observations at the time of the event that triggered the investigation, and the subsequent testing at the distributor site. The second branch is relatively detailed, breaking down the investigation according to the physical structure of the mechanical assembly, in order to examine the potential contribution of factors such as the material properties of the components involved, and other non-physical factors such as incorrectly fitted parts. Evidence that supports or detracts from each hypothesis is examined and where relevant, attached to corresponding nodes in the tree. This action has the associated effect of tagging the evidence item with the corresponding ontology entity, enriching the metadata stored for the item and further increasing the scope of ontology search (refer steps D and E during *Knowledge Gathering and Generation* in Figure 1).

Free text comments may be attached to nodes to record brief summaries of users' thoughts. Meetings called to discuss selected hypotheses for

Figure 4. Propagating a search for similar information to different document and media types by re-formulating the original image feature search to include also ontology-based search, using metadata derived from the user's prior interaction with their knowledge space. (See also Figure 3.)

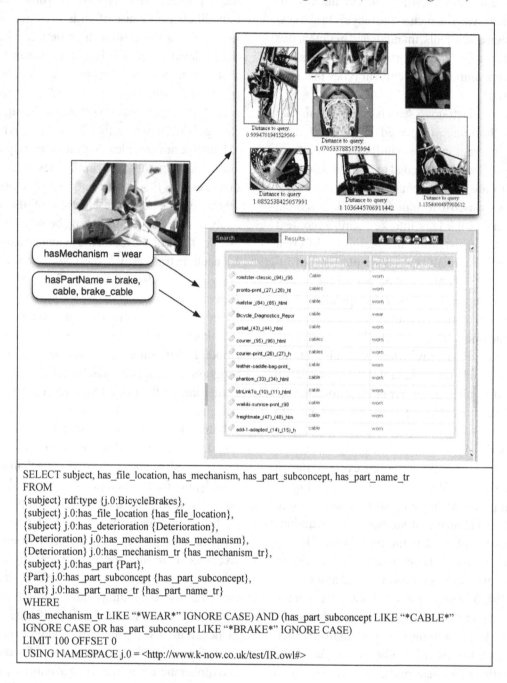

```
SELECT subject, has_file_location, has_mechanism, has_part_subconcept, has_part_name_tr
FROM
{subject} rdf:type {j.0:BicycleBrakes},
{subject} j.0:has_file_location {has_file_location},
{subject} j.0:has_deterioration {Deterioration},
{Deterioration} j.0:has_mechanism {has_mechanism},
{Deterioration} j.0:has_mechanism_tr {has_mechanism_tr},
{subject} j.0:has_part {Part},
{Part} j.0:has_part_subconcept {has_part_subconcept},
{Part} j.0:has_part_name_tr {has_part_name_tr}
WHERE
(has_mechanism_tr LIKE "*WEAR*" IGNORE CASE) AND (has_part_subconcept LIKE "*CABLE*"
IGNORE CASE OR has_part_subconcept LIKE "*BRAKE*" IGNORE CASE)
LIMIT 100 OFFSET 0
USING NAMESPACE j.0 = <http://www.k-now.co.uk/test/IR.owl#>
```

Figure 5. The root cause analysis for the failure of the brake system on a bicycle being performed within the X-Media knowledge framework. Evidence collected during the investigation is attached to relevant nodes in the analysis tree, as alternative hypotheses for the root cause are investigated. A dialog, top, right, is used to record additional notes on the current status of the hypothesis with the focus. The information created during or imported into the graphical root cause analysis is (transparently) formalised according to the underlying ontologies and stored in the shared semantic knowledge repository

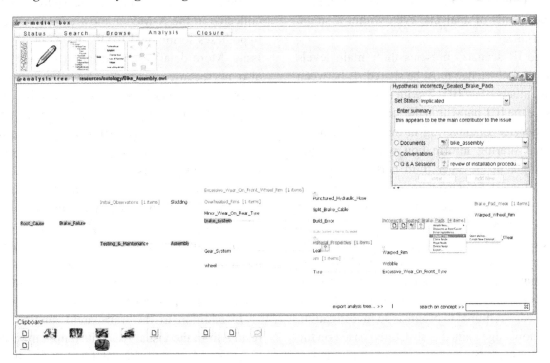

the root cause may have their minutes recorded using custom objects attached to the hypotheses (nodes) of interest. The context of the investigation is therefore saved, allowing (interim) conclusions drawn to be reviewed at any point in time, within the context in which the decisions were made. Figure 5 illustrates a relatively advanced stage in the RCA for the brake failure investigation.

Because the RCA is built on the structure of the domain ontology its output is easily formalised and captured to the shared semantic repository. New knowledge may also feed into ontology evolution. This makes both the knowledge contained in legacy data and the implicit knowledge gained by individual users through experience in RCA and other related activities available to the wider community. The RCA tool provides analysts with

the resources to support increasingly exhaustive investigations that converge to the most likely root cause; the analysis tree prompts the investigation of potentially relevant hypotheses for the root cause by retrieving related entities from the backing ontologies that correspond to each hypothesis formulated for the root cause. This reveals paths of inquiry that may not otherwise have been recognised. The knowledge contained within the domain ontologies is also helpful in resolving conflicting information (Gruber, 1995) a not uncommon occurrence.

Knowledge Sharing & Reuse

The KM lifecycle is completed when the knowledge generated and/or enriched is formalised and stored such that it can be effectively shared with different communities and reused in other scenarios and activities in the same or related domains. A major stumbling block to knowledge sharing and reuse, however, is the differences in information requirements, tasks and the end use of the results of analysis, even within a single organisation.

The IR scenario presents three main levels at which knowledge must be shared: 1. between the members of an IPT, 2. with interested parties outside the IPT but within the same organisation, e.g., Service Engineering in the manufacturing domain sharing information with Design and Development, 3. other third parties, including the customers or consumers of an end product. What should be shared and how is influenced by the target audience: the IPT will have the least restricted access to the knowledge generated by its members, in order to synthesise the information collected, resolve conflicts, perform collaborative analysis and extract or generate the knowledge required to progress an investigation. The knowledge gained is structured based on the domain ontology, to ensure it is correctly understood and reused, especially outside the IPT. The formalised information on the different types of users, communities and tasks provides the layer necessary to ensure that knowledge is presented to each community from the perspective(s) most appropriate to them. Within the X-Media framework we refer to this layer as a *knowledge lens*; different lenses or perspectives guide the selection of analysis tools and methods for presenting the results of analysis. See also Bonifacio et al. (2002), Wenger (2004), who discuss the importance of supporting the different points of view of CoPs.

A recognised limitation in activities such as IR is difficulty accessing and reusing the knowledge obtained and the lessons learnt in previous investigations, employing traditional methods for information retrieval and use. The context in which decisions are made is often lost, especially where intuition and previous experience – implicit

knowledge – contribute to the analysis of the information collected, as this type of knowledge is seldom formally recorded.

As previously described, the intuition (derived from the experience) of members of an IPT is captured to comments/notes attached to evidence collected in the X-Media knowledge space and hypotheses formulated for the root cause of an issue. More detailed conversation threads may also be recorded using the XMediaBox, with references to other knowledge objects that support the statements made. In order to enhance the output of users' regular work without increasing their cognitive load all such input mirrors informal note-taking by using free text. TR is used to extract key terms from the input; these are mapped to ontology concepts, generating metadata that allows subsequent ontology search to retrieve not just matching documents but also the corresponding comments and other knowledge objects – the conversation threads and action lists – that record users' thought processes.

In addition to the transparent tagging that results from the visual RCA, its output may also be exported to a variety of forms, including a snapshot of the graph and a formatted report that details the hypotheses formulated and the evidence supporting or detracting from each. While these allow easy inspection of each user's analysis the knowledge derived from the RCA must also be exported to the semantic repositories in order to allow wider sharing and reuse. Hypotheses that map directly to entities in the (backing) ontologies are easily formalised and stored in the semantic repositories. However, where ontology entities do not exist that encapsulate users' analysis and the causes that may contribute to an issue, user-defined terms may be used to grow the RCA tree. For such nodes additional analysis is required to translate and/or break down the hypotheses and formalise the knowledge encapsulated, before storing it in the semantic repositories. This information is mapped to existing entities (as synonyms, variants or abbreviations of concepts and instances), and where necessary the ontology is extended to capture new knowledge. As existing knowledge is updated and enriched the semantic knowledge base continues to grow, in what may be described as an enlarging spiral of increasingly richer knowledge, rather than just a simple closing of the knowledge lifecycle.

We summarise next the evaluation of the X-Media knowledge framework, as a prelude to a detailed discussion of the challenges encountered in supporting KM with SW technology, and the steps we take to ensure that the valuable knowledge generated here is correctly interpreted during subsequent sharing and reuse.

EVALUATION

Each independent module integrated into the XMediaBox underwent scientific testing, to obtain measures of the robustness of the techniques developed both for the target domains and wider use. The integrated system was then reviewed by usability experts working with aerospace engineers, using an iterative cycle of design and development, to ensure that the framework was able to support the IR process in practice.

Two major usability evaluations were carried out with target users in aerospace engineering, one at the end of each phase of the X-Media project. The first started with a pilot involving three participants, all domain experts with some degree of familiarity with X-Media. This was followed by a formal evaluation with twelve experts from three different departments: Design, Development and Service Engineering. While only service engineers regularly carry out issue investigation, development engineers may perform IR during the testing of new gas turbines (more commonly known as jet engines). Design engineers occasionally act as experts during issue investigation. The evaluation focused on support for defining issues strictly according to the structure of the domain ontologies,

basic ontology search and the initial visual RCA tool. The results, described in (Dadzie, Lanfranchi, & Petrelli, 2009), were overall very positive, and fed into a review of the user requirements and the redesign and extension of the initial prototypes.

The second major evaluation involved one domain expert, who had also been involved in X-Media, taking part in the pilot. Eleven participants from the same departments carried out the formal usability evaluation, none of whom participated in the first usability evaluation. As for the first, they worked in pairs, to simulate more closely the loose collaboration of an IPT during issue investigation in the field. A scenario that simulated a real IR case, built based on actual cases (as for the bike brakes case we describe in this chapter) was used to step the participants through the evaluation. This covered the full range of tools developed to support the IR process as the project neared its conclusion, integrated into the knowledge framework discussed. This allowed a more complete assessment of the use of the domain ontology in different analysis activities and as the main medium for information exchange between tools and users. The participants carried out four main sets of tasks:

1. issue definition and initial legacy data search (based on the issue report and other related information available at the start of the investigation);
2. directed information retrieval and browsing of the knowledge repository;
3. root cause analysis;
4. export of the results of the investigation (using pre-formatted report templates).

The most clearly recognised benefit, noted by all participants, was the "intelligence" seen in the system – the knowledge captured to the domain ontology – that guided the performance of the tasks set.

While they did not explicitly evaluate the large-scale IE used to populate the semantic repository the effect on reducing the load associated with information retrieval was clearly recognised by the participants. User feedback reported the advantages in being able to quickly retrieve related information across different corpora and media types, and collate and analyse it in a single workspace. The added value in the technology that used the (shared) ontology to highlight links across data was also recognised. While this was a common theme across all tools, it was most visible to the participants during the ontology-based search supported by TR, browsing through the legacy corpora, knowledge object tagging and RCA. The participants valued the capability to retrieve not just direct matches to their input keywords, but also, a wider set of matches using domain-specific terms and variants, and synonyms of the input. For the RCA participants especially valued the suggestions provided (from the domain ontology) for paths to follow, in addition to the ability to attach evidence to the investigation to provide context for the decisions taken, and the visual, permanent reminder of this).

The ability to export the results to formal reports was also seen to be valuable, especially for sharing their knowledge content outside investigations. Additionally, support for saving investigations such that the knowledge gained could be retrieved and applied to other scenarios was seen to have great potential. This underscores the importance of correctly encoding the knowledge generated within the X-Media framework and storing this in ways that promote its reuse.

This evaluation, which concluded the project, provided a measure of the extent to which we had been able to meet the challenges to effective KM in complex environments. The next section takes a detailed look at these challenges, and the research done in X-Media to handle them.

CHALLENGES IN SEMANTIC KNOWLEDGE MANAGEMENT

We have discussed the benefits of supporting KM with SW technology. These include richer knowledge capture and more effective sharing and (re)use. However a number of challenges exist; effective management of these is necessary in order to reap the full benefits of our approach. We assess first those faced in providing effective support for semantic KM for the different users and CoPs that share data and processes in related sub-domains. We then discuss the implications these have for ontology evolution and the corresponding update of the semantic (knowledge) repositories.

Knowledge Sharing within Communities of Practice

The creation of dynamic teams to resolve specific issues or simply to share knowledge is increasingly the norm in knowledge-intensive organisations (Bonifacio et al., 2002, Wenger, 2004). An example is the IPTs formed to determine the root causes of issues that arise in a domain, which comprise members with different skills and expertise, often crossing traditional organisational boundaries. This brings multiple perspectives to each investigation, ensuring a wider point of view and a more exhaustive investigation. However what is a benefit may also pose a challenge; the differences in users, their skills, regular activities and environments may result in conflicts and/or ambiguity in the interpretation of information and tasks. For the same reason the results of analysis may be incorrectly interpreted.

We tackle this challenge by using ontologies to extract, in the first instance, the knowledge contained in legacy data corpora, with their context of use, to semantic knowledge repositories. The formal, agreed definitions of the knowledge that result, especially for domain-specific information, should aid correct interpretation (Gruber, 1995), and the generation of new knowledge through further interaction with and contextualisation of the information. This new knowledge is easily encoded using the same ontologies, ensuring that further reuse continues to build an increasingly richer, more complete knowledge base.

A second challenge is defining users in different CoPs and the activities they perform. Using a modular ontology provides a simple, yet effective solution; a sub-ontology is used to define the main user types in an organisation and the skills each community typically has. Additional (sub-) ontologies define the activities different user types regularly perform, and other important but less frequently performed tasks. The task ontology also defines the resources and artefacts users employ. The information here is especially useful to novices and even domain experts performing tasks with which they are unfamiliar, as well as the end users of the results of analysis. Understanding the aim of a task, and the resources used to complete it, helps to ensure that the resulting knowledge is effectively interpreted and (re)used.

A third challenge is the sub-languages typically developed within sub-cultures in an organisation (Butters & Ciravegna, 2008, Berners-Lee et al., 2001). Variations in terminology, including the use of acronyms and abbreviations, synonyms and conversely, homonyms, and varying degrees of abstraction or generality in naming, contribute to ambiguous and/or incorrect interpretation of input data and the results of analysis (see, among others, Golder & Huberman, 2006, Iria, 2009). This is further compounded by incompleteness of data, inconsistency and errors such as misspellings. Data dictionaries, taxonomies and ontologies help to resolve the challenges posed. Domain lexicons are also used, where available, to support especially automated IE and TR, and guide information retrieval. We focus predominantly on the use of domain ontologies, starting with concepts that encapsulate the agreed, formal descriptions of users, activities and artefacts. These are supplemented

with instances of the concepts that provide refinements of the more general descriptions, and a list of known synonyms. Relations between concepts in each ontology and mappings across ontologies help end users to recognise the inter-relationships within data.

A final challenge is ensuring that flexible, customisable solutions are provided via interfaces that support the work of different users and CoPs. Those tools developed as part of the X-Media project, for information extraction and retrieval, and knowledge capture and analysis, make use of appropriate SW technology to enable semantic KM. Each tool incorporates design that allows its output to be captured to RDF, according to the domain ontology, to a shared semantic repository.

Contributing to the challenges faced in designing UIs that support effectively the work of multiple CoPs are the obstacles typically faced in the adoption of new tools and ways of working, predominantly due to the steep learning curves often encountered. The XMediaBox interface was designed to ensure that the user's normal activities could continue unimpeded, but enhanced by their ability to retrieve and make use of existing knowledge and generate new, richer knowledge. The IR scenario in the X-Media context provides a case in point: a number of knowledge retrieval and sharing tools support different stages in the KM lifecycle. The original design required end users to define new issue investigation cases and the results of analysis using forms that mapped strictly to key ontology concepts, and explicitly annotate all free text input (in comments, for e.g.) using the ontologies. The structured methods for capturing users' input translated directly to the encoding and formalisation of the knowledge contained. However end users found this approach to knowledge capture to be too rigid. First of all it required them to translate their interpretation of issues and the implicit knowledge they brought to the analysis to what was initially a large, complex, monolithic ontology that captured an organisation-wide schema defined at a fairly high level. Further, where the ontology did not map directly to the work of a specialised CoP or cover (new) areas being explored it was difficult for end users to encode properly new knowledge gained.

Improvements to the design of the X-Media knowledge framework include the use of simple forms that, while still backed by relevant subsections of the domain ontology, capture information using free text. A semi-automatic approach, using TR to extract key words and terms from users' free text input, is now used to encode the knowledge represented. Users may verify and correct the extraction, after which it is translated (via the ontologies in use) into a formal representation, and stored in the shared semantic repositories.

Following the same approach, data categorisation and annotation are obtained as a by-product of users' interaction with their *knowledge spaces*. For instance, the graphical hypothesis investigation automatically tags evidence and comments with the corresponding ontology entities for the nodes in the analysis tree to which they are attached. This allows users and CoPs to maintain their personal interpretation of the data and knowledge they interact with while a formalised, shareable translation is captured to the semantic knowledge repositories.

Ontology Evolution

In order to support effective, semantic KM the domain ontology must evolve to capture the new knowledge created as end users interact with data and information during their normal working activity. Static ontologies rapidly diverge from the users' changing needs (Tempich et al., 2006), leading to the eventual abandonment of expensive systems.

The RCA, which is constructed on the spine of the domain ontology, is one of the main sources of new knowledge within the IR scenario. Domain ontologies are neither exhaustive nor complete (Brewster et al., 2007); during RCA, therefore, end users may formulate (new) hypotheses out-

side those defined in the existing ontology. New hypotheses may map to new concepts or instances of existing concepts, or synonyms, variants or abbreviations of existing entities. Further, the RCA may lead to the definition of new relations between previously unconnected entities.

The ontology-based tagging using the framework also leads to a simpler form of ontology evolution. This action generates new instances of existing concepts or synonyms, variants and abbreviations of existing instances.

Multiple sources of information are analysed as part of the RCA and the investigation as a whole, and new knowledge is discovered throughout the investigation process. The information retrieved from one document may support existing knowledge which is contradicted by another source. Resolving such conflicts is a significant challenge to ensuring that valid, correctly formalised knowledge is fed into ontology evolution.

This work has made us very aware of two challenges which need to be tackled to support ontology evolution. While a number of tools exist for ontology engineering there is a lack of technical solutions suitable for domain experts. A significant challenge in the ontology evolution process is the validation of the knowledge generated, in order to prevent incorrect information being encoded as new knowledge. There is therefore the need to support the definition of change control policies which address the trade off between the need to maintain high quality ontologies and limited human resources for maintenance (Zablith, Sabou, d'Aquin, & Motta, 2008).

Until recently most ontology design tools have assumed a single editor (Castro et al., 2006). This has begun to be tackled, with systems being produced that aim to support distributed teams of ontology engineers, e.g., Palma et al. (2008). While this is relevant to the challenge, because such systems tackle issues such as the detection of inconsistency, they do not address the user interface requirements of domain experts, who are typically expert in the use of numerical software and, in our experience, are not necessarily comfortable with ontology editing tools (see also Ernst & Storey, 2003). In the use case discussed in this chapter, ontology changes are produced as a side effect of the IR process. Engineers want to focus on their main task, and not be distracted by machine requests to check some inconsistency or approve minor changes. Therefore, we foresee a scenario in which changes are made locally, allowing each IPT or CoP the freedom to explore different possibilities when looking for the root cause of an issue, much as in Castro et al. (2006), Tempich et al. (2006). Then, before local knowledge is shared more widely, appointed gatekeepers will validate proposed changes to the ontology.

Ernst and Storey (2003), Castro et al. (2006), among others, have carried out research into the use of graphical representations to support ontology management, by mapping the structure of ontologies to a spatial representation. The visual, ontology-backed approach to RCA described is one route we continue to explore as a means of supporting intuitive ontology evolution. While the visual tree represents the end user's view on their analysis, the translation and formalisation of its knowledge content according to the ontology provides a shareable, reusable version to be captured to the semantic repositories. Further, the context, i.e., supporting evidence, for each new concept is also made available. Using the formalised, shareable view the gatekeeper is more easily able to (correctly) interpret each user's analysis, and merge common knowledge before submitting changes to the ontology evolution process.

Combining the gatekeeper scenario with the modular design of the ontology, we have a situation in which different gatekeepers may validate different modules of the ontology. To maintain consistency in large organisations, the gatekeepers would need a clearly defined policy for change control (see also Tempich et al., 2006, who describe a similar approach to managing the evolution of local and shared ontologies for distributed CoPs). Changes can affect any part of

the ontology. However in our current discussions we have identified two areas in which changes are expected to be common in KM scenarios: extension of classes with new instances and the design of new data structures, such as forms.

Semantic Repository Update

The update of the semantic repository is triggered by three main events: (1) the capture of new knowledge, (2) updates or corrections to existing knowledge and (3) ontology evolution. It is important to ensure that only correct, validated information is encoded as new knowledge in the semantic repositories. Capturing new knowledge to the repositories is relatively straightforward, especially where users' activities are aligned to the domain (or other relevant) ontologies. However, even for new knowledge that falls outside the domain ontology it may still be useful to make this available to users before validation is completed, albeit with a flag, as such knowledge often provides a refinement of existing concepts and/or captures information not available in the validated version of the ontology.

Again using the IR scenario as an example, we have previously discussed avenues for ontology-guided knowledge creation. The simple, ontology-backed forms used to capture the description of an issue, and the conclusions drawn and the lessons learnt when an issue investigation is closed provide information that is fed directly into populating the semantic repository. Metadata composed of the key terms and concepts automatically extracted from the free text descriptions, once verified, is encoded into formal knowledge via the underlying ontologies and stored in the shared semantic repositories.

Updating existing knowledge however introduces a level of complexity. It is necessary to identify which new statements concern the same real world entities. Within the X-Media system a unique URI is generated for each new knowledge object created. However, multiple copies of the same document created outside the system and imported into a user's knowledge space, for instance, are more difficult to resolve. The current solution generates a URI for each new import, and maps this to the (absolute) location of the entity at the time of import – this may be a location on a file system or a Web URL (Uniform Resource Locator). While this approach is the simplest and most effective for data storage dependent on a file system, moving the same (unedited) file to a different location will result in the inability to locate a previously referenced resource, or duplication if the document is then imported from the new location. An additional challenge is that new statements about entities in the repository, generated based on new information discovered, may conflict with existing statements. We use fusion (Nikolov, Uren, Motta, & de Roeck, 2008) as the first step in handling such conflicts.

Finally, before attempting to update the semantic repository it is necessary to decide how updates are to be made to existing statements, e.g., adding new metadata for a document reference. Where inconsistencies or errors have been identified in existing metadata, decisions must be made as to whether these should simply be corrected, or new statements inserted to flag and correct these errors. The latter has the advantage of providing a complete history for each element in the repository, but also increases complexity and the danger of retrieving inconsistent information.

FUTURE RESEARCH DIRECTIONS

The value that structuring knowledge intensive activities around domain ontologies brings to end users in complex environments was clearly seen in the evaluation of the X-Media knowledge framework. To build on this we continue to study target end user groups, in order to obtain a more complete understanding of the environments in which they work and the artefacts employed in their normal work. This will give us a more solid grounding from which to improve the design of the knowledge framework developed.

End users found visual hypothesis analysis backed by an ontology to provide a clear, structured method for root cause analysis. The context driven, ontology based approach also provided good support for other tasks in the IR scenario. We continue to explore and evaluate alternative perspectives, both visual and using other methods for the presentation of users' analysis, to support the variations in requirements of different users and tasks.

There is a very clear link between the quality and level of support our approach to semantic KM provides to users and the evolution of the ontology and the semantic repositories to capture new knowledge, both from the overall organisational perspective and the individual, customised views of various CoPs. We must improve support for the human gatekeepers that control ontology evolution, to ensure that the process is sustained, without placing a large burden on the gatekeepers. Brewster et al. (2007), among others, discuss techniques for supporting dynamic ontology evolution; the approach proposed is in line with the work described in Iria (2009), who argues for a move from semi-supervised to (at least initial) fully automatic IE for very large scale data. The degree of success here will impact significantly on the sustainability of semantic KM, which promises more effective methods for unearthing the valuable knowledge that often remains hidden in the very large legacy data stores dealt with on a regular basis in today's information-rich organisations.

Finally, we focus on the ontologies built to capture descriptions of specific domains. While we do make use of other more general ontologies (e.g., Dublin Core[7]) this is only at a relatively basic level. We continue to look into linking across ontologies outside the small set of custom ontologies for each domain, in order to support more intuitive linking to and cross-referencing of external, related information.

CONCLUSION

We have looked at the challenges to semantic knowledge management highlighted by the investigation process carried out to determine the root cause of issues in complex scenarios. This involves teams of experts analysing different aspects of an issue to identify its potential root causes.

We take an approach to Knowledge Management that harnesses the power of Semantic Web technology to enable richer knowledge discovery, exploration and capture, that focuses on the knowledge content of data rather than on just the data. We have designed a knowledge framework that integrates a number of tools, each of which supports a specific aspect of the analysis required in complex scenarios, by providing alternative perspectives on data, customised to suit different users and tasks across multiple communities of practice. We use domain ontologies to guide users in data exploration and analysis, and support the contextualisation and codifying of the information retrieved into knowledge, supporting more effective information and knowledge retrieval, as well as analysis that is woven into users' normal working activities.

We have evaluated our knowledge framework with end users in the aerospace engineering domain, using a simulation of an IR case. User observation and an analysis of the quantitative results of the evaluation confirmed the power of SW technology to increase intuition and ability during complex issue investigation. The participants found that the ontology-guided hypothesis exploration and investigation aided the contextualisation of information, leading to an increase in the confidence with which they came to conclusions about the simulated issues.

There remain other open issues, including the need to support more effective and accurate automated annotation, to reduce the large burden associated with manual annotation, especially where this must be updated regularly to cope with evolving ontologies across multiple corpora. We continue to investigate new methods and techniques that support both automated knowledge acquisition on a very large scale from heterogeneous data repositories, and the design of intuitive interfaces that support end users in converting data into knowledge. Further work should lead to richer, higher quality semantic repositories and improve the support that SW technology provides to what still remains invaluable human analytical and reasoning capability.

ACKNOWLEDGMENT

The research described in this chapter was funded by the X-Media project, sponsored by the European Commission (EC) as part of the Information Society Technologies programme under EC grant number ISTFP6-026978.

REFERENCES

Berners-Lee, T., Hendler, J., & Lassila, O. (2001). *The Semantic Web*. Scientific American Magazine.

Bhagdev, R., Chakravarthy, A., Chapman, S., Ciravegna, F., & Lanfranchi, V. (2008). Creating and using organisational Semantic Webs in large networked organisations. In *ISWC '08: Proc., 7th International Conference on The Semantic Web* (pp. 723–736). Springer-Verlag.

Bonifacio, M., Bouquet, P., & Cuel, R. (2002). Knowledge nodes: The building blocks of a distributed approach to knowledge management. *Journal for Universal Computer Science, 8*(6), 652–661.

Brewster, C., Iria, J., Zhang, Z., Ciravegna, F., Guthrie, L., & Wilks, Y. (2007). Dynamic iterative ontology learning. In *RANLP '07: Proc., the Recent Advances in Natural Language Processing Conference*.

Butters, J., & Ciravegna, F. (2008). Using similarity metrics for terminology recognition. In *LREC'08: Proc., 6th International Conference on Language Resources and Evaluation* (pp. 2817–2822).

Castro, A. G., Rocca-Serra, P., Stevens, R., Taylor, C., Nashar, K., Ragan, M. A., & Sansone, S.-A. (2006). The use of concept maps during knowledge elicitation in ontology development processes - the nutrigenomics use case. *BMC Bioinformatics, 7*(267).

Ciravegna, F., & Staab, S. (2005). *Large scale cross-media knowledge acquisition, sharing and reuse in X-Media.* In EWIMT 2005: The 2nd European Workshop on the Integration of Knowledge, Semantics and Digital Media Technology (pp. 407–408).

Dadzie, A.-S., Iria, J., Petrelli, D., & Xia, L. (2009). The XMediaBox: Sensemaking through the use of knowledge lenses. In L. Aroyo, et al. (Eds.), *ESWC 2009: The Semantic Web: Research and Applications, Proc., 6th European Semantic Web Conference* (pp. 811–815).

Dadzie, A.-S., Lanfranchi, V., & Petrelli, D. (2009). Seeing is believing: Linking data with knowledge. *Information Visualization, 8*(3), 197–211. doi:10.1057/ivs.2009.11

Ernst, N. A., & Storey, M.-A. (2003). *A preliminary analysis of visualization requirements in knowledge engineering tools. (Tech. Rep.).* CHISEL, University of Victoria.

Gennari, J. H., Musen, M. A., Fergerson, R. W., Grosso, W. E., Crubézy, M., & Eriksson, H. (2003). The evolution of Protégé: An environment for knowledge-based systems development. *International Journal of Human-Computer Studies, 58*(1), 89–123. doi:10.1016/S1071-5819(02)00127-1

Giovannetti, E., Marchi, S., Montemagni, S., & Bartolini, R. (2008). Ontology learning and semantic annotation: A necessary symbiosis. In *LREC'08: Proc., 6th International Conference on Language Resources and Evaluation* (pp. 2079–2085).

Golder, S. A., & Huberman, B. A. (2006). Usage patterns of collaborative tagging systems. *Journal of Information Science, 32*, 198–208. doi:10.1177/0165551506062337

Grau, B. C., Parsia, B., Sirin, E., & Kalyanpur, A. (2006). Modularity and Web ontologies. In P. Doherty, J. Mylopoulos, & C. A. Welty (Eds.), *KR2006: Proc., 10th International Conference on Principles of Knowledge Representation and Reasoning* (pp. 198–209).

Gruber, T. R. (1995). Toward principles for the design of ontologies used for knowledge sharing. *International Journal of Human-Computer Studies, 43*(5-6), 907–928. doi:10.1006/ijhc.1995.1081

Hayes, P., Eskridge, T. C., Saavedra, R., Reichherzer, T., Mehrotra, M., & Bobrovnikoff, D. (2005). Collaborative knowledge capture in ontologies. In *K-CAP '05: Proc., 3rd International Conference on Knowledge Capture* (pp. 99–106). ACM.

Hoffman, R. R., Shadbolt, N. R., Burton, A. M., & Klein, G. (1995). Eliciting knowledge from experts: A methodological analysis. *Organizational Behavior and Human Decision Processes, 62*(2), 129–158. doi:10.1006/obhd.1995.1039

Iria, J. (2009). Automating knowledge capture in the aerospace domain. In *K-CAP '09: Proc., 5th International Conference on Knowledge Capture* (pp. 97–104). ACM.

Katifori, A., Halatsis, C., Lepouras, G., Vassilakis, C., & Giannopoulou, E. (2007). Ontology visualization methods—a survey. *ACM Computing Surveys, 39*(4), 10. doi:10.1145/1287620.1287621

McShane, M., Nirenburg, S., Beale, S., & O'Hara, T. (2005). Semantically rich human-aided machine annotation. In *CorpusAnno '05: Proc., Workshop on Frontiers in Corpus Annotations II* (pp. 68–75).

Mödritscher, F. (2009). Semantic lifecycles: Modelling, application, authoring, mining, and evaluation of meaningful data. *International Journal of Knowledge and Web Intelligence, 1*(1/2), 110–124. doi:10.1504/IJKWI.2009.027928

Mularz, D., & Lyell, M. (2004). Integrating concept mapping and Semantic Web technologies for knowledge management. In *DEXA2004: Proc., 15th International Workshop on Database and Expert Systems Applications* (pp. 449–453).

Mutton, P., & Golbeck, J. (2003). Visualization of semantic metadata and ontologies. In *INFOVIS 2003: Proc., 7th International Conference on information visualization* (pp. 300–305).

Navarro, B., Marcos, R., & Abad, P. (2005). *Semantic annotation and inter-annotators agreement in Cast3LB corpus*. In TLT 2005: 4th Workshop on Treebanks and Linguistic Theories.

Nikolov, A., Uren, V., Motta, E., & de Roeck, A. (2008). Integration of semantically annotated data by the KnoFuss architecture. In *EKAW 2008: Proc., 16th International Conference on Knowledge Engineering: Practice and Patterns* (pp. 265–274).

Palma, R., Haase, P., Corcho, O., Gómez-Pérez, A., & Ji, Q. (2008). An editorial workflow approach for collaborative ontology development. In *ASWC 2008: Proc., 3rd Asian Semantic Web Conference* (pp. 227–241).

Petrelli, D., Dadzie, A. S., & Lanfranchi, V. (2009). Mediating between AI and highly specialized users. *AI Magazine, 30*(4), 95–102.

Staab, S., Studer, R., Schnurr, H.-P., & Sure, Y. (2001). Knowledge processes and ontologies. *IEEE Intelligent Systems, 16*(1), 26–34. doi:10.1109/5254.912382

Tempich, C., Pinto, H. S., & Staab, S. (2006). Ontology engineering revisited: An iterative case study. In Y. Sure & J. Domingue (Eds.), *ESWC 2006: The Semantic Web: Research and Applications, Proc., 3rd European Semantic Web Conference* (pp. 110–124).

Wenger, E. (2004). Knowledge management is a donut: Shaping your knowledge strategy with communities of practice. *Ivey Business Journal, 68*(3), 1–8.

Xia, L., & Iria, J. (2008). An approach to modeling heterogeneous resources for information extraction. In *LREC '08: Proc., 6th International Conference on Language Resources and Evaluation* (pp. 2768–2772).

Zablith, F., Sabou, M., d'Aquin, M., & Motta, E. (2008). *Using background knowledge for ontology evolution*. In International Workshop on Ontology Dynamics (IWOD) at the International Semantic Web Conference (ISWC 2008).

Zhang, Z., Xia, L., Greenwood, M. A., & Iria, J. (2009). Too many mammals: Improving the diversity of automatically recognized terms. In *RANLP '09: Proc., International Conference on Recent Advances in Natural Language Processing*.

ADDITIONAL READING

Alavi, M., & Leidner, D. E. (2001). Review: Knowledge Management and Knowledge Management Systems: Conceptual Foundations and Research Issues. *Management Information Systems Quarterly, 25*(1), 107–136. doi:10.2307/3250961

Berners-Lee, T., Hendler, J., & Lassila, O. (2001). *The Semantic Web*. Scientific American Magazine.

Gruber, T. R. (1995). Toward principles for the design of ontologies used for knowledge sharing? *International Journal of Human-Computer Studies*, *43*(5-6), 907–928. http://www.w3.org/standards/semanticweb/ontology. doi:10.1006/ijhc.1995.1081

http://www.w3.org/standards/semanticweb

Nonaka, Ik., & von Krogh, G. (2009). Perspective--Tacit Knowledge and Knowledge Conversion: Controversy and Advancement in Organizational Knowledge Creation Theory. *Organization Science*, *20*(3), 635–652. doi:10.1287/orsc.1080.0412

Shneiderman, B., Plaisant, C., Cohen, M., Jacobs, S. (2009) Designing the User Interface: Strategies for Effective Human-Computer Interaction, 5ed, Pearson Education

Siemieniuch, C. E., & Sinclair, M. A. (1999). Organizational aspects of knowledge lifecycle management in manufacturing. *International Journal of Human-Computer Studies*, *51*(3), 517–547. doi:10.1006/ijhc.1999.0274

KEY TERMS & DEFINITIONS

Community of Practice: Wenger (2004) provides the most cited definitions of a *community of practice*: "Communities of practice are social structures that focus on knowledge and explicitly enable the management of knowledge to be placed in the hands of practitioners." "Communities of practice are groups of people who share a passion for something that they know how to do, and who interact regularly in order to learn how to do it better."

Knowledge Lifecycle: Closely related to KM, the Knowledge Lifecycle is the iterative, increasingly richer cycle of knowledge creation and capture, retrieval, enrichment in use, sharing and re-use, that results in the generation of yet richer and/or new knowledge. (See also: Wenger, E. (2004). Knowledge management is a donut: shaping your knowledge strategy with communities of practice. Ivey Business Journal, 1–8.

Knowledge Management: The activities involved in monitoring the creation and effective use of shared knowledge in an organisation. KM involves both the management of the processes followed and the actual knowledge that results from combining experience with the insight obtained through the use of information retrieval and analysis tools.

Ontology: Ontologies provide formal, structured specifications of a domain, the entities within it and the relationships between those entities. The W3C provide a more detailed definition of a *vocabulary*, and compare this to the more formal *ontology*: "On the Semantic Web, vocabularies define the concepts and relationships (also referred to as "terms" used to describe and represent an area of concern. " An *ontology* is then described as a "formal collection of terms", and by Berners-Lee et al., (2001) as "collections of information".

Semantic Web: Formally defined by the W3C (the World Wide Web Consortium) in 2001 - http://www.w3.org/2001/sw: "The Semantic Web provides a common framework that allows data to be shared and reused across application, enterprise, and community boundaries. It is a collaborative effort led by W3C with participation from a large number of researchers and industrial partners. It is based on the Resource Description Framework (RDF)."

Semantic Web Technology: A range of technologies built based on or incorporating W3C standards, to provide methods for expressing information and knowledge formally, and enable effective use and storage. The most well-known and widely used SW technologies are ontologies and the languages RDF and OWL for publishing data and ontologies, respectively, and SPARQL for querying the "web of data". Berners-Lee et al., (2001) begin the article *The Semantic Web* with a statement encompassing the potential of SW-based technology: "A new form of Web content that is meaningful to computers will unleash a revolution of new possibilities".

User-Centred Design: User-Centred design (UCD) goes beyond the notion of *user-friendliness*, to incorporate an intensive study of end users, their environments and work practices, in order to collaborate with users to design and build truly effective systems and interfaces that cater to their (varied) requirements. UCD is an important contributor to the adoption and continued use of especially new, leading edge technology.

Visual Analytics: Visual Analytics (VA) is a relatively new field of practice that grew out of Information Visualisation. VA is often seen to cater more closely to the special requirements of visualisation in real-world analysis applications. Thomas et al., (2005) provide the formal definition: "Visual analytics is the science of analytical reasoning facilitated by interactive visual interfaces." (J.J. Thomas and K.A. Cook, eds. (2005) Illuminating the Path: The Research and Development Agenda for Visual Analytics, IEEE CS Press.)

ENDNOTES

[1] The X-Media Project: http://www.x-media-project.org

[2] Time Ontology in OWL: http://www.w3.org/TR/owl-time

[3] See the GIRL (General Image Representation Library) web site: http://girl.labri.fr/xmedia.html

[4] Flickr (online photo management and sharing): http://www.flickr.com

[5] Del.icio.us (social bookmarking): http://delicious.com

[6] Resource Description Framework (RDF): http://www.w3.org/RDF; see also the associated suite of W3C Recommendations at http://www.w3.org/standards/techs/rdf#w3c_all

[7] Dublin Core Metadata Initiative: http://dublincore.org

Section 3
Emerging Trends in Ontology Learning and Knowledge Discovery

Chapter 12
Automated Learning of Social Ontologies

Konstantinos Kotis
University of the Aegean, Greece

Andreas Papasalouros
University of the Aegean, Greece

ABSTRACT

Learned social ontologies can be viewed as products of a social fermentation process, i.e. a process between users who belong in communities of common interests (CoI), in open, collaborative, and communicative environments. In such a setting, social fermentation ensures the automatic encapsulation of agreement and trust of shared knowledge that participating stakeholders provide during an ontology learning task. This chapter discusses the requirements for the automated learning of social ontologies and presents a working method and results of preliminary work. Furthermore, due to its importance for the exploitation of the learned ontologies, it introduces a model for representing the interlinking of agreement, trust and the learned domain conceptualizations that are extracted from social content. The motivation behind this work is an effort towards supporting the design of methods for learning ontologies from social content i.e. methods that aim to learn not only domain conceptualizations but also the degree that agents (software and human) may trust these conceptualizations or not.

INTRODUCTION

Although Semantic Web has lately moved closer to its pragmatic realization, a critical mass of semantic content is still missing. Web users can only find few well-maintained and up-to-date

DOI: 10.4018/978-1-60960-625-1.ch012

domain ontologies. Only a small number of Web users, typically members of the Semantic Web community, build and publish ontologies. To assist and motivate humans in becoming part of the Semantic Web movement and contribute their knowledge and time to create or refine/enrich useful ontologies, there is need to advance semantic content creation by providing Web users with a "starting point of assistance" i.e. with automatically learned kick-off (starting-up) ontologies.

Traditionally, the learning of ontologies involves the identification of domain-specific conceptualizations that are extracted from text documents or other semi-structured information sources e.g. lexicons or thesauruses. Such learned ontologies do not utilize any available social data that may be related to the domain one e.g. information ownership details (contributor, annotator or end-user), tags or argumentation/dialogue items that have been used to comment, organize or disambiguate domain-specific information, querying information related to user clicks on retrieved information. Recently, the learning of ontologies also concerns social content that is mainly generated within Web 2.0 applications. Social content refers to various kinds of media content, publicly available, that are produced by Web users in a collaborative and communicative manner. Such content is associated to social data that has been produced as a result of the *social fermentation* process. The most popular social data in Web 2.0 content is tags, which are often single words listed alphabetically and displayed with a different font size or color to capture its importance. Tags are usually hyperlinks that lead to a collection of items that each tag is manually or automatically associated with. Such social data can be processed in an intelligent way towards shaping social content into ontologies. Since social data is created as part of the social fermentation process, that is, tags are introduced in a collaborative and communicative manner; it can be argued that the learned ontologies produced from such a process encapsulate some degree of agreement and trust of the learned conceptualizations.

Social content generation (SCG) refers to a conversational, distributed mode of content generation, dissemination, and communication among communities of common interest (CoI). Social intelligence (SI) aims to derive information from social content in context-rich application settings and provide solution frameworks for

applications that can benefit from the "wisdom of crowds" through the Web. Within this setting, a social ontology can be defined as: *an explicit, formal and commonly agreed representation of knowledge that is derived from both domain-specific and social data*. In the context of this chapter, the meaning of the term "social ontology" must be clearly distinguished from the meaning that is used in social sciences. A representative definition in the context of social sciences is given by T. Lawson of the Cambridge Social Ontology Group[1]: "...the study of what is, or what exists, in the social domain; the study of social entities or social things; and the study of what all the social entities or things that are have in common".

Formally, an ontology is considered to be a pair $O=(S, A)$, where S is the ontological signature describing the vocabulary (i.e. the terms that lexicalize concepts and relations between concepts) and A is a set of ontological axioms, restricting the intended interpretations of the terms included in the signature (Kalfoglou & Schorlemmer, 2003; Kotis et al, 2006). In other words, A includes the formal definitions of concepts and relations that are lexicalized by natural language terms in S. In this chapter, we extend such model by adding a social dimension (equal to *social semantics*) that is inspired by the definition of the "Actor-Concept-Instance model of ontologies" (Mika, 2007) formulated as a generic abstract model of semantic-social networks. This extended model is build on an implicit realization of emergent semantics, i.e. meaning must be depended on a community of agents. According to the extended model, a social ontology is defined as a triple $O=(C, S, A)$, where C is the set of collaborated contributors that have participated in a *SCG* task, from which S and A have been derived using the *SI* found in C. The range however of C over both S and A at the same time is not guaranteed, i.e. S may have been derived from C, but not A, which may have been automatically derived from external information sources such as a general ontology or lexicon, e.g. from WordNet.

The automated learning of social ontologies can be seen as a two-dimensional problem. The first dimension concerns the automated creation of ontologies from content (social and domain-specific), and the second, the social dimension, concerns the collaboration and communication aspects (the *social fermentation*) that are related to the creation of the content. Since automation is also involved and human agents do not participate in the conceptualizations' agreement process, a key issue (due to its importance for the exploitation of the learned ontologies) is the trust on the extracted ontological agreement from social data i.e. the estimation of the degree of certainty that contributors of shared conceptualizations about a specific domain have agreed on a common understanding about the domain i.e. that such an agreement is successfully extracted in an automated fashion from social data (e.g. in open Web agents' world where agents must trust each others conceptualizations about the domain of discourse in order to be able to collaborate within an agreed context). In terms of trusting content, the chapter follows the assumption that the content used as input in an ontology learning process is a social one (or content that is indirectly involved in a social fermentation process), thus it is, at least in some degree, agreed and trusted. Blogs, (Semantic) Wikis, Folksonomies and other more sophisticated Web 2.0 applications such as Yahoo! Answers or Fixya.com, provide reputation-based trust by using personal experience or the experiences of others, possibly combined, to make a trust decision about an entity, or voting mechanisms for their content. Other types of content such as Web users' query logs provide a kind of trusting content, based on the "majority vote of user clicks" on Web search results.

By the time this chapter is being authored and to the best of our knowledge that is mainly based on recent literature review (Artz & Gil, 2007; O'Hara et al, 2004; Tang et al., 2009), there is no mean to automatically discover and attach uncertainty values on learned social ontologies' signature (S)

and axioms (A). This chapter, in addition to the presentation of a novel method for learning social ontologies, introduces a model that represents trust for such an ontology i.e. an ontology of the form $O = \{C, S, A\}$. Such a model is formed as a meta-ontology which represents meta-information related to each element of a social ontology i.e. classes, properties, instances and contributors. Such meta-information is related to social data (e.g. contributors' details, voting information) that is in turn related to the content represented in the domain ontology. The definition of $O = \{C, S, A\}$ is then extended by also introducing trust-related representations.

BACKGROUND

Ontology learning is an important research area for the Semantic Web realization. Many research efforts have been contributing in this area during the past few years. However, much of these efforts focus on the extraction of concepts and simple relations (mainly hierarchical) from text, especially from large collections of text documents. For instance, an early work (Maedche & Staab, 2001) proposes an ontology learning framework that integrates data mining approaches (such as hierarchical cluster and association rule) and some background knowledge to learn concepts, hierarchical relations, and associative relations from text. An alternative approach (Han & Elmasri, 2003) proposed the extraction of domain ontologies from Web pages based on HTML tags, lemmatization tags, and conceptual tags. Other efforts have focused on the measuring of the accuracy of the learned ontologies (evaluation problem of learning ontologies e.g. OntoEval systems (Dellschaft & Staab, 2006)). The text-corpora-related efforts, to the best of our knowledge, do not involve, directly or indirectly, social data i.e. the learned ontologies cannot be considered as social ones, and they do not encapsulate any kind of agreement and trust.

Recently, several research efforts have provided methods for the learning of ontologies from user created social data e.g. folksonomies (collaborative social tagging). Such methods mainly propose the learning of a domain ontology using tag clouds that are generated during the tagging of Web content within social networking authoring environments. The learned ontology is, or at least should be, a compromise between a formal ontology and a freely created folksonomy (Gruber, 2007). A few algorithms have been proposed for learning synonym and hypernym relations between tags. Some other efforts try to generate clusters of highly related tags and associate each cluster to a concept of an existing ontology. Other efforts propose unsupervised methods for exploring the hierarchical relations between tags but without considering the different types of relations (e.g., hypernym, synonym, and others) between tags. A recent method (Tang et al, 2009) discovers synonym, hypernym and some other relations between tags, without to require prior knowledge about the domain. Such an approach can learn an ontology hierarchy from any social tagging application. In conclusion, the methods that have been so far proposed for learning ontologies from tags integrate social data in a direct way so that social data is not implied. Such integration is important since it "moves" an already agreed organization of information (folksonomy) into a new formal organization (ontology) that it works well in applications only if this organization is commonly agreed.

Trusting of ontological specifications and the path to ontological agreement is a key issue to the automated learning of social ontologies due to its importance for successful exploitation. Ontological agreement (or ontological commitment) states that some conceptualizations about a specific domain have been shared among certain contributors and that they have agreed on a common understanding about the domain. Such an agreement can only be achieved through social fermentation – discussion and argumentation in a collaborative and democratic fashion (e.g. argumentation dialogues and voting). Trust refers to the degree of confidence that contributors may have or not on the shared ontologies. Such confidence is usually measured using reputation values for the specified conceptualizations, derived from social data that is associated to them. Based on these facts, we conjecture that the following definitions can hold: a) an agreement on a conceptualization can be trusted by all contributors (trusted agreement) or not, and b) a confidence/reputation/uncertainty value can be computed based on the (degree of) agreement or disagreement between contributors upon specific conceptualizations (consensus trust).

Although several types of input for a decision on trust have been proposed, i.e. direct experience, categorization (generalization to or from something known), reasoning (application of common sense or rules to verify truth), and reputation, *the problem of how content's trust may be derived and how it may be automatically captured and used on the Semantic Web is still an open topic.* Intelligent social network analysis and mining for automatically extracting - from humans' opinions and voting - trust over information they own or information owned by others is mainly based on reputation information. Reputation-based trust uses personal experience or the experiences of others, possibly combined, to make a trust decision about an entity. Any statements contained in the Semantic Web must be considered as claims rather than facts, until trust, a method of dealing with uncertainty, can be established (Artz & Gil, 2007). Social network analysis and mining are important for the direct or indirect representation of (consensus) trust of shared domain conceptualizations. Software agents must be enabled to use context and reputation to determine what information to trust in the Semantic Web. By providing agents with social ontologies i.e. content, context and its reputation in a formal (e.g. uncertainty values in the range of 0 to 1 interval "attached to" semantic relations between classes of learned ontologies) and/or associative manner (e.g. ontology elements "linked to" networks of trust: people say how much they trust other people in a formal way), is a hit in the "heart of the Semantic Web vision" (O'Hara et al, 2004).

LEARNING SOCIAL ONTOLOGIES

Learning Ontologies from Query Logs

The method, introduced in (Kotis & Papasalouros, 2010), explores the automated learning of social ontologies from query logs. Such a method is not depended on other ontology engineering tasks (e.g. merging with other ontologies), it is a fully automated method, and finally, it analyzes and utilizes unstructured information without utilizing any social data directly. The social dimension of the learning process is somehow 'hidden' into the nature of the input content (i.e. Web users' query logs) and into the organization of single queries into clusters of relevant queries prior to the ontology learning process (majority vote of user clicks).

Method Description

A number of single Web queries that have been recorded in a Web search engine's log file are first clustered into query sets, based on domain relevance. The clustering method utilizes the links to Web documents returned by the search engine and selected (clicked) by users. The clustered queries are analyzed in a batch fashion (POS tagging, occurrence frequency measuring, relation extraction) using NLP techniques (term-to-query and term-to-query-Set analysis) and are then transformed into a starting (kick-off) lightweight ontology. The final ontology is an enrichment of the kick-off one using additional semantics from WordNet lexicon (extracted using term-to-synset mapping techniques). The method has been evaluated by manually examining the learned OWL ontologies

in the context of an ontology engineering lifecycle (by knowledge engineers) and also by automatically comparing them against gold ontologies using a common ontology evaluation method.

The main aim of this method is not to focus on the usefulness of kick-off query-ontologies in terms of ontology-based applications e.g. Semantic Search engines, such as in Spiliopoulos et al. (2008). This method, in contrast to other related approaches, aims to provide evidences that query logs, when combined with general lexicons or other external knowledge resources, can be used to automatically learn not only lightweight ontologies but also richer ontologies that are more useful in the kick-off phase of an ontology development lifecycle of a collaborative and human-centered ontology engineering methodology for devising evolving ontologies. An empirical evaluation (user interviews, questionnaires, usability testing) of the approach that engages end-users, provides such preliminary evidences. The chapter aims to present a method that learns kick-off social ontologies with richer semantics and vocabulary than the lightweight versions of related approaches (disjoint axioms, equivalent classes and individuals). This method extends the one presented in Spiliopoulos et al. (2008) in the following ways:

1. The approach deals with the mining of sets of queries, instead of single queries,
2. The learned ontology is richer in terms of semantics (e.g. disjoint classes, individuals, synonyms), and
3. A different vector-based space model method is used in the disambiguation process of query terms, due to the utilization of more than one query in the computation of the vicinity of query terms (bag of words used with the Latent Semantic Indexing method in order to map query terms to WordNet senses).

The approach meets the following specific requirements:

1. Learn kick-off domain ontologies to advance the SW content creation, integrating ontology-learning-related tasks in HCOME O.E. methodology
2. Learn such ontologies from domain-specific query logs. The approach can take input of query logs from the open Web, e.g. Search Engines query logs, given that a pre-processing step is performed for the classification of queries in domain-specific query sets (clustering method)
3. Learn semantically rich ontologies using semantics that are extracted from external sources such as lexicons
4. Automate the learning process

Query logs reflect knowledge workers' domain-specific search interests. Knowledge workers query information spaces, searching for domain-related information. Such queries are recorded in query logs, usually without linking them to meta-information concerning the precision and recall of the returned information. The query logs may contain queries that have been already placed in the past in different forms and also may contain queries from different knowledge workers. (see Figure 1)

The first step of the proposed method is to analyze the query set and identify the important terms i.e. terms that occur frequently (more than one time). In addition to this, the neighbour terms of each term (called the vicinity of a term) in every query are identified. Stop words are excluded from the vicinity of each term. Such information is needed for the disambiguation of terms using Latent Semantic Indexing (LSI) method to map key terms to WordNet senses (Kotis et al, 2006). The analysis of a domain-specific query log is based on the assumption that all queries are related to a unique domain and thus, their terms should be somehow related between each other. We conjecture that such a relation, a domain-related one, is present not only between terms of an individual query but also between terms of every query of a particular domain-specific query log. Formally, the vicinity of each query term is computed as follows:

1. For a term t_i that occurs only in one query $q_j = \{t_1, t_2, ..., t_k\}$ of the query set $Q = \{q_1,$

Figure 1. Architecture of the proposed approach

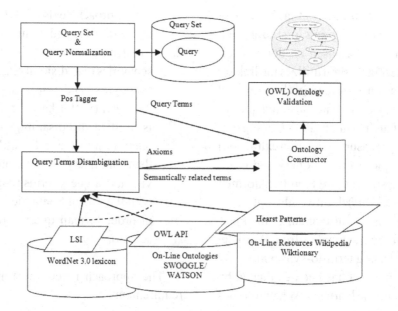

$q_2, \ldots, q_n\}$, the vicinity V_{t_i} of t_i comprises the rest terms of q_j, i.e. $V_{t_i} = q_j \setminus \{t_i\}$.

2. For a term t that occurs in more than one queries (i.e. an important term), its vicinity V_t comprises the rest terms of all queries that the important term is contained i.e.

$$V_t = \bigcup_{t \in q_j} q_j \setminus \{t\}.$$

LSI method maps bags of query terms to WordNet synsets. Doing so, the method computes a mapping between each of these terms and a "hidden intermediate" ontology (Kotis et al. 2006b). This mapping is computed by the LSI method which assumes that there is an underlying latent semantic space that it estimates by means of statistical techniques using an association matrix (n×m) of terms-documents: Documents in our case correspond to WordNet senses. The use of a latent semantic space helps to deal with problems of imprecise and vague descriptions of queries, as well as with cases of polysemy and synonymy that other traditional techniques such as Vector Space Models (VSM) cannot handle. LSI is implemented via Latent Semantic Analysis (LSA) which computes the arrangement of a k-dimensional semantic space to reflect the major associative patterns in the data. This is in particular done by deriving a set of k uncorrelated indexing factors. Then, each term and document is represented by its vector of factor values, indicating its strength of association with each of these underlying latent "concepts". By virtue of dimension reduction from the N terms space to the k factors space, where k<N, terms that did not actually appear in a document may still end up close to the document, if this is consistent with the major patterns of association in the data.

The second step of the proposed ontology learning method is to identify the part of speech (POS) for each query term of each query, using a general POS tagging algorithm such as the Stanford tagger[2]. Future work on this step will focus on alternative techniques to POS identification to avoid incorrect tagging due to tagger's

inability to perform well with very small queries (information absence). This step identifies mainly nouns, verbs, and adjectives in order to be able to apply simple heuristics e.g. for the identification of object properties.

The third step is the core step of the proposed approach since it takes as input the first and second step and a mapping method to assign WordNet senses to query terms, and returns in the output a set of semantically related query terms. The output of this step is used by an ontology construction module to transform such information into a W3C standard OWL (Ontology Web Language). In Figure 2 the algorithm for the main (WordNet-based) functionality of the proposed approach is presented. The proposed algorithm discovers subsumption, synonym and disjoint relations between query terms (using WordNet Hypernym/Hyponym, Synonym and Antonym relative semantic relations between senses). Individual objects are also discovered using functionality provided by the WordNet API[3].

It must be pointed out that the learned ontology is not just a projection of a WordNet termi-

Figure 2. Algorithm for the main (WordNet-based) functionality of the proposed approach

```
1.   (Perform query set pre-processing)
2.   For each query q
3.     For each key query term t
4.       POS tag t,
5.       disambiguate t using neighbor terms of queries that have a t
6.       occurrence
         return the mapped WordNet sense s
7.       If t.POS is Noun
8.         If s is Instance
9.           find its concept's hypernym ch from WordNet
10.          add ch in the ontology
11.          add s in the ontology as an individual of class ch
12.        End if
13.        Else (* s is a class *)
14.          add s in the ontology as a class
15.          add any synonyms of s as label of the class
16.          add any hypernyms up to depth UPPER_DEPTH (>=0)
17.          add any hyponyms up to depth LOWER_DEPTH (>=0)
18.        Else if t.POS is Verb
19.          add s in the ontology as a class
20.          add any synonyms of s as label of the class
21.          add any antonym of s as a disjoint class
22.          add any hypernyms up to depth UPPER_DEPTH (>=0)
23.        End if
24.      End for
25.   End for
```

nological subset, although currently it is heavily depended on it, since non-WordNet terms are also handled by the method (not depicted in the algorithm of Figure 2 for presentation reasons). Such terms may be: a) single terms that have no entry in WordNet and b) compound terms. For instance, a query term lexicalized by the word "ecology-car" is transformed by the proposed algorithm to a class "ecology-car" classified under an introduced class "car". Furthermore, a class "Ecology" will be introduced that will be related with class "ecology-car" via a generic role "related_to". Different forms of compound terms are also handled by the algorithm, using heuristic rules. For instance, terms such as "ecology_car", "ecology-car", 'ecologyCar" are also identified equally as compound terms. (see Figure 3)

Finally, it must be accentuated that, in extend to other approaches (e.g. Spiliopoulos et al. 2008; Cimiano et al. 2007), the constructed ontology utilizes a set of queries (a domain specific subset of a query log) and the interrelation of their terms

in order to learn a single ontology (many queries to one ontology mapping, m:1). An extension for future work is the learning of a kick-off ontology for a single query (one query to one ontology mapping, 1:1) using terms from other "related" queries of the domain-specific subset of the query log that the query belongs to.

Due to space limitations, the auxiliary preprocessing method of mining of query logs for organizing queries into clusters is not presented in this chapter. Please refer to an earlier publication of this line of research (Kotis and Papasalouros, 2010).

Related Work

In Sekine & Suzuki (2007), although focusing on the acquisition of ontological knowledge from queries, authors do not report on issues related to the automatic learning of ontologies. Evaluation of the approach was extensive; however the usefulness of the learned ontologies in real

Figure 3. Learned ontology specifications in RDF triples form for a subset of "car repair" domain query log (query terms in bold and underlined form indicate correspondence with the presented triples)

Queries	RDF triples form (< Subject, **predicate**, Object >)
car engine **fix** in **Australia**	\<Repair **rdf:subClassOf** Improvement> \<Repair **rdfs:label** Fix>
replace her broken **car** **window**	... \<Country **rdfs:subClassOf** Thing>
repair a busted **car** **window**	\<Australia **rdf:type** Country>
auto mobile **repair**, instructions for breaks	... \<Break **rdf:subClassOf** Destroy> \<Break **owl:disjointWith** Repair>
ecology-car **repair** instructions	... \<Window **rdf:subClassOf** Opening>
not-in-wordnetTerm car seat repair	\<Car-window **rdf:subClassOf** Window>
	... \<Car **rdf:subClassOf** Motor_vehicle> \<Ecology-car **rdf:subClassOf** Car>
	... \<Related_to **rdfs:domain** Ecology-car> \<Related_to **rdfs:range** Ecology>
	... \<Term **rdfs:subClassOf** Thing> \<wordnetTerm **rdfs:subClassOf** Term> \<not-in-wordnetTerm **rdfs:subClassOf** wordnetTerm>
	... \<Seat **rdfs:subClassOf** Support> \<Car-Seat **rdfs:subClassOf** Seat>

SW applications as well as the comparison with gold-ontologies is not reported. Another related work concerns the mining of query logs to assist ontology learning from relational databases (Zhang et al, 2006), based on Formal Concept Analysis (FCA). The approach is heavily depended on the schema extracted from the database since it is used as input in the mining of the query log. Evaluation of the constructed hierarchies is done manually. More importantly, the usefulness of the learned ontologies is not measured in terms of evaluating them in real SW applications. In Gulla et al (2007), an unsupervised key-phrase extraction system has been used to speed up the construction of search ontologies. The learned ontologies are verified manually by domain experts and concepts are related to each other with various hierarchical and associative relationships appropriately (manual work is needed to complete the hierarchies and possibly add more abstract concepts that link everything together in complete ontologies). Evaluation of the usefulness of the learned ontologies in real applications is not reported. In Park et al (2003), a method for building ontologies on demand from scientific queries by applying text mining technologies is presented. The approach is heavily based on the analysis of the returned documents, even if they are incorrectly returned by the search engine. Furthermore, the constructed ontology does not utilize a set of queries and the interrelation of their terms, as it is proposed in this chapter, but rather it only formalizes a single query using information only from the query itself. In ORAKEL (Cimiano et al, 2007), a similar approach to the one proposed in this chapter is presented. However, a target corpus must be available to construct custom lexicons that will then assist the learning method of lightweight ontologies. Furthermore, the constructed ontology does not utilize a set of queries and the interrelation of their terms, as it is proposed by the presented approach in this chapter.

SOCIAL DIMENSION OF THE LEARNED ONTOLOGIES

Web queries reflect Web users' search interests. By clustering such interests into domains using the method described in Kotis and Papasalouros (2010), it is their wisdom (clicks on similar Web pages) that classifies specific common interests in specific domains. Such common interests can be considered as an agreement on terminology that will be used to lexicalize the conceptualizations i.e. the signature S represented in a learned ontology $O=\{C, S, A\}$. Furthermore, it can be conjectured that the majority vote of user clicks is an indication of the relevance of results. By analysing user logs one can measure the reputation of clicked results and consequently the trust on the content that has been related to a specific query. Such trusted content is then used in a variety of ways in the learning process e.g. to cluster queries in a query log, to disambiguate queries, etc., thus it contributes to the acceptance (trust degree) of the learned ontology by the knowledge contributors C.

Web users are self-trained (by experience) to choose query terms that are meaningful and less ambiguous (focused on the domain). Such queries, indirectly capture human knowledge since they inquire *"what is already known"* (common knowledge), and convey knowledge in the querying process. As stated in Pasca (2007), query logs convey knowledge through queries that may be answered by the knowledge asserted in expository text of document collections.

Evaluation of Method

The method has been evaluated in several ways: a) comparing learned ontologies against gold ones, b) manually examining the learned ontologies, c) evaluating the learned ontologies within an ontology development lifecycle. The preliminary results are quite promising.

The tight integration of an ontology learning task to OE methodologies has been recognized by the research community as a very important challenge for ontology engineering and evaluation and as a crucial invest in the development of new ontology engineering methodologies which will be able to integrate the results of ontology learning systems in the OE process, keeping at the same time user involvement at a minimum level while concerned with the maximization of the produced ontologies' quality (with respect to a particular domain) (Cimiano et al, 2006). Thus, the ontologies learned from the proposed ontology learning method were put in the context of the HCOME methodology and in the loop of an ontology development lifecycle by selected users with different experience/role (both knowledge workers and knowledge engineers). Users were asked to assess the quality of the ontologies in terms of how well they reflect the domain of the query set and in terms of the consistency of the formal conceptualizations. More importantly, they were asked to assess the usability of the learned kick-off ontologies within an ontology development lifecycle. To do so, they were given both the learned ontology and the query set that the ontologies have been learned from. Four different ontologies/query-set pairs, with a variety of length (in terms of query number and number of learned ontology elements/axioms), were put in HCOME ontology development lifecycle as kick-off ontologies. The feedback from this evaluation process was taken in two ways: a) by a personal interview, b) by a questionnaire. The evaluators were Web users with an academic training in ontology engineering: familiar with the HCOME methodology and with ontology development tools such as Protégé and HCONE. The questionnaire was given to the evaluators, together with the related material (learned ontologies and query-sets of Yahoo! and Google). A qualitative and quantitative examination of the filled questionnaires has been conducted. The results are summarized in the following:

- The usefulness of an automatically learned kick-off ontology in ontology-based applications such as semantic annotation, knowledge viewing, and semantic search has been accentuated by the evaluators: Questioned about the usefulness of query-ontologies in ontology-based applications, evaluators reported that using these ontologies to annotate documents that they want to query is of high usefulness; they reported that using ontologies in order to reformulate/enrich queries in order to retrieve information is also of high usefulness.

- The usefulness of an automatically learned kick-off ontology in ontology development lifecycle has been accentuated by the evaluators: they stated that they would use a kick-off ontology in order to compare it with their own ontology and copy parts of it in their own ontology. In addition, they stated that they would use a kick-off ontology also as a consultation for constructing their own ontology. Consequently, it can be generally stated that users find kick-off ontologies useful in the ontology development process.

Learned ontologies were also compared with gold ones. Such an evaluation was conducted using the Dellschaft and Staab's approach (Dellschaft and Staab, 2006), re-using the OntEval system[4]. The approach takes two ontologies defined in OWL formats as input, one of which is assumed the Gold Standard (reference) ontology (O_r) and the other as the machine computed ontology (O_c); then we performed evaluation by computing measures such as Lexical Precision (LP), Lexical Recall (LR), Taxonomic Precision (TP), Taxonomic Recall (TR), F-Measure (TF). The lexical precision and recall reflect how good the learned lexical terms cover the target domain. Results over 70% for each distinct measure were encouraging for continuing in this research direction. The ontology learning method has been evaluated using Yahoo! and a Google query datasets.

Impact to the Semantic Web

The learned ontologies, reflecting the domain-specific search interests, are the best candidates for Semantic Search applications. Semantic search systems such as SAMOS (Spiliopoulos et al, 2008) exploit query-ontologies (i.e. ontologies learned from queries) to retrieve Semantic Web documents (SWD) using ontology alignment techniques. Beyond the accuracy of the matching algorithms, the efficiency of the system is heavily influenced by the quality of the learned ontology. Although experiments have been already conducted and preliminary results are promising, further steps must be followed in order to measure the impact of increasing the agreement of the learned ontologies to the applications' performance i.e. test the impact of larger query logs that are produced by different number of users in different time sequences.

FUTURE RESEARCH DIRECTIONS

Learning Ontologies from Web 2.0 Question/Answers Applications

Extending the work conducted using query logs as input to a social ontology learning process, a novel social ontology learning method is proposed in this chapter, with the ultimate objective to be used for the evaluation of a framework for trusting the learning of social ontologies from Web 2.0 content. As a case study the Web 2.0 application of Yahoo! Answers community (and Fixya.com as an alternative) has been selected. Yahoo! Answers (http://answers.yahoo.com/) is a shared place where people collaborate and communicate by asking and answering questions on any topic. The aim of such a social fermentation is to build an open and commonly agreed knowledge base for the benefit of the community. Organized in

topics (simple thematic category hierarchies), questions are posted by the users of the social network, expecting several answers that will eventually satisfy their knowledge acquisition needs. A voting for the best answer mechanism ensures that an agreed (by the majority) and trusted (by the number of "for" voters) answer is related to a question. Professional knowledge can also be shared within the community by *knowledge partners*. Such knowledge supplements the answers received from the community by answering questions in a specialized field, drawing on partners training, their professional experiences, and other appropriate resources. As a benefit, knowledge partners may mention their products or services, where relevant, in an answer, for advertisement reasons. Such a mutual benefit (for partners and community users) can guarantee a live social network that is difficult to "die" and at the same time it can guarantee a strong building of trust for the content that all stakeholders are sharing.

The content of Yahoo! Answers is similar to the content of query logs. *Questions* in Yahoo! Answers has a correspondence to Web queries and *answers* have a correspondence to Search Engines Web pages returned as results. Based on this fact, the learned ontologies, reflecting the domain-specific search interests as in the query-logs-based ontology learning method, are the best candidates for using them in Semantic Search applications. The proposed method utilizes the following inputs:

1. A question/answer document which contains the following information:
    - the topic of the question (and the more general/specific categories of the topic hierarchy). Topics are pre-defined by Yahoo! Answers application
    - user information: who posted the question, who posted an answer, who voted against or for
    - the question and the associated answers in natural language: users can post a title and a comment for the

question, and only comments for their answers
- the best answer and the votes for it
- the votes for all other answers
- other related questions, resolved or open, on the same topic

2. WordNet lexicon. It will be used to enrich the ontology with additional semantics (entities, semantic relations, individuals)

The processing of the proposed social ontology learning method is performed in the following steps (Figure 4):

- **Step 1:** The method learns the starting RDF triples from the types of the pre-defined hierarchy that the topic of the posted question is classified under.

- **Step 2:** The posted question (both title and comment) is analyzed using an NLP API (e.g. GATE5) in order to identify parts of speech (POS) and perform tokenization.

- **Step 3:** Since context is known (from Step-1) and some text analysis has been done (in Step-2), important terms can be identified and semantic relations between them can be recognized (Kotis & Papasalouros, 2010). The following techniques can be used in combination: a) Hearst patterns, b) Simple heuristic rules that utilize knowledge from the POS tagging.

- **Step 4:** Semantics are enriched using WordNet. Mapping of terms to WordNet senses is performed automatically using a statistical technique from Information Retrieval to compute latency of terms in term-document spaces (Kotis et al, to appear).

- **Step 5:** Steps 2 to 4 are repeated for the best (voted) posted answer. The ontology elements extracted from this step (classes, properties, instances) are assigned the uncertainty value 1.0 (representing the uncertainty of this element in respect to the

Figure 4. The architecture of the proposed learning method

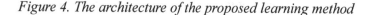

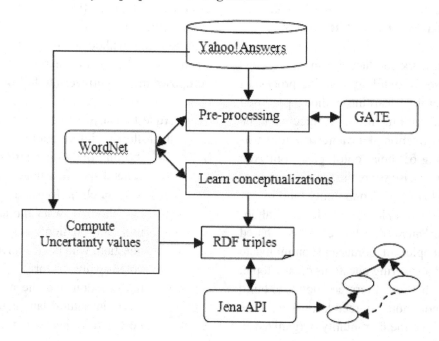

community trust of the commonly agreed "best answer").

- **Step 6:** Steps 2 to 4 are repeated for the rest posted answers. To keep the size of the learned ontology small (and to avoid noise) only important terms (most frequent terms) are introduced as classes of the learned ontology. The importance of terms is a threshold value that can be empirically set at '2'. However, in large sized answers (more than one paragraph of text) such value must be set higher. Other techniques should be also tested to avoid noise of large answers (e.g. to first locate important partitions of the text, applying n-grams analysis for instance, and then extract important terms from there). The ontology elements extracted from this step (classes, properties, instances) are assigned an uncertainty value (normalized) between the interval 0 and 0.9.
- **Step 7:** The generated RDF triples from Step-2 to Step-6 are transformed into a consistent OWL model. The development proposed is based on Jena API and Pellet.

The output of the method is a learned ontology with uncertainty weights attached to its elements (classes, properties, instances).

The voting mechanism integrated in Yahoo!Answers provides social data that is used to relate content i.e. a posted answer to some other content, i.e. to a posted question. Such relation can be interpreted as agreement or disagreement on users' opinion and eventually as a trust value to the shared knowledge that is encapsulated in the most agreed opinion (best voted answer). Trusted more or less, the related-to-a-topic knowledge is shaped into a domain ontology where each element is associated with an uncertainty value that is computed directly from the social data associated with the represented content.

Professional knowledge can also be shared within the community by Knowledge Partners.

Such knowledge supplements the answers received from Answers community. Since this kind of knowledge is contributed by experts, it can also be considered as highly trusted.

Furthermore, as already stated, the mutual benefit of knowledge partners and community users (advertisement and expertise knowledge contribution) plays a key role to "truth telling" when it comes to partners' answers in community users' posts. This can guarantee a live social network with strong roots of trust for the content that both stakeholders are sharing.

Relatively to ontology learning from query logs method, this method can be trusted in a higher degree since social data is both directly and indirectly associated with the content represented in the ontology.

The proposed method is under development. Although input data has been gathered and organized, there is no any evaluation conducted yet. However, some initial experiments have been conducted with a manual processing of input data, i.e. manually extracting knowledge from input documents and building experimental ontologies. Such a manual process simulates the automatic learning approach as much as possible.

TRUSTING THE LEARNING OF SOCIAL ONTOLOGIES

Representing Trust in Social Ontologies

This chapter also proposes a model that represents trust for an ontology $O = \{C, S, A\}$. More specifically, O is formed as a meta-ontology which represents meta-information related to each element of a social ontology i.e. classes, properties, instances, contributors. Such meta-information is related to social data (e.g. contributors' details, voting information) that is in turn somehow related to the content represented in the domain ontology. The definition of $O = \{C, S, A\}$ is then extended by introducing trust T for C, S and A such as $T = \{u, v_a, v_f\}$ where: u specifies the uncertainty value computed for a given instance of C, S or A, v_a specifies the number of votes that do not trust an instance of C, S or A, and v_f specifies the number of votes that do trust an instance of C, S or A. In other words, some trusted (with some degree of uncertainty) contributors C are trusting (with some degree of uncertainty) a particular class, property or instance (i.e. an instance of S ontological signature) or an axiom (i.e. an instance of A axioms) that is learned from C's contributed content. Although the computation of u *(uncertainty value)* reflects the trust in C, S or A within a social network of C contributors, values v_a and v_f are reflecting the absolute *number of agreement* between the members of C for a given instance of C, S or A.

Integrate Trust in HCOME-3O Meta-Ontologies Framework

Ontologies are *evolving* and *shared* artefacts that are collaboratively and iteratively developed, evolved, evaluated and discussed within communities of common interest (CoI), shaping domain-specific information spaces. To enhance the potential of information spaces to be collaboratively engineered and shaped into ontologies within and between different communities, these artefacts must be escorted with *all* the necessary meta-information concerning the conceptualization they realize, implementation decisions and their evolution. In HCOME-3O framework (Vouros et al, 2007), the integration of three (meta-) ontologies that provide information concerning the conceptualization and the development of domain ontologies, the atomic changes made by knowledge workers, the long-term evolutions and argumentations behind decisions taken during the lifecycle of an ontology, has been proposed (and evaluated via its utilization in later work). This involves ontology engineering tasks for a *domain* ontology and its versions *(domain knowledge)*, i.e. editing, argumentation, exploiting and inspect-

ing, during which meta-information is captured and recorded (*development ontologies*) either as information concerning a simple task or as information concerning the interlinking of tasks. This framework has been proposed in the context of HCOME collaborative engineering methodology (Kotis & Papasalouros, 2010).

Recently, HCOME methodology has been extended with ontology learning tasks (Kotis & Papasalouros, 2010) in order to capture knowledge that is automatically extracted from content and learned in the domain ontology. In such a new dimension of the methodological aspect of ontology engineering, agent agreement on automatically learned conceptualizations may be assisted by integrating representations of already computed uncertainty values in the following way: collaborating knowledge contributors consult uncertainty values of the learned conceptualizations and agree or disagree on the conceptualizations.

The integration of the proposed model into the HCOME-3O framework can be easily achieved by merging its semantics with the Administration meta-ontology (Vouros et al, 2007), which mainly records instances of domain conceptualizations (classes, properties, individuals) and contributors of such conceptualizations, in the following way (Figure 2): a) add trust-related datatype properties ("uncertainty_value", "votes_against", "votes_for") of the trust model to the Administration meta-ontology, Administered_Item class), b) add object properties (has_superClass, has_Domain, has_Range, has_Type) to the corresponded ontology elements, extending the Administration meta-ontology, in order to facilitate the assignment of trust on (simple) axioms (*A)* also. (see Figure 5)

A *Formal Item* (a Class, a Property or an Individual item of the domain ontology) is recorded in the meta-ontology as domain knowledge that is contributed by a specific Contributor. Trust-related properties are attached to formal items, represented with the data type properties: *uncertainty_value, votes_against, votes_for*. Such properties are inherited to all formal items of the

Figure 5. The proposed trust meta-ontology that have been integrated in the HCOME-3O Administration meta-ontology

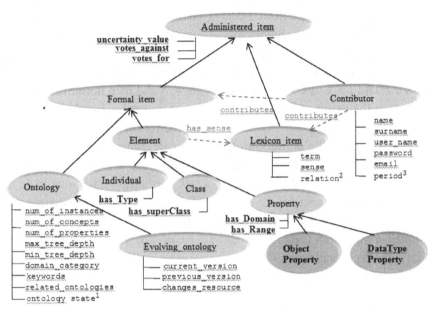

1. It specifies whether an ontology is personal, shared or agreed
2. It specifies the semantic relation between the term that lexicalizes the concept and the lexicon/thesaurus term entry (e.g. synonym, more specific, more general)
3. A period starts when a personal ontology is send to the shared space and ends when a version of this ontology is in the agreed state.

extracted signature S of the domain ontology. Furthermore, the trust-related properties are also attached (inherited via the Administered Item specification) to the Contributor. Such information is necessary in order to keep record of trusted (by others) people also. A similar conceptualization for trusting people is provided in Trust ontology of MindSwap (http://trust.mindswap.org/trustOnt. shtml) however it is not interlinked with trust-aware domain conceptualizations that these people may contribute. On the other hand, several other efforts have been lately presented (see related work section) for modeling trusted conceptualizations; however they are not interlinked with the trust-aware recording of their contributors. Having said that, since the Administration meta-ontology is part of a wider meta-information framework (that is HCOME-3O framework), the 'range' of the trust-related properties can be expanded to other meta-information also such as

the changes that are recorded between each new version that contributors are developing, the argumentation dialogue items (arguments, issues, positions) that are recording during the collaborative evaluation/development of ontologies, etc. As a result of this effect, the model can provide answers to more complex queries such as '*give me all changes that were made between version O_i and version O_{i+1} of the ontology O, for all contributors with trust $T = \{0.6, 4, 5\}$*' or '*give me all suggesting positions (argumentation items) that were made by the community for classes of the domain ontology with a trust $T = \{0.6, 4, 5\}$.*'

For a detailed description of the Administration meta-ontology and its role in the HCOME-3O framework please refer to the related article (Vouros et al, 2007).

Trust for axioms can be also extracted since they also comprise domain knowledge that can be found in social content. Trust of axioms however can be easily inferred from already trusted upper level classes and axioms of the learned ontology. Consider for instance axioms that have been used "as found" in a simple pre-defined topic hierarchy as in Yahoo!Answer Web 2.0 application: If class *A*, class *B* and class *C* are trusted with value "1.0" and the axioms $A \sqsubseteq B$ and $B \sqsubseteq C$ are also trusted with value "*1.0*", then the axiom $A \sqsubseteq C$ can be also trusted.

Concluding the paragraph, the definition of the social ontology can now be reformulated as follows: $O = \{T, C, S, A\}$ where $T = \{u, v_a, v_f\}$ is the trust function (uncertainty, votes against, votes for) for ontological signature *S* and axioms *A* that a set of collaborated contributors *C* participated in a task of social content generation (SCG) have derived using their social intelligence (SI).

Computation of Uncertainty Values

For a Web social application that uses a voting system to trust (or not) some content (e.g. in Yahoo!Answers application where users vote for or against a posted answer to a Yahoo!Answers community question), the uncertainty value *u* for this piece of content can be computed using the simple formula $u = V_f - V_a$, i.e. the number of votes after subtracting the votes against (V_a) from the votes for (V_f). The vector of the voting values computed for some content, $VVV = (u_1, u_2 ... u_n)$ where *n* represents the number of content chunks that have been related to the voting system (e.g. in the Yahoo!Answers application *n* is the number of answers *a* posted for a question *q*), is then normalized to the interval *[0, 1]*. The normalization will work well if data is positive or zero. If data contains some negative numbers, for example, *-1*, *3* and *4*, then the sum is 6. If it is normalized by the maximum value we get *-1/6*, *½*, and *2/3*. The sum of the three values is still *1* but now a negative number (*-1/6*) is part of the index. The following general solution may be however applied: Shift data by adding all numbers with the absolute of the most negative (minimum value of data*)* such

that the most negative one will become zero and all other numbers become positive. Then data is normalized using any common normalization method for zero or positive numbers. For example, if data is *-1*, *3* and *4*, the most negative number is -1, thus we add all numbers with +*1* to become: *0*, *4*, *5* and then normalize it.

A general normalization solution is described in the following lines. Suppose we have a range or scale from *A* to *B* and we want to convert it to a scale of *1* to *10*, where *A* maps to *1* and *B* maps to *10*. Furthermore, we want to do this with a linear function, so that for example the point midway between *A* and *B* maps to halfway between *1* and *10*, or *5.5*. Then the following (linear) equation can be applied to any number *x* on the *A-B* scale:

$$y = 1 + (x - A) * (10 - 1) / (B - A) \qquad (1)$$

Note that if $x = A$, this gives $y = 1 + 0 = 1$ as required, and if $x = B$, $y = 1 + (B - A) * (10 - 1) / (B - A) = 1 + 10 - 1 = 10$, as required. One can use this equation even if $A > B$. In our case, the scale will be *0.0* to *1.0* for every *x*, where $x \in \{u\}$.

Related work on the uncertainty of learned ontologies (Lau et al, 2007; Tho et al, 2006) defines the notion of Fuzzy set and Fuzzy Relation to represent knowledge with uncertainty. We use two definitions (taken from the related literature) in order to distinguish the presented work with the related ones:

- **Definition 1 (Fuzzy Set)** A fuzzy set F consists of a set of objects drawn from a domain X and the membership of each object x_i in *F* is defined by a membership function $\mu F: X \rightarrow [0, 1]$. If *Y* is a crisp, that is non-fuzzy, set, $\varphi(Y)$ denotes a fuzzy set generated from the traditional set of items *Y*.

- **Definition 2 (Fuzzy Relation)** A fuzzy relation is defined as the fuzzy set *G* on a domain $X_X Y$ where *X* and *Y* are two crisp sets.

Both related approaches (Lau et al, 2007; Tho et al, 2006) view an uncertain ontology from the text mining perspective. According to this perspective, a discovered keyword is an object and it belongs to different concepts (a linguistic class) with various memberships. The subsumption relations among linguistic concepts are often uncertain and are characterized by the appropriate fuzzy relations. Consequently, a *fuzzy ontology is defined* as $Ont = < X, C, RXC, RCC >$, where X is a set of objects and C is a set of concepts. The fuzzy relation $RXC: X_X C \rightarrow [0, 1]$ maps the set of objects to the set of concepts by assigning the respective membership values, and the fuzzy relation $RCC: C_X C \rightarrow [0, 1]$ denotes the fuzzy taxonomy relations among the set of concepts C.

The work presented in this chapter does not follow this perspective. Uncertainty in the learned ontologies is not captured as an effect of a "good" or "bad" text mining technique. Rather, uncertainty results from the social fermentation process during the creation of social content (social data and domain-specific content). This is an important distinction to the related work since it is in-line with the social dimension of the automatic learning ontology process. Nevertheless, it seems to be the right approach when referring to social ontology learning (not just ontology learning). However, the text-mining uncertainty dimension may be also of some importance when combined with a social one: A "gold" approach towards trusting automated learning of social ontologies can serve as a merger of both dimensions i.e. the text-mining and the social one. Intuitively, the average uncertainty of the two values can be considered the "gold" uncertainty value u_g of the formulae $T = \{u, v_a, v_f\}$ of our approach, where $u_g = (u+u_{RXC})/2$ *and for the taxonomy relations* $u_g = (u+u_{RCC})/2$. However, more sophisticated formulas may be proposed, if based, for instance, on the work of learning trust decision strategies in agent-based reputation exchange networks (Fullam & Barber, 2006; O'Hara, 2004). Assuming that a pessimistic strategy is followed (O'Hara, 2004), where agents do not trust each other unless there is a reason to do so, u_{RXC} should be weighted more than u.

To apply the proposed framework on a queries-to-ontology learning method, an important assumption must be made since a voting mechanism is not integrated. The formula of $T = \{u, v_a, v_f\}$ must be reduced to $T = \{u\}$ since in this case v_a and v_f are zero. The computation of u for a Web query q is based on the reputation of the query in a particular context. Such reputation is reflected by the number of clicks on resulted documents for a particular query (reflecting that users' interests have been found in this query). Since this value can be considered as the reputation of a particular query, it can also be considered as the reputation of the learned conceptualizations from the particular query that a contributor C provided, i.e. the query-related signature S and axioms A of the learned ontology. Thus, the formula $O = \{T, C, S, A\}$ is valid for this use case. Low reputation values will be computed for queries that have a smaller number of clicked documents associated with them i.e. many Web users did not find search results to be much related to the query (they did not clicked on them). An additional step to this approach may be the analysis of history of queries: measuring the frequency of similar queries placed for the same context. This is left for other lines of future research.

To apply the proposed framework on question-Answers-to-ontology learning method, and to respect the formula $O = \{T, C, S, A\}$, the learned ontology must be recorded in the extended Administration meta-ontology of the HCOME-3O model, interlinking the trusted conceptualizations with trusted contributors. In this use case, the contributors are Yahoo!Answers voters, members of the Yahoo! community, for which trust values can be also computed using a) a point system that is provided by the application in order to represent the reputation in the community, and b) their experience in the community (time of registration).

CONCLUSION

This chapter discusses issues related to the automated learning of social ontologies. More specific it presents a novel method and preliminary evaluation results of automatically learning social ontologies. In addition, due to its importance for a successful exploitation of the learned ontologies, it introduces a first approach towards modeling the trust on learned conceptualizations, as part of a social fermentation process between users that belong in communities of common interests (CoI), in open, collaborative and communicative environments. The chapter specifies the requirements for a devising a method for the automated learning of social ontologies and furthermore reports on the interlinking of agreement, trust and the learned domain conceptualizations that are extracted from social data of Web applications. The reported work can be used as a consultation for the design of future methods that concern the learning of ontologies from social data. Such methods need to be capable of learning not only domain conceptualizations but also the degree that agents (humans or software) may trust them (and also their contributors) or not. The contribution of the presented work to the Semantic Web realization is focused on the semantic content creation bottleneck. The technology presented is aiming to ease the development of ontologies by encouraging Web users to participate and contribute in the semantic content creation process.

REFERENCES

Artz, D., & Gil, Y. (2007). A survey of trust in computer science and the Semantic Web. *Journal of Web Semantics: Science. Services and Agents on the World Wide Web, 5*, 58–71. doi:10.1016/j. websem.2007.03.002

Cimiano, P., Haase, P., & Heizmann, J. (2007). Porting natural language interfaces between domains – a case study with the ORAKEL system. In *Proceedings of the International Conference on Intelligent User Interfaces* (IUI), (pp. 180–189).

Cimiano, P., Völker, J., & Studer, R. (2006). Ontologies on demand? - A description of the state-of-the-art, applications, challenges and trends for ontology learning from text. *Information. Wissenschaft und Praxis, 57*(6-7), 315–320.

Dellschaft, K., & Staab, S. (2006). *On how to perform a gold standard based evaluation of ontology learning.* International Semantic Web Conference, (pp. 228-241).

Fullam, K., & Barber, S. (2006). *Learning trust strategies in reputation exchange networks.* AAMAS'06, May 8-12, 2006, Hakodate, Hokkaido, Japan

Gruber, T. (2007). Ontology of Folksonomy: A mash-up of apples and oranges. *International Journal on Semantic Web and Information Systems, 3*(2).

Gulla, J., Borch, H., & Ingvaldsen, J. (2007). Ontology learning for search applications. In Meersman, R., & Tari, Z. (Eds.), *OTM 2007, part I, (LNCS 4803)* (pp. 1050–1062).

Han, H., & Elmasri, R. (2003). *Ontology extraction and conceptual modeling for Web information. Information modeling for Internet applications* (pp. 174–188). Hershey, PA: IGI Global.

Kalfoglou, Y., & Schorlemmer, M. (2003). Ontology mapping: The state of the art. *The Knowledge Engineering Review, 18*(1), 1–31. doi:10.1017/S0269888903000651

Kotis, K., & Papasalouros, A. (2010). *Learning useful kick-off ontologies from query logs: HCOME revised.* 4th International Conference on Complex, Intelligent and Software Intensive Systems (CISIS-2010).

Kotis, K., Vouros, G., & Stergiou, K. (2006). Towards automatic merging of domain ontologies: The HCONE-merge approach. [JWS]. *Journal of Web Semantics*, *4*(1), 60–79. doi:10.1016/j. websem.2005.09.004

Lau, R., Li, Y., & Xu, Y. (2007). *Mining fuzzy domain ontology from textual databases*. IEEE/WIC/ACM International Conference on Web Intelligence, 2007.

Maedche, A., & Staab, S. (2001). Ontology learning for the Semantic Web. *IEEE Intelligent Systems*, *16*(2), 72–79. doi:10.1109/5254.920602

Mika, P. (2007). Ontologies are us: A unified model of social networks and semantics. *Journal of Web Semantics*, *5*, 5–15. doi:10.1016/j. websem.2006.11.002

O'Hara, K., Alani, H., Kalfoglou, Y., & Shadbolt, N. (2004). Trust strategies for the Semantic Web. In *Proceedings of Workshop on Trust, Security, and Reputation on the Semantic Web, 3rd International Semantic Web Conference*, 2004.

Park, Y., Byrd, R., & Boguraev, B. (2003). Towards ontologies on demand. *Proceedings of Workshop on Semantic Web Technologies for Scientific Search and Information Retrieval, In Conjunction with the 2nd International Semantic Web Conference*.

Sekine, A., & Suzuki, H. (2007). *Acquiring ontological knowledge from query logs*. WWW 2007, May 8-12, 2007, Banf, Canada.

Spiliopoulos, V., Kotis, K., & Vouros, G. A. (2008). Semantic retrieval and ranking of SW documents using free-form queries. *International Journal of Metadata. Semantics and Ontologies*, *3*(2), 95–108. doi:10.1504/IJMSO.2008.021888

Tang, J., Leung, H., Luo, Q., Chen, D., & Gong, J. (2009). *Towards ontology learning from Folksonomies*. JCAI-09, Pasadena, California, USA, 11th - 17th July 2009.

Tho, Q. T., Hui, S. C., Fong, A. C. M., & Tru Hoang, C. (2006). Automatic fuzzy ontology generation for Semantic Web. *IEEE Transactions on Knowledge and Data Engineering*, *18*(6), 842–856. doi:10.1109/TKDE.2006.87

Vouros, G., Kotis, K., Chalkiopoulos, C., & Lelli, N. (2007). *The HCOME-3O framework for supporting the collaborative engineering of evolving ontologies*. ESOE 2007 International Workshop on Emergent Semantics and Ontology Evolution, ISWC 2007.

Zhang, J., Xiong, M., & Yu, Y. (2006). *Mining query log to assist ontology learning from relational database. (LNCS 3841)* (pp. 437–448). Springer – Verlag.

KEY TERMS AND DEFINITIONS

Communities of Interest (CoI): CoIs are communities that aim to bring together members from different communities of practices (CoPs) to solve a particular (design) problem of common concern.

Social Fermentation (as a knowledge process): a process of knowledge creation and exchange between users that belong in communities of common interests (CoI), in open, collaborative and communicative environments.

Social Data: data usually related to content ownership details (contributor, annotator or end-user), tags or argumentation/dialogue items that have been used to comment, organize or disambiguate domain-specific information, querying information related to user clicks on retrieved information, etc. Social data is usually created as a result of social fermentation. The most popular social data in Web 2.0 content is tags, which are (often) single words listed alphabetically and with a different font size or color (to capture its importance).

Social Intelligence (SI): aims to derive actionable information from social data in context-rich application settings and provide solution frameworks for applications that can benefit from the "wisdom of crowds" through the Web.

Kick-Off Ontology: A lightweight ontology, usually representing only concepts and some simple/basic axioms such as inclusion - an initial (starting) stage of definition of conceptualizations, prior to refinement and enrichment.

Social Ontology: an explicit, formal and commonly agreed representation of knowledge that is derived from both domain-specific and social data.

Social Content Generation (SCG): a conversational, distributed mode of content generation, dissemination, and communication among communities of common interest (CoI).

Trusted Social Ontology: An ontology O = {T, C, S, A} where T = {u, v_a, v_f} is the trust function (uncertainty, votes against, votes for) for ontological signature S and axioms A that a set of collaborated contributors C participated in a task of social content generation (SCG) have derived using their social intelligence (SI).

ENDNOTES

[1]   T. Lawson, A Conception of Ontology, The Cambridge Social Ontology Group, 2004, http://www.csog.group.cam.ac.uk/A_Conception_of_Ontology.pdf

[2]   http://nlp.stanford.edu/software/tagger.shtml

[3]   http://lyle.smu.edu/cse/dbgroup/sw/jaws.htm

[4]   http://nlp.shef.ac.uk/abraxas/onteval.html

[5]   http://gate.ac.uk/

Chapter 13
Mining Parallel Knowledge from Comparable Patents

Bin Lu
City University of Hong Kong, Hong Kong

Benjamin K. Tsou
City University of Hong Kong, Hong Kong & Hong Kong Institute of Education, Hong Kong

Tao Jiang
ChiLin Star Corporation, China

Jingbo Zhu
Northeastern University, China

Oi Yee Kwong
City University of Hong Kong, Hong Kong

ABSTRACT

In recent years, the field of ontology learning from text has attracted much attention, resulting in a wide variety of approaches on mining knowledge from textual data. Since patent documents usually contain a large amount of technical terms, it is possible to acquire technical vocabularies from patents and to learn the relation between the technical terms.

In this chapter, the authors address some major issues of mining parallel knowledge from comparable Chinese-English patents which contain both equivalent sentences as well as much noise. Based on a Chinese-English comparable corpus of patents, the authors attempt to mine two kinds of parallel knowledge which are parallel sentences and parallel technical terms, and investigate the application of the mined knowledge on statistical machine translation.

The extracted parallel sentences and technical terms could be a good basis for further acquisition of term relations and the translation of monolingual ontologies, as well as for statistical machine translation systems and other cross-lingual information access applications.

DOI: 10.4018/978-1-60960-625-1.ch013

1. INTRODUCTION

Ontology learning from text has been attracting more attention from different research communities, such as natural language processing, machine learning, knowledge representation/engineering and user interface design (Brewster et al., 2003; Cimiano, 2006; Buitelaar and Cimiano, 2007; Hjelm, 2009; Wong, 2009). Ontologies could be used by computers to reason over the terms and relations, as well as to deduce new information that might not be found explicitly in the ontologies. The constructed ontologies would finally contribute to the realization of the Semantic Web (Berners-Lee et al., 2001; Shadbolt et al., 2006).

Patent documents containing a large amount of technical terms could be a good source for learning technical terms and their relations, and multilingual patents would be useful further for learning not only monolingual ontologies but also multilingual ontologies. Little work on ontology learning from patent documents has been done, and even less on ontology learning from multilingual parallel or comparable patents.

In this chapter, we present our experimental work on mining parallel sentences and technical terms from comparable Chinese-English patent documents. Part of the current chapter is based on our previously published work (Lu et al, 2009; Lu & Tsou, 2009). When compared to *comparable* patents, a *parallel* corpus of matched equivalent sentences is an invaluable resource for many applications, such as multilingual ontology learning, machine translation, and cross-lingual information retrieval. However, obtaining a large-scale parallel corpus is much more expensive than obtaining a comparable bilingual corpus. From our corpus of about 7,000 Chinese-English comparable patents with titles, abstracts, claims and full texts, we try to address the following three issues:

1. Parallel sentence extraction: alignment of only parallel sentences in the comparable patents by combining three quality measures,

thereby deriving a useful parallel corpus of sentences. The experiments show that high-quality parallel sentences can be obtained by aligning sentences and filtering sentence alignments with the combination of different quality measures.

2. Bilingual term extraction: identification of bilingual technical terms by combining both linguistic and statistical information under an SVM classifier. Based on the high-quality parallel sentences extracted, bilingual technical terms, including both single-word terms and multi-word ones can be readily identified by combining Part-of-Speech (POS) patterns and statistical scores given by a word alignment tool. Meanwhile, linguistic and statistic features can further improve the performance of bilingual term extraction via the machine learning approach (i.e. an SVM classifier).

3. Chinese to English Statistical Machine Translation (SMT): automatic translation of patents from Chinese to English based on an SMT engine trained on the mined parallel sentences. An SMT engine trained on the parallel sentences achieves promising BLEU scores.

Given the relative paucity of parallel patent data, the use of such comparable corpus for mining parallel knowledge would be a helpful step towards multilingual ontology learning and other cross-lingual access applications in the patent domain, such as MT, cross-lingual information retrieval. The extracted parallel sentences and technical terms could be a good basis for further acquisition of attributes, term relations, as well as for the translation of monolingual ontologies since most current ontologies are monolingual.

In the next section we introduce the background of the research. Then the comparable Chinese-English patent corpus and its preprocessing are described in Section 3. Our approaches on parallel sentence extraction, bilingual term extraction and the SMT experiment are presented in Section 4, 5 and 6, respectively. Discussion is given in Section 7, and we conclude in Section 8.

2. BACKGROUND

An ontology constitutes a formal, explicit specification of a shared conceptualization, and ontologies are "*fundamental to the success of the Semantic Web as they enable software agents to exchange, share, reuse and reason about concepts and relations using axioms*" (Wong, 2009, pp. 13-14). Ontology learning from text is "*the process of identifying terms, concepts, relations and optionally, axioms from natural language text, and using them to construct and maintain an ontology*" (Wong, 2009, pp. 14).

Patents are the legal documents which represent "*a government grant to an inventor assuring him the sole right to make, use, and sell his invention for a limited period*" (Collins English Dictionary[1]). Patents are important indicators of innovation. Sun (2003) stated "*As the economy is globalized, patenting increasingly becomes an international activity*", and more firms, especially multinational ones, are investing more and more money on intellectual property (especially patents) to protect their own technologies, and filing patents in foreign countries. There have been many legal cases involving the claims of patent infringement, such as Nokia vs Apple, Cisco vs. Huawei, Intel vs AMD, and the DVD manufacturers in China vs. the dvd6c licensing group. The companies may be interested in monitoring and analyzing the patents filed in different languages, such as English, Chinese, Japanese, Germany, etc. The traditional practice for monitoring patents filed in foreign languages is usually to involve translation companies to manually translate patents into a relevant language, which is slow, time-consuming, costly, and the quality is often inconsistent.

Meanwhile, patent applications are increasing very quickly, especially for the Chinese ones filed in China (Sun, 2003). The patent application numbers filed in the top leading patent offices from 1996 to 2008 are shown in Figure 1, from which we can observe that in about 12 years, the patent application number grows by 10 times in China and doubles in USA. The increasing trend of patent applications also impose more workload for the manual translation which demands more advanced machine translation engines and more parallel data to help us handle this problem.

Given the large amount of technical terms in patents and the increasing patent applications, patents are a good source for learning technical terms and their relations, and multilingual patents would further be useful for learning not only monolingual ontologies but also multilingual ontologies. This chapter addresses the issues of extracting parallel sentences and terms from a comparable Chinese-English patent corpus.

In the following parts, we will introduce the related work on *parallel sentence extraction, bilingual term extraction*, and *statistical machine translation*, respectively.

2.1 Parallel Sentence Extraction

Parallel sentences can be extracted from parallel corpora or from comparable corpora. Since parallel corpora are bilingual text collections consisting of the same content in two or more different languages, it would be easier to find parallel sentences or parallel terms. However, comparable corpora contain bilingual texts that are not exact translations but closely related or taken from the same text domain in two or more different languages, which raises further challenges for finding parallel sentences or terms.

To get parallel sentences from parallel corpora, different approaches can be used, which can be based on a) the information of sentence length in bilingual sentences, b) lexical information in bilingual dictionaries, c) statistical translation model, or d) the composite of more than one approach. The sentence-length-based approach (Brown et al. 1991; Gale and Church, 1991) aligns sentences

Figure 1. Patent application numbers by the top leading patent offices Source: WIPO: Patent Applications by Office²

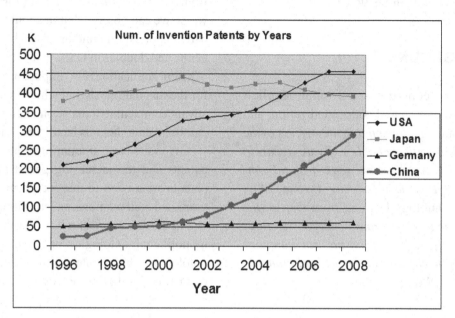

based on the number of words or characters in each sentence. Dictionary-based techniques use extensive online bilingual lexicons to match sentences. For instance, Ma (2006) described Champollion, a lexicon-based sentence aligner designed for robust alignment of potential noisy parallel text, and increased the robustness of the alignment by assigning greater weights to less frequent words.

Statistical translation model is also used for sentence alignment. Chen (1993) constructed a simple statistical word-to-word translation model on the fly during sentence alignment and then found the alignment that maximizes the probability of generating the corpus. Simard and Plamondon (1998) and Moore (2002) both used a composite method in which the first pass does alignment at the sentence length level and the second pass uses IBM Model-1.

Comparable corpora are also used to mine parallel sentences. For instance, Resnik and Smith (2003) introduced the STRAND system for mining parallel text on the Web for low-density language

pairs. Munteanu and Marcu (2005) presented a method for discovering parallel sentences in large Chinese, Arabic, and English comparable, non-parallel corpora based on a maximum entropy classifier. Wu and Fung (2005) exploited Inversion Transduction Grammar to retrieve truly parallel sentence translations from large collections of highly non-parallel docuements. Zhao and Vogel (2002) investigated the mining of parallel sentences from bilingual Web news collections which may contain much noise. Utiyama and Isahara (2003) aligned articles and sentences from noisy parallel news articles, then sorted the aligned sentences according to a similarity measure, and selected only the highly ranked aligned sentence alignments.

2.2 Bilingual Term Extraction

The traditional way of manually constructing monolingual or bilingual dictionaries is time-consuming and labor-intensive. Therefore, automatic and semi-automatic approaches for constructing such dictionaries have been proposed to reduce the burden of manual construction.

Automatic extraction of monolingual terms is "*to determine whether a word or phrase is a term which characterizes the target domain*" (Wong, 2009). It can be further decomposed to reveal two critical notions, namely *unithood* and *termhood*. Unithood is defined as "*the degree of strength or stability of syntagmatic combinations and collocations*" (Kageura and Umino, 1996), while termhood refers to "*the degree that a linguistic unit is related to domain-specific concepts*" (Kageura and Umino, 1996). For example, Frantzi and Ananiadou (1997; 1999) proposed to use the measures CValue and NCValue for extracting multi-word terms by incorporating contextual information.

Bilingual term extraction is to extract parallel terms from bilingual domain-specific corpora, and it is crucial for many NLP fields, such as Machine Translation, bilingual lexicography, cross-language information retrieval, and bilingual ontology extraction. Many researchers have done bilingual term extraction, such as Kupiec (1993), Vintar (2001), Daille et al. (2004), Piperidis and Harlas (2006), and Ha et al. (2008).

Much research has been conducted on the construction of bilingual dictionaries from parallel corpora (Erdmann, 2009), which could be accomplished with the same methods used for machine translation (Brown et al., 1990; 1993). For example, Wu and Xia (1994) proposed to extract English-Chinese translation lexicon through statistical training on a large parallel corpus. However, obtaining a large-scale parallel corpus is more expensive than obtaining a comparable corpus. Recently, some researchers have pursued the idea of using Wikipedia as a corpus for bilingual terminology extraction (Erdmann et al., 2009; Yu and Tsujii, 2009), which uses the inter-language link information in Wikipedia.

2.3 Statistical Machine Translation

Machine translation (MT) is the automatic translation from one natural language into another using computers, and statistical MT (SMT) is an approach to MT that is characterized by the use of statistical and machine learning methods. SMT has made tremendous strides in two decades (Brown et al., 1991; 1993; Och and Ney, 2003; 2004; Chiang, 2005; 2007), and new ideas are constantly introduced (Chiang et al., 2009; Liu et al., 2009; Wang et al., 2010). SMT treats the translation of natural language as a machine learning problem, and SMT algorithms automatically learn how to translate by examining many samples of human-produced translations (Lopez, 2008).

Brown et al. (1990; 1993) proposed the groundbreaking IBM approach, which introduced many of the common problems in translation modeling and has continued to influence the field of SMT. The IBM models are word-based models and represent the first generation of SMT models. Later comes the second generation of SMT models called phrase-based models (Och and Ney, 2004; Koehn, 2004) in which translation unit may be any contiguous sequence of words, called a phrase. Please note that the term *phrase* here has no specific linguistic sense. Phrase-based translation is implemented in the Pharaoh toolkit (Koehn, 2004) and its open-source successor Moses[3] (Koehn et al., 2007). They are widely used in the SMT research community because phrase-based models produce better translations than word-based models. We in this chapter also use Moses for the SMT experiments. Currently, more researchers are taking advantage of syntax-based models (Chiang et al., 2005; Chiang, 2007; Wang et al., 2007), in which researchers attempt to incorporate syntax into word-base/phrase-based models.

3. THE COMPARABLE PATENTS AND ITS PREPROCESSING

Our work is based on about 7,000 Chinese-English comparable patents with about 6000 of them containing full texts. The patents were first filed in the China Patent Office with Chinese as the original language. They were translated into English, and then filed in *USPTO* (United States Patent and Trademark Office).

We first get access to the English patents filed in USPTO, and then their Chinese corresponding patents were identified by using the priority information described in the *USPTO* patents (Lu et al., 2009). The priority information is actually the application number of the Chinese patent. Therefore we can get the sections for Chinese patents by searching on the website of the State Intellectual Property Office (SIPO) of the People's Republic of China[4] or the website of China Intellectual Property Net[5].

3.1 Data Description

Each patent application consists of different parts, namely, *bibliographical data (including title, abstract), claims, description*, etc. Since we focus on the text in the patent applications, only *title, abstract, claims and description*s are used in the experiments discussed in this chapter. From the legal perspective, the *claims* section is the most important part in a patent application, because it defines the coverage that the applicant wants to claim. The *description* section gives the technical details of the patent involved, and the descriptions of some patents also have subdivisions, such as *Field of the Invention, Background of the Invention, Objects of the Invention, Summary of the Invention, Brief Description of the Drawings, Detailed Description of the Invention, Detailed Description of the preferred Embodiment*, etc. In general, claims are listed one by one, which may mean that the claims would be easier to align than the description section.

Utiyama and Isahara (2007) used only the "*Detailed Description of the Preferred Embodiments*" and "*Background of the Invention*" part in the description section of each patent to find parallel sentences because they found these two parts have more literal translations than others. However, since our corpus has much less Chinese-English patent pairs, we use all parts of each patent to find parallel sentences. In total, there are about 730K Chinese sentences and 1,080K English sentences in the comparable patents. The detailed statistics for each section are shown in Table 1.

3.2 Problem of Loose Translation

Our observation indicated loose translations in Chinese-English comparable patents to be very common. We consider such patents comparable or noisy parallel, which are not parallel in the strict sense but still closely related because almost the

Table 1. Statistics for each section

Sections	Chinese		English		Ratio	
	#Chars	#Sents	#Words	#Sents	#CN Chars/ #En Words	#EN Sent/ #CN Sent
Title	89K	7K	49K	7K	1.8	1
Abstract	1.5M	29K	1.0M	32K	1.5	1.1
Claim	6.4M	145K	5.9M	201K	1.1	1.3
Description	27.7M	557K	20.9M	840K	1.3	1.4
Total	35.7M	738K	27.9M	1,080K	1.2	1.4

same information is conveyed (Zhao and Vogel, 2002).

To evaluate the translations, the *abstract* sections of 100 patent pairs were taken from our patent data, and a bilingual annotator was asked to judge whether the abstracts are a) *literally translated*: most components of English sentences are literally translated from the Chinese ones; b) *loosely translated:* only some components of the supposedly parallel English and Chinese sentences overlap; c) *rewritten:* the whole abstract is totally rewritten, and it is difficult to find any parallel sentences.

The results showed their empirical distribution to be 55%, 26% and 19% respectively. This means that a large proportion of the abstracts are not literally translated. There may be two major explanations for this phenomenon of common loose translations in these patents:

1. The field of intellectual property is highly regulated and different stylistic conversions exist for patents in different countries. Thus the translation may be highly influenced by the stylistic differences in the individual countries.

2. For protection of intellectual property, the patent applicants may intentionally change some technical terms or the patent structure to broaden the patent coverage when a new version is produced in another language and country.

3.3 Data Preprocessing

English sentences were tokenized and POS-tagged by the POS-tagger developed at Stanford NLP lab

(Toutanova and Manning, 2000; Toutanova et al., 2003). The tagger uses Penn Treebank POS tagset, including the tags for the following content words: JJ (adjective), NN (noun), VB (verb), RB (adverb).

The Chinese sentences were word-segmented and POS-tagged by using a Chinese lexical analyzer ICTCLAS[6]. The Chinese POS tag set of ICTCLAS contains 22 first-level POS tags, in which the tags for content words include n (noun), v (verb), a (adjective), b (adjectives to describe difference, e.g. 急性/*acute* vs 慢性/*chronic*), z (adjective to describe status, e.g. 优良/*excellent*), and d (adverb). The English words are stemmed by using Porter Stemmer. The statistics of word tokens and words types in the Chinese and English patents are given in Table 2.

4. PARALLEL SENTENCE EXTRACTION

In this section, our work on extracting parallel sentences from comparable patents is introduced. We first compared and evaluated three publicly available sentence aligners and chose one of them to align the sentences in the comparable patents. Because of loose translation in comparable patents, the results include a large proportion of incorrect alignments. To filter out the incorrect sentences, we compared and evaluated three individual measures and different ensemble techniques. The three measures are the length-based score, the dictionary-based score, and the translation probability score.

Although Utiyama and Isahara (2007) extracted parallel sentence from the Japanese-English comparable patents, we have made the

Table 2. Word statistics

	#Word Tokens	#Word Types	#Content Word Types	#Pairs of Word and POS
EN	27.9M	84K	41K	96K
CN	25.6M	64K	17K	64K

following improvements on the basis of our data: 1) all sections of the patents, instead of only two parts in the description section, were used to find sentence alignments; 2) for sentence filtering, we integrated three individual measures, including the dictionary-based one (Utiyama and Isahara, 2007), and the experiments showed the combination of measures could improve the performance of sentence filtering.

4.1 Preliminary Sentence Alignment

To choose a sentence aligner, we first compare three publicly available sentence aligners, namely Champollion (Ma, 2006), Hunalign (Varga et al., 2007), and Microsoft Bilingual Sentence Aligner (MS aligner) (Moore, 2002), based on the manually aligned Chinese-English parallel corpus included in Champollion. For the bilingual dictionary needed by Champollion and Hunalign, we combine LDC_CE_DIC2.0[7] constructed by LDC, bilingual terms in HowNet[8] and the bilingual lexicon in Champollion. Since the MS aligner only extracts 1-1 sentence matches, we use only the 3,005 manually aligned 1-1 matches in the evaluation corpus so as to compare the three aligners on the same basis. The performance in terms of Precision (P), Recall (R) and F-score, is shown in Table 3.

Because of its better performance than Hunalign and MS aligner, Champollion is chosen as the sentence aligner for our subsequent experiment to extract sentence pair candidates in the relevant sections of the comparable patents. In total, 352K sentence pair candidates are extracted, including 1-1, 2-1, 1-2, 1-3, 3-1, 1-4 or 4-1 alignments. This means more than 48.6% of Chinese sentences or 32.6% of English sentences find their corresponding ones in the other language. The breakdown of sections is shown in Table 4. The pairs of titles are considered parallel sentence candidates. The repeated sentence pairs in different sections are counted only once for the total numbers.

To assess the quality of the sentence alignments, we randomly sampled 1,000 pairs from them. Two Chinese-English bilingual annotators were asked to separately classify them into three categories: a) *correct*: the English sentence is exactly the literal translation of the Chinese one, or the content overlap between them are above 80% with no need to consider phrasal reordering during the translation; b) *partially correct*: the Chinese sentence and the English one are not the literal translation of each other, but the content of each sentence can cover more than 50% of the other; c) *incorrect*: the contents of the Chinese sentence and the English one are not related, or more than 50% of the content of one sentence is missing in the other.

The *correct* ones are the most valuable resources for MT and other NLP applications, but the *partially correct* ones may also be useful for some NLP applications, such as bilingual term extraction or word alignment. Then we compute the inter-annotator agreement among the two annotators, which is 91.5%, showing the high consistency between our annotators and also the task is well-defined. For the 85 disagreements, two annotators discussed and then resolved the final category for each sentence pair. The final numbers for sentence pairs of *correct*, *partially correct*, and *incorrect* are 448 (44.8%), 114 (11.4%) and 438 (43.8%), respectively.

Table 3. Performance of aligners on a small corpus

	P (%)	R (%)	F-score (%)
Champollion	98.4	98.3	98.4
Hunalign	82.9	97.1	89.4
MS Aligner	95.4	92.5	93.9

Table 4. Numbers of sentence pair candidates

Section	Title	Abstract	Claim	Desc.	Total
#Candidate	7K	16K	57K	276K	352K

The above evaluation on the sentence alignments from the comparable patents shows that a large proportion of aligned sentences are incorrect because of noise in the patents and in the system. To get truly parallel sentence pairs, filtering out the misaligned sentences is quite necessary; otherwise, they may adversely affect the subsequent NLP applications.

4.2 Filtering of Parallel Sentence Candidates

To filter out incorrect alignments, we sort all sentence pairs based on a scoring metric so as to remove those with lower scores as incorrect alignments. Here we compare and evaluate three individual measures and different ensemble techniques for sentence filtering.

Suppose we are given a sentence pair, namely the Chinese sentence S_c and its English counterpart S_e, and l_c and l_e respectively denote the lengths of S_c and S_e in terms of the number of words. Three kinds of measures for scoring aligned sentences are introduced as follows.

The *length-based score* P_l (Len): we consider the length ratio between S_c and S_e have a normal distribution with mean μ and variance σ^2 (Gale and Church, 1991). The formula for p_l is as follows:

$$p_l(S_c, S_e) = p_l(l_c / l_e) = 2 * (1 - \frac{1}{\sqrt{2\pi}} \int_{-\infty}^{\delta} e^{-z^2/2} dz)$$

(1)

where $\delta = (l_e - l_c \mu) / \sqrt{l_c \sigma^2}$. The parameters μ and σ^2 are estimated on the basis of preliminary sentence pairs obtained in Section 4.1.

The *dictionary-based score* P_d: the score is computed based on a bilingual dictionary as follows (Utiyama and Isahara, 2003):

$$p_d(S_c, S_e) = \frac{\sum_{w_c \in S_c} \sum_{w_e \in S_e} \frac{\gamma(w_c, w_e)}{\deg(w_c) \deg(w_e)}}{l_e + l_c / 2}$$

(2)

where w_c and w_e are respectively the word types in S_c and S_e; and $\gamma(w_c, w_e) = 1$ if w_c and w_e is a translation pair in the bilingual dictionary or are the same string, otherwise 0; and

$$\deg(w_c) = \sum_{w_e \in S_e} \gamma(w_c, w_e)$$

(3)

Here, to alleviate the coverage problem of the bilingual dictionary, we propose a modified version, *the normalized dictionary-based score (DictN)*, in which l_c and l_e denote the numbers of words occurring in the bilingual dictionary in S_c and S_e respectively.

The *bidirectional translation probability score* P_t (Tran): it combines the translation probability value of both directions (i.e. Chinese->English and English->Chinese), instead of using only one direction (Moore, 2002; Chen, 2003). It is computed as follows:

$$p_t(S_c, S_e) = \frac{\log(P(S_e | S_c)) + \log(P(S_c | S_e))}{l_c + l_e}$$

(4)

where $P(S_e | S_c)$ denotes the probability that a translator will produce S_e in English when presented with S_c in Chinese, and vice versa for $P(S_c | S_e)$.

A wide variety of ensemble methods have been used in various fields (Polikar, 2006; Wan, 2008). Before the ensemble of individual scores, we first need to normalize the scores into the range between 0 and 1 according to their distributions: the length-based and dictionary-based scores are already within the range; the translation score are normalized according to its roughly linear distribution. We evaluate the following ensemble methods:

1. Average (*Avg*): the average of the individual scores;
2. Multiplication (*Mul*): the product of the individual scores;
3. Linear Combination (*LinC*): the weighted average by associating each individual score with a weight, indicating the relative confidence in the value;
4. *Filter*: use P_t for sorting, but if P_d or P_t of a sentence pair is lower than a predefined threshold, that pair will be moved to the end of the sorting list. The thresholds can be empirically set based on the data.

4.3 Empirical Evaluation

To assess the performance of individual measures and ensemble methods, the randomly selected 1,000 sentence pairs are used as the test data, and their final manual categories mentioned in Section 4.1 and the gold standard. Each method sorts these 1,000 sentence pairs in descending order according to their corresponding scores given by that method. For the evaluation metrics of each sorted list, we use the 11-point interpolated average precision (*P11*) and MAP (Mean Average Precision) which are commonly used in Information Retrieval. The baseline method does not sort sentence pairs, and its precision is 44.8% if only the 448 correct alignments are considered correct (*case 1*); while its precision is 56.2% if we include the 448 correct pairs and the 114 partially correct ones (*case 2*).

For *DictN*, we use the combined bilingual dictionary mentioned in Section 4 to compute the scores. For *Tran*, we use the preliminarily aligned sentences mentioned in Section 4 as the training data and compute the word alignment probability score given by the default training process of Giza++ (Och and Ney, 2003), which is based on IBM Model 4 (Brown et al., 1993). The weights for *Tran, Len, DictN* are empirically set as 99, 30 and 16, respectively. We empirically set the un-

normalized thresholds of *Len* and *DictN* to 0.25 and 0.0075, respectively. The results for *case 1* and *case 2* are shown in Table 5, from which we can observe:

1. *Len* performs the worst among the three measures although it is much better than the baseline method. The reason is that it alone is not reliable for comparable data because of lack of lexical evidence. The performance of *DictN* is worse than that of the translation probability score because it can not fully cover the large amount of technical terms in patents.
2. *Tran* shows much better performance than the other two measures, which may be explained by the fact that the translation model can leverage the probabilistic information of both lexical and length information, and hence generally performs well. However, *TRAN* tends to be error-prone for the highest ranked sentence pairs. The possible explanation is that the training data itself contain some incorrectly aligned sentences, which lead to some bad parameters in the translation model.
3. All ensemble methods outperform individual measures in terms of P11 and MAP, which shows that each individual measure has its own strength in identifying the correct sentence pairs. Thus fusing the evidence together could improve the performance of the sorted list.
4. *LinC* and *Filter* achieve better performance than *Avg* and *Mul*, showing that we can achieve better performance using some delicate fusing strategies than simply using average or multiplication. *Filter* is shown to be the best among all ensemble methods, which can be explained by the good filtering effects of *Len* and *DictN* for misaligned sentences among the highly ranked sentence pairs in the sorted list of *Tran*.

Table 5. Performance of sentence filtering

Measures & Ensemble Methods		Case 1		Case 2	
		P11 (%)	MAP (%)	P11 (%)	MAP (%)
Baseline		44.8	44.8	56.2	56.2
Individual	Len	70	68.5	79.0	77.8
	DictN	73.9	71.8	82.9	83.1
	Tran	85.1	84.3	89.0	88.7
Ensemble	Avg	**89.2**	89.7	92.7	94.7
	Mul	88.0	**89.8**	**92.9**	**95.0**
	LinC	**91.5**	**92.2**	**93.4**	**95.5**
	Filter	**92.0**	**93.4**	**94.7**	**96.6**

4.4 Final Corpus of Parallel Sentences

To generate the final corpus of truly parallel sentences, we first evaluate the precision of the 352K sentence pair candidates by sorting them in descending order using the ensemble method *Filter*. We randomly selected 100 samples from each of the 12 blocks ranked at the top 240,000 sentence pairs (each block has 20,000 pairs). An annotator classified them into *correct (Cor)*, *partially correct (PaC)*, and *incorrect (IC)* just as in Section 4. The results of evaluation are given in Table 6.

The table shows that the number of IC's increases rapidly as the rank increases. This demonstrates that the ensemble method *Filter* can distinguish the correct alignments from the incor-

rect ones. Then, we choose the top 160K alignments as the final parallel corpus, in which the average precision of correct and partially correct sentences is about 90.0% based on the samples above. We give some basic statistics of the corpus in Table 7.

We also compare the sentence pair candidate numbers among different sections in the final corpus. The result in Table 8 shows that the title and claims sections have two highest precisions: 74.4% and 64.8% respectively; while the abstract and description sections show lower precisions: 45.2% and 40.9% respectively. This shows that it is more difficult to find parallel sentences in the description or abstract section than in the title or claim sections, and that a large proportion of the patent titles are parallel.

Table 6. Rank vs judgment

Range	1 -	20001 -	40001 -	60001 -	80001 -	100001 -	
#Cor	98	98	96	91	92	88	
#PaC	1	0	2	5	2	1	
#IC	1	2	2	4	6	11	
Range	120001 -	140001 -	160001 -	180001 -	200001 -	220001 -	Total
#Cor	77	73	64	37	34	32	880
#PaC	6	7	7	7	6	8	52
#IC	17	20	29	56	60	60	268

Table 7. Basic statistics of the final parallel corpus

#Patents	#Sentence Pairs	#Word Tokens		#Word Types	
		EN	CN	EN	CN
7K	160K	4,168K	4,130K	46K	44K

5. BILINGUAL TERM EXTRACTION

In this section, our work on extracting bilingual terms from comparable patents is introduced (Lu and Tsou, 2009). Generally speaking, there are two possible options to find parallel terms from comparable corpora: 1) first find parallel sentences in comparable corpora, and then extract parallel terms from the parallel sentences; 2) directly find parallel terms from in comparable documents by computing the similarity of bilingual terms using co-occurrence statistics without the process of extracting parallel sentences.

The former is characterized by high precision and low recall since it could make use of the parallel sentences extracted which may already eliminate much noise and hence improve the precision of extracted parallel terms. The latter has the characteristics of low precision and high recall since it may find more term candidates from the comparable documents.

Here we just choose the former one, i.e. extract bilingual terms from parallel sentences which are already identified in Section 4. The steps used in this chapter include:

1. Extracting of monolingual term candidates in monolingual patents;

2. Finding parallel term candidates from parallel sentences extracted in the previous section;

3. Identifying *"true"* parallel terms from the less likely ones using an SVM classifier by integrating both linguistic and statistical information.

Here what do we mean by *"true"* parallel terms? By deeming a pair of words/phrases as *true parallel*, we mean that it has two properties: a) the translation is correct, i.e. the Chinese side and English side have equivalent meaning; b) both the Chinese side and English side should be domain-specific technical terms. As patents contain many technical terms, patent is treated as a specific domain, in contrast with other domains such as news, legal text, or medical records. The parallel terms extracted from comparable patents should be patent-specific, and should express or represent concepts that characterize various aspects of the patent domain.

The experimental results show that our method can well identify true parallel terms from comparable patents, and the SVM classifier can further improve its performance. We obtain more than 70K bilingual terms and the sampled precision is over 80%.

Table 8. Selected percentages of different sections

Section	Title	Abstr.	Claims	Desc.	Total
#Candidates	7,029	15,755	56,667	275,737	352K
#Final Pairs	5,232	7,119	36,722	112,812	160K
Selected (%)	**74.4**	45.2	**64.8**	40.9	45.4

5.1 Identification of Monolingual Term Candidates

Monolingual terms could be single-word or multi-word. According to Nakagawa and Mori (2002), 85% of domain-specific terms are multi-word in nature. Therefore, for single-word terms, we can just use content words as candidates, while the selection of multi-word terms is more complicated and will be introduced below.

5.1.1 Monolingual Multi-Word Term Candidates

There are many methods to extract monolingual multi-word term candidates from texts. We just consider noun phrases as term candidates, and extract English and Chinese noun phrases from parallel sentences extracted from comparable patents by using regular expressions (Friedl, 2002). The number of words within one phrase is limited to five.

As mentioned earlier in Section 3.3, both Chinese and English patents are POS-tagged with POS tag sets defined by Penn English Treebank and the Chinese lexical analyzer ICTCLAS. We use POS-tag based regular expressions to extract noun phrases from Chinese and English patents.

The English POS regular expression for noun phrases is *JJ*NN+*, in which *JJ* and *NN* are the POS tags mentioned earlier, respectively representing adjective and noun, the * symbol matches zero or more occurrences of the preceding POS tag, and the + symbol is similar but matches one or more. Two examples of English noun phrases are "coverage/NN area/NN" and "effective/NN power/NN factor/NN".

The Chinese POS regular expression for noun phrases is *(n|v|a|z|b|d)*(n|v)+*, in which the letters denote the POS tags mentioned in Section 3.3, the | symbol match either one of the POS tags inside the group denoted by the characters (and). It is similar to the ones in (Zhao and Huang, 1999) or (Zhao et al., 2000). The reason to include *v*

(verb) in the regular expression is that: 1) many verbs can be used as nouns in Chinese; 2) verbs are usually tagged as verbs, even if they are used as nouns in Chinese; 3) we want to improve the recall of Chinese term candidates. Examples of Chinese noun phrases include "离子/n 化合物/n"(ion compound), "摆动/v 装置/n" (swing means), "按摩/v 治疗/v" (massage treatment), "氧化/v 隔离/v 结构/n"(oxide isolation structure).

Since monolingual terms are not the focus of this study, these term candidates will not be filtered by some statistic or linguistic measures. They are just used for the next step of extracting parallel terms.

5.2 Extraction of Bilingual Term Candidates

Based on the 160K parallel sentences mentioned earlier, we perform word alignment with Giza++ (Och and Ney, 2003) which combines IBM models (Brown et al., 1994) and Hidden Markov Model. The bilingual corpus is aligned bi-directionally, i.e. we first align words from English to Chinese and then from Chinese to English. The two alignments are combined to form the final word alignment with the heuristics used in the Moses toolkit (Koehn et al., 2007).

From the final word alignments, we extract phrasal translation pairs that are consistent with the word alignment. This means that Chinese phrase and English phrase in a phrase pair are only aligned to each other, without non-aligned words. The maximum word number of a phrase in our experiment is five. Meanwhile, we remove as noise those word/phrase pairs with translation

Table 9. Statistics of term candidates

	#N-gram	#Candidates of Term Candidates
EN	26.8M	695K
CN	29.1M	2,690K

probability at either direction (Chinese->English or English->Chinese) lower than 0.1, which is empirically set and demonstrated to be quite effective to eliminate noise in our following experiment.

5.2.1 Bilingual Single-Word Term Candidates

Based on the final word alignments, we extract a table of lexical translations, in which both sides of a translation pair are single words, rather than multi-word phrases. For these single-word translations, we use the combined bilingual dictionary mentioned in Section 4.1 to filter the common words and consider the remaining ones as term candidates. After removing those in the combined dictionary, 9093 bilingual single-word pairs with translation probability higher than 0.1 are remained in the translation table. We manually verified these single-word term candidates, and 48.5% of them are marked as true parallel terms. Some examples of single-word parallel terms are shown in Table 10.

The first and second columns respectively show the English and Chinese terms; the third the translation probability of the Chinese word to the English word; and the fourth vice versa. From Table 10, we can see that these terms are quite technical and usually used in technology-specific texts, and therefore are not collected in the combined bilingual dictionary, whose entries are mostly frequently used general words.

5.2.2 Bilingual Multi-Word Term Candidates

To extract multi-word term candidates, we already have three lists: 1) the English term candidates; 2) the Chinese term candidates; 3) bilingual phrasal translation pairs extracted from the final word alignments of the parallel sentences. First, we extract the bilingual translation pairs whose English side strings are in the list of English term candidates, and denote these pairs as *EBil*. Then we filter out from *EBil* those pairs whose Chinese side strings are not in the list of Chinese term candidates, and denote the remaining candidates as *ECBil*.

In total, we find about 5,310K bilingual phrasal pairs, out of which 1,236K (23.3%) pairs have greater probability than 0.1 at both directions (CN->EN and EN->CN), and *EBil* comprises 71,621 (5.4% out of 1,236K) pairs. Table 11 shows several samples of extracted bilingual phrasal pairs. The first column shows the English terms; the second Chinese terms; the third the translation probability of the Chinese phrase to the English phrase; and the fourth vice versa.

We sampled 2,000 patents to evaluate the performance of these extracted pairs. In sum, 30,224 phrasal pairs of *EBil* occurs in the 2,000 patents; 24,458 (80.9% of 30,224) of these pairs also exist in *ECBil*. We ask Chinese-English bilingual annotators to mark each of these pairs as *correct* or *wrong* according to the parallelism of

Table 10. Examples of single-word parallel terms

English Term	Chinese Term	CN->EN Prob.	EN->CN Prob.
Acclimation	驯化	0.33	0.33
Accompaniment	伴唱	0.43	0.4
Accordion	手风琴	0.92	0.52
Accountant	会计	0.5	0.36
Acetic	醋酸	0.35	0.32
Acetochloral	三氯乙醛	0.33	0.5
Acetone	丙酮	0.63	0.63

the translation pairs, as well as the termhood of the Chinese terms and English terms. Finally, 81.2% of the 30,224 pairs in *EBil* are marked as *correct*, while 85.2% of the 24,458 pairs in *ECBil* are marked as *correct*. We may conclude that:

1. the method used can find true parallel terms, whose precision is higher than 80%;
2. English noun phrases are good indicators for technical terms, and it alone can achieve the precision of 81.2%;
3. Filtering with Chinese term candidates can further improve the precision of extracted bilingual term candidates from 81.2% to 85.2%, but the recall drops from 100% to 84.9% (=85.20%*24458/(81.20%*30224)) when considering the recall of *EBil* as 100%.

The results seem quite good in comparison to other language pairs, such as Spanish and English in Ha et al., (2008). The reasons here could be: 1) the criterion used to extract phrasal translation, i.e. the Chinese phrase and English phrase in a phrase pair are only aligned to each other without non-aligned words, is quite strict, and thus remove many wrongly aligned phrases, 2) the cross validation of Chinese term candidates and English term candidates when extracting parallel terms help filter out many unlikely terms (or general words); 3) the patent domain may cover many other technical domains, such as chemistry, electronics, transportation, electronics, and it could contain more technical terms than other individual domains.

5.3 Identification of Correct Bilingual Terms

In this section, we investigate whether we can improve the precision of extracted bilingual multi-word terms by using machine learning techniques. An SVM classifier is used to help distinguish between true parallel terms and less likely words/phrases. To build the classifier, we first need to find the useful features for the differentiation of true parallel terms and wrong terms. The features used by our SVM classifier could be categorized as linguistic features and statistic features:

1. **Linguistic features:** Chinese monolingual term candidates (CMC): a binary feature indicating whether the Chinese side of the bilingual pair is in the list of Chinese term candidates.

    Statistic features: (the first three features are got by using Moses) Lexical weighting probability (LWP, Koehn et al., 2007): the probability of lexical translation $\phi(c, e)$. The formula used here is as follows:

$$\phi(c, e) = \log(lex(\text{e} \mid c)) + \log(lex(\text{c} \mid e))$$

Table 11. Bilingual multi-word term examples

English Term	Chinese Term	CN->EN	EN->CN
AC converter	AC 转换器	0.67	0.71
AC input	AC 输入	0.33	1
AC load	AC 交流负载	1	0.14
Acceptance message	接受 消息	1	0.25
access ability	接入 能力	0.33	0.5
access API	接入 API	1	1
Access apparatus	接入 装置	0.5	0.55

where $lex(e \mid c)$ and $lex(c \mid e)$ are the lexical weights.

CN->EN phrase translation probability (CEP, Koehn et al., 2007): a numeric feature ranging from 0 to 1;

EN->CN phrase translation probability (ECP): similar with CEP, but the translation direction is reversed;

Frequency ratio (FR): ratio between lower and higher frequency of phrases in the pair:

For the SVM classifier, we use LIBSVM (Change and Lin, 2001), and 5-fold cross-validation is used. Here we consider true parallel terms as the positive class and others as the negative class. Since the data is unbalanced, we train the classifier with different penalties for the negative class and the penalty for the positive class is just set as 1. The penalties tried for the negative class include 1, 2, 2.5, 3, and 5. The comparison of performance is shown in Table 12, from which we can observe:

1. The SVM classifier can improve the precision significantly from 0.812 to 0.908 with penalty 5 for the negative class; while the recall drops from 100% to 61.7%.
2. The SVM classifier with penalty 2.5 for the negative class outperforms ECBil on both precision and recall, showing that the

linguistic and statistical features are useful for the identification of true parallel terms.

In the following part, we investigate the contribution of each feature on the overall performance. First we build a balanced data set by using all the *wrong* pairs and the same number of *correct* pairs. The features are compared and evaluated one by one and the performances are shown in Table 13. We can observe that: CMC is the best one among individual features, followed by LWP; the combination of CMC and LWP achieves better performance than any individual features; and the combination of all features achieves the best performance among any individual features and other combinations.

6. SMT EXPERIMENTS

SMT performance on the Japanese-English patent translation has been tested at NTCIR-7 (Fujii et al., 2008). But currently there is no publicly available Chinese-English parallel patent corpus, and no publicly presented SMT experiments on the Chinese-English patent translation task.

We conduct SMT experiments based on the parallel sentences extracted above from comparable patents. The 352K sentence pair candidates are divided into the training and test data sets like the scenario in (Fujii et al. 2008). Since the most recent English patents in our data were filed in

Table 12. SVM classifier's performance on bilingual multi-word term candidates

	Precision	Recall	F1
EBil	0.812	**1.000**	0.896
ECBil	0.852	0.849	0.830
1:1	0.817	0.995	**0.897**
2:1	0.847	0.911	0.878
2.5:1	0.865	0.860	0.862
3:1	0.876	0.789	0.830
5:1	**0.908**	0.617	0.735

Table 13. SVM performance for different feature combinations

Combinations	Precision	Recall	F1
CMC	0.581	0.882	0.701
LWP	0.673	0.665	0.669
CEP&ECP	0.550	0.825	0.660
FR	0.531	0.711	0.608
CMC&LWP	0.681	0.737	0.708
All	0.688	0.743	0.715

2008, we use those filed in 2008 in *USPTO* to produce the test data consisting of about 35K sentence pair candidates, and other patents filed before 2008 to produce the training data, which consists of about 320K Chinese-English sentence pair candidates.

Although the experiment in Section 4 shows that sentence filtering can help identify really parallel sentences, we may wonder whether the sentence filtering actually leads to better SMT performance. Therefore, we also evaluate the impact of sentence filtering on SMT. The Moses toolkit (Koehn et al., 2007) was used to conduct

Chinese->English SMT experiments, and BLEU and NIST scores are used as the evaluation metrics. We followed the instruction of the baseline system for the shared task in the 2008 ACL workshop on SMT.

All the sentence pairs are sorted using the *Filter* ensemble method mentioned earlier in Section 4. We choose the top ranked 2000 Chinese-English sentence pairs in the test data as the test set, and compare SMT performance by using different percentages of the sorted sentence pair candidates in the training data to train the translation model. Note, from Table 6, we can see that in general

Figure 2. BLEU scores for percentages

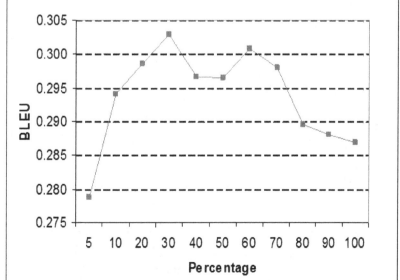

the quality of lower ranked sentence pairs is not as good as that of higher ranked ones. The SMT results are shown in Figure 2 and Figure 3, from which we can observe that:

1. The BLEU and NIST scores for the highest ranking 10%-90% sentence pairs of the training data are higher than those of 100%. Even if we only use the highest ranking 10% of the training data, we can get better BLEU and NIST scores than using the highest ranking 80%, 90% or 100%. This shows that sentence filtering can identify really parallel sentences, which in turn improve SMT performance.
2. Performance peaks for the highest ranking 30% and 60% of the training data in terms of BLEU and NIST scores show that filtering out too many or too few sentence pair candidates cannot get the best performance. Performance is worst at 5% of the training data, demonstrating that a training corpus of very small size cannot achieve good performance for SMT.
3. The possible explanation for the two peaks of performance in the figures could be that there may be some data between 50% and 70% of the training data which may be more relevant to the test data, and thus lead to better performance than at 40% and 50%.

The highest BLEU score of the SMT engine trained on the parallel sentences extracted is above 0.3 on the test set. The results show that the parallel sentences extracted are in good quality for the SMT engine to learn a good model, and it also shows that our proposed method for parallel sentence extraction can help identify parallel sentences in comparable patents since filtering out misaligned sentence actually leads to better SMT performance.

7. DISCUSSION

As mentioned earlier, *"true"* parallel terms have two properties: a) the translation is correct, i.e. the Chinese side and English side have equivalent

Figure 3. NIST scores for percentages

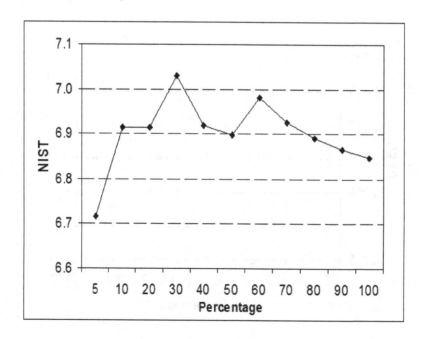

meaning; b) both the Chinese side and English side should be patent-specific technical terms. Here we give some analysis on the real cases in our experiment. For the wrong word pairs, there are mainly three kinds: 1) word/phrase pairs with non-parallel meaning; 2) verb phrases, e.g. *module locates*/模块会维持; 3) uncommon paraphrasing which may lead to errors if the translation is used directly, for example, *high voltage*/电压高. For the correct cases (i.e. the true parallel terms), it is more complicated and the following kinds have been found: 1) Apparently true parallel terms such as the examples in Table 11; 2) Chinese translations which, though missing specific details, are generally understood to refer to the English one. For example, both *high voltage*/高电压 and *high voltage*/高压 are considered correct; 3) General *adjective + noun* phrases, which are likely to be used in a context with specific technical meaning, e.g. *simple form*/简单形式; 4) Some terms followed by a noun phrase, and it could be a verb or a noun depending on the context, e.g. *access routers*/接入路由器; 5) Some uncommon form of Chinese translations, which may sound appropriate in certain contexts but not in other situations, e.g. *active application*/当前应用; 6) Chinese translations containing Roman letters which cannot be translated, for example, *V-shaped*/V型.

But some problems have been found for bilingual term extraction. The first problem here is the definition of term itself. Since the terms dealt with in this chapter refer to the technical terms in the patent domain, we would consider a word/phrase as a term as long as it is relevant to the patent domain. Still different people may have different answers towards the question whether a word/phrase is a term in a specific domain. For example, our annotators disagree on whether the following phrases are patent-specific terms or not: 1 *top block*/上横梁, 2) *frame*/框体, 3) *mask*/掩模, since they are polysemous and quite ambiguous when considered independently out of context. Thus it would be a little difficult to judge whether they are terms or not.

The second problem here is loose translation, rewriting of Chinese phrases or paraphrasing. Many non-literal translations can be found in comparable patents. For example, *inner ring* means 内环 in Chinese, but instead 启闭环 is used as equivalence in the corresponding Chinese patent. The literal translation of 非线性非树状选单 is *non-linear and non-tree-shaped menu*, but *OSD menu* is used in the corresponding English patent.

Last but not least, as for term extraction, patent is treated as a specific domain, in contrast with other domains such as news, legal text, or medical records. Meanwhile, patents may cover a wide range of other technical domains, such as chemistry, biomedicine, electronics, vehicle, etc. Therefore, patents also have the potential to simultaneously find terms for the mentioned technical domains, which

What is interesting here is the very concept of translations being "parallel". The commonly used BLEU and NIST scores in SMT evaluation just reduce the concept of parallelism to a rather technical mapping of language units. But it is well known that high-quality human translations often do not keep sentence units of the source language. Therefore, we may need more elaborate schemes to better evaluate the quality of machine translation, and the field of translation studies (Munday, 2001) could be a possible source to consult. Note the concept parallel corpora has been used ambiguously in NLP or computational linguistics: it could be corpora of parallel documents (Koehn, 2005) or corpus of parallel sentences (Utiyama and Isahara, 2007), and in this study we use the latter one.

8. CONCLUSION AND FUTURE WORK

In this chapter, we investigate the issues of mining parallel knowledge from comparable patents from the following perspectives: 1) Parallel sentence extraction: we propose to combine three measures to filter out misaligned sentences extracted from comparable patents; 2) Bilingual term extraction: we identify true parallel terms by integrating the monolingual term candidates in Chinese and English patents, and phrasal translations found in extracted parallel sentences, and then try to combine both linguistic and statistical information into an SVM classifier; 3) Chinese-English SMT: it is conducted based on the parallel sentences mined. The experiments show that the proposed combination and approach show good performance for parallel sentence extraction and bilingual term extraction, and the SMT engine trained on the mined parallel sentences gives promising results.

Monolingual term extraction and the mutual influence of monolingual and bilingual term extraction are ongoing now. The usefulness of the extracted bilingual terms and their influence on SMT is also our interest. Relation acquisition, as an important aspect of ontology learning, is to extract semantic relations between pairs of entities from texts. Since we have extracted bilingual terms, the semantic relation between the terms could be quite interesting to be learned from comparable patents.

Since different (sub-)sections (namely, title, abstract, claims, description, and subsections in the description part) in patents have their own writing styles which may influence the word choice and syntactic structure of the sentences, as well as patents cover many technical domains (such as chemistry, biomedicine, electronics, vehicle, etc.), experiments on cross-section and cross-IPC machine could be enlightening for further understanding the characteristics of the technical domains and the sections. For example, claims have legal effect, and tend to use more relative clauses to modify head words.

Given the relative paucity of parallel patent data, the use of such comparable corpus for mining parallel knowledge would be a helpful step towards multilingual ontology learning and other cross-lingual access applications in the patent domain, such as MT, cross-lingual information retrieval. The extracted parallel sentences and technical terms could be a good basis for further acquisition of attributes, term relations, as well as for the translation of monolingual ontologies since most current ontologies are monolingual.

REFERENCES

Berners-Lee, T., Hendler, J., & Lassila, O. (2001). The Semantic Web. *Scientific American*, 34–43. doi:10.1038/scientificamerican0501-34

Brewster, C., Ciravegna, F., & Wilks, Y. (2003). Background and foreground knowledge in dynamic ontology construction. In *Proceedings of the SIGIR Semantic Web Workshop*.

Brown, P. F., Cocke, J., Pietra, S. A. D., Pietra, V. J. D., Jelinek, F., & Lafferty, J. D. (1990). A statistical approach to machine translation. *Computational Linguistics*, *16*(2), 79–85.

Brown, P. F., Lai, J. C., & Mercer, R. L. (1991). Aligning sentences in parallel corpora. In *Proceedings of the Annual Meeting of the Association of Computational Linguistics (ACL)*. (pp. 169-176).

Brown, P. F., Pietra, S. A. D., Pietra, V. J. D., & Mercer, R. L. (1993). Mathematics of statistical machine translation: Parameter estimation. *Computational Linguistics*, *19*(2), 263–311.

Buitelaar, P., & Cimiano, P. (Eds.). (2008). *Ontology learning and population: Bridging the gap between text and knowledge*. Amsterdam, The Netherlands: ISO Press.

Chang, C. C., & Lin, C. J. (2010). *LIBSVM: A library for support vector machines*. Retrieved from http://www.csie.ntu.edu.tw/cjlin/libsvm

Chen, S. F. (1993). Aligning sentences in bilingual corpora using lexical information. In *Proceedings of the Annual Meeting of the Association of Computational Linguistics (ACL)*. (pp. 9-16). Columbus, OH.

Chiang, D. (2005). A hierarchical phrase-based model for statistical machine translation. In *Proceedings of the Association for Computational Linguistics (ACL)*. (pp. 263-270).

Chiang, D. (2007). Hierarchical phrase-based translation. *Computational Linguistics, 33*(2), 201–228. doi:10.1162/coli.2007.33.2.201

Chiang, D., Wang, W., & Knight, K. (2009). 11,001 new features for statistical machine translation. In *Proceedings of NAACL-HLT*, (pp. 218–226).

Cimiano, P. (2006). *Ontology learning and population from pext: Algorithms, evaluation and applications*. New York, NY: Springer.

Daille, B., Gaussier, É., & Langé, J. M. (1994). Towards automatic extraction of monolingual and bilingual terminology. In *Proceedings of the 15th Conference on Computational Linguistics*.

Erdmann, M., Nakayama, K., Hara, T., & Nishio, S. (2009). Improving the extraction of Bilingual terminology from Wikipedia. *ACM Transactions on Multimedia Computing. Communications and Applications, 5*(4), 1–17.

Frantzi, K. T., & Ananiadou, S. (1997). Automatic term recognition using contextual cues. In *Proceedings of the IJCAI Workshop on Multilinguality in Software Industry: the AI Contribution,* Japan.

Frantzi, K. T., & Ananiadou, S. (1999). The C-Value/NC-Value domain independent method for multi-word term extraction. *Journal of Natural Language Processing, 6*(3), 145–179.

Friedl, J. E. F. (2002). *Mastering regular expressions* (2nd ed.). Sebastopol, CA: O'Reilly Media.

Fujii, A., Utiyama, M., Yamamoto, M., & Utsuro, T. (2008). Overview of the patent translation task at the NTCIR-7 workshop. In *Proceedings of the 7th NTCIR Workshop Meeting on Evaluation of Information Access Technologies (NTCIR)*. (pp. 389-400). Tokyo, Japan.

Gale, W. A., & Church, K. W. (1991). A program for aligning sentences in bilingual corpora. In *Proceedings of the Annual Meeting of the Association of Computational Linguistics (ACL)*. (pp. 79-85).

Ha, L. A., Fernandez, G., Mitkov, R., & Corpas, G. (2008). Mutual bilingual terminology extraction. In *Proceedings of the Sixth International Language Resources and Evaluation (LREC)*. (pp. 1818-1824).

Hjelm, H. (2009). *Cross-language ontology learning: Incorporating and exploiting cross-language data in the ontology learning process*. Unpublished doctoral dissertation, Stockholm University, Sweden.

Kageura, K., & Umino, B. (1996). Methods of automatic term recognition: A review. *Terminology, 3*(2), 259–289. doi:10.1075/term.3.2.03kag

Koehn, P. (2004). Pharaoh: A beam search decoder for phrase-based statistical machine translation models. In *Proceedings of the Conference of the Association for Machine Translation in the Americas (AMTA)*.

Koehn, P. (2005). Europarl: A parallel corpus for statistical machine translation. In *Proceedings of MT Summit X*.

Koehn, P., Hoang, H., Birch, A., Callison-Burch, C., Federico, M., & Bertoldi, N. ... Herbst, E. (2007). Moses: Open source toolkit for statistical machine translation. In *Proceedings of the Annual Meeting of the Association of Computational Linguistics (ACL) Demo Session*. (pp. 177-180).

Kupiec, J. (1993). An algorithm for finding noun phrase correspondences in bilingual corpora. In *Proceedings of the 31st Annual Meeting of the Association for Computational Linguistics* (ACL).

Liu, Y., Lü, Y., & Liu, Q. (2009). Improving tree-to-tree translation with packed forests. In *Proceedings of ACL/IJCNLP*, (pp. 558-566).

Lopez, A. (2008). Statistical machine translation. *ACM Computing Surveys*, *40*(3), 1–49. doi:10.1145/1380584.1380586

Lu, B., & Tsou, B. K. Y. (2009). Towards bilingual term extraction in comparable patents. In *Proceedings of the 23rd Pacific Asia Conference on Language, Information and Computation (PACLIC)*. (pp. 755-762). Hong Kong. December, 2009.

Lu, B., Tsou, B. K. Y., Zhu, J., Jiang, T., & Kwong, O. Y. (2009). The construction of a Chinese-English patent parallel corpus. In *Proceedings of MT Summit XII 3rd Workshop on Patent Translation*. Ottawa, Canada.

Ma, X. (2006). Champollion: A robust parallel text sentence aligner. In *Proceedings of the 5th International Conference on Language Resources and Evaluation (LREC)*. Genova, Italy.

Moore, R. C. (2002). Fast and accurate sentence alignment of bilingual corpora. In *Proceedings of AMTA*. (pp. 135-144).

Munday, J. (2001). *Introducing translation studies: Theories and applications*. Oxon, UK: Routledge.

Munteanu, D. S., & Marcu, D. (2005). Improving machine translation performance by exploiting non-parallel corpora. *Computational Linguistics*, *31*(4), 477–504. doi:10.1162/089120105775299168

Nakagawa, H., & Mori, T. (2002). A simple but powerful automatic term extraction method. In *Proceedings of the International Conference on Computational Linguistics (COLING)*.

Och, F. J., & Ney, H. (2003). A systematic comparison of various statistical alignment models. *Computational Linguistics*, *29*(1), 19–51. doi:10.1162/089120103321337421

Och, F. J., & Ney, H. (2004). The alignment template approach to machine translation. *Computational Linguistics*, *30*(4), 417–449. doi:10.1162/0891201042544884

Piperidis, S., & Harlas, I. (2006). Mining bilingual lexical equivalences out of parallel corpora. *Lecture Notes in Computer Science, Advances in Artificial Intelligence*.

Polikar, R. (2006). Ensemble based systems in decision making. *IEEE Circuits and Systems Magazine*, *6*(3), 21–45. doi:10.1109/MCAS.2006.1688199

Resnik, P., & Smith, N. A. (2003). The Web as a parallel corpus. *Computational Linguistics*, *29*(3), 349–380. doi:10.1162/089120103322711578

Simard, M., & Plamondon, P. (1998). Bilingual sentence alignment: Balancing robustness and accuracy. *Machine Translation*, *13*(1), 59–80. doi:10.1023/A:1008010319408

Sun, Y. (2003). Determinants of foreign patents in China. *World Patent Information*, *25*, 27–37. doi:10.1016/S0172-2190(02)00086-8

Toutanova, K., Klein, D., Manning, C., & Singer, Y. (2003). Feature-rich part-of-speech tagging with a cyclic dependency network. In. *Proceedings of HLT-NAACL*, *2003*, 252–259.

Toutanova, K., & Manning, C. D. (2000). Enriching the knowledge sources used in a maximum entropy part-of-speech tagger. In *Proceedings of the Joint SIGDAT Conference on Empirical Methods in Natural Language Processing and Very Large Corpora (EMNLP/VLC-2000)*, (pp. 63-70).

Utiyama, M., & Isahara, H. (2003). Reliable measures for aligning Japanese-English news articles and sentences. In *Proceedings of the Annual Meeting of the Association of Computational Linguistics (ACL)*. (pp. 72–79).

Utiyama, M., & Isahara, H. (2007). A Japanese-English patent parallel corpus. In *Proceeding of MT Summit XI*. (pp. 475–482).

Varga, D., Halacsy, P., Kornai, A., Nagy, V., Nemeth, L., & Tron, V. (2005). Parallel corpora for medium density languages. In *Proceedings of RANLP 2005 Conference*.

Vintar, Š. (2001). *Using parallel corpora for translation-oriented term extraction. Babel Journal*. John Benjamins Publishing.

Wan, X. (2008). Using bilingual knowledge and ensemble techniques for unsupervised Chinese sentiment analysis. In *Proceeding of EMNLP 2008*. (pp. 553-561).

Wang, C., Collins, M., & Andkoehn, P. (2007). Chinese syntactic reordering for statistical machine translation. In *Proceedings of EMNLP-CoNLL*. (pp. 737-745).

Wang, W., May, J., Knight, K., & Marcu, D. (2010). Re-structuring, re-labeling, and re-aligning for syntax-based statistical machine translation. *Computational Linguistics*, *36*(2). doi:10.1162/coli.2010.36.2.09054

Wong, W., Liu, W., & Bennamoun, M. (2008). Determination of unithood and termhood for term recognition. In Song, M., & Wu, Y. (Eds.), *Handbook of research on text and Web mining technologies*. Hershey, PA: IGI Global. doi:10.4018/9781599049908.ch030

Wong, W. Y. (2009). *Learning lightweight ontologies from text across different domains using the Web as background knowledge*. Unpublished doctoral dissertation, University of Western Australia, Australia.

Wu, D., & Fung, P. (2005). Inversion transduction grammar constraints for mining parallel sentences from quasi-comparable corpora. In *Proceedings of IJCNLP 2005*.

Wu, D., & Xia, X. (1994). Learning an English-Chinese lexicon from a parallel corpus. In *Proceedings of the First Conference of the Association for Machine Translation in the Americas*.

Yu, K., & Tsujii, J. (2009). Bilingual dictionary extraction from Wikipedia. In *Proceedings of Machine Learning Summit XII*.

Zhao, B., & Vogel, S. (2002). Adaptive parallel sentences mining from Web bilingual news collection. In *Proceedings of Second IEEE International Conference on Data Mining (ICDM'02)*.

Zhao, J., & Huang, C. N. (1999). The model for Chinese baseNP structure analysis. *Chinese Journal of Computer*, *22*(2), 141–146.

Zhao, T., Yang, M., Liu, F., Yao, J., & Yu, H. (2000). Statistics based hybrid approach to Chinese base phrase identification. In *Proceedings of the Second Workshop on Chinese Language Processing*. (pp. 73-77).

Zhou, L. (2007). Ontology learning: State of the art and open issues. *Information Technology Management*, *8*(3), 241–252. doi:10.1007/s10799-007-0019-5

Zhu, Q., Inkpen, D., & Asudeh, A. (2007). Automatic extraction of translations from Web-based bilingual materials. *Machine Translation*, 2.

ADDITIONAL READING

Alani, H., Kim, S., Millard, D. E., Weal, M. J., Hall, W., Lewis, P. H., & Shadbolt, N. R. (2003, Jan./Feb.). Automatic Ontology-Based Knowledge Extraction from Web Documents. *IEEE Intelligent Systems*, 2–9.

Bourigault, D., Jacquemin, C., & L'Homme, M.-C. (Eds.). (2001). *Recent Advances in Computational Terminology*. Amsterdam, Netherlands: John Benjamins Publishing Company.

Cabre, M. T., Castellvi, M. T. C., Sager, J. C., & DeCesaris, J. A. (Eds.). (1998). *Terminology: Theory, Methods and Applications*. Amsterdam, Netherlands: John Benjamins Publishing Company.

Cheung, L., Lai, T., Luk, R., Kwong, O. Y., Sin, K. K., & Tsou, B. K. (2002). Some considerations on guidelines for bilingual alignment and terminology extraction. In *Proceedings of the first SIGHAN workshop on Chinese Language*.

Daille1, B., & Morin, E. French-English Terminology Extraction from Comparable Corpora. In *Lecture Notes in Computer Science: Vol. 3651. Natural Language Processing - IJCNLP 2005* (pp. 707-718). Springer Berlin / Heidelberg.

Fung, P. (1998). A Statistical View on Bilingual Lexicon Extraction: From Parallel Corpora to Non-Parallel Corpora. In *Lecture Notes in Computer Science: Vol. 1529. Machine Translation and the Information Soup* (pp. 1-17). London: Springer Publisher.

Gaussier, É. (2001). *General considerations on bilingual terminology extraction*. Recent Advances in Computational Terminology.

Hearst, M. A. (1992). Automatic Acquisition of Hyponyms from Large Text Corpora. In *Proceedings of the 14th International Conference on Computational Linguistics (COLING)*. pp.539-545.

Higuchi, S., Fukui, M., Fujii, A., & Ishikawa, T. (2001). A system for multi-lingual patent retrieval. In *Proccedings of MT Summit VIII* (pp. 163–167). PRIME.

Hippisley, A., Cheng, D., & Ahmad, K. (2005). The Head-modifier Principle and Multilingual Term Extraction. *Natural Language Engineering, 11*(2), 129–157. doi:10.1017/S1351324904003535

Jiang, T., Tsou, B. K., & Lu, B. (2010). Part-of-speech model for N-best list reranking in experimental Chinese-English SMT. In *Proceedings of 1st International Workshop on Advances in Patent Information Retrieval*. Milton Keynes, UK.

Kit, C., & Liu, X. (2008). Measuring Monoword Termhood by Rank Difference via Corpus Comparison. *Terminology, 14*(2), 204–229. doi:10.1075/term.14.2.05kit

Maedche, A., & Staab, S. (2004). Ontology Learning. In Staab, S., & Studer, R. (Eds.), *Handbook on ontologies*. Berlin, Germany: Springer-Verlag.

Ozdowska, S. (2004). Identifying correspondences between words: An approach based on a bilingual syntactic analysis of French/English parallel corpora. In *Proceedings of COLING 04 Workshop on Multilingual Linguistic Resources*.

Rapp, R. (1999). Automatic Identification of Word Translations from Unrelated English and German Corpora. In *Proceedings of the Annual Meeting of the Association for Computational Linguistics (ACL)*.

Resnik, P., & Smith, N. A. (2003). The Web as a Parallel Corpus. *Computational Linguistics, 29*(3). doi:10.1162/089120103322711578

Sadat, F., Yoshikawa, M., & Uemura, S. (2003). Bilingual Terminology Acquisition from Comparable Corpora and Phrasal Translation to Cross-language Information Retrieval. In *Proceedings of the 41st Annual Meeting of the Association for Computational Linguistics (ACL)*. pp. 141-144.

Shadbolt, N., Hall, W., & Berners-Lee, T. (2006). The Semantic Web revisited. *IEEE Intelligent Systems*, (May/June): 96–101. doi:10.1109/MIS.2006.62

Tsujii, J., & Ananiadou, S. (2005). Thesaurus or Logical Ontology, Which One Do We Need for Text Mining? *In Language Resources and Evaluation. Springer Science and Business Media B.V., 39*(1), 77–90.

Valderrabanos, A.S., Belskis, A., & Moreno, L.I. (2002). Multilingual Terminology Extraction and Validation.

Wong, W., Liu, W., & Bennamoun, M. (2009). Acquiring Semantic Relations Using the Web for Constructing Lightweight Ontologies. In Theeramunkong, T. (Eds.), *PAKDD 2009, LNAI 5476* (pp. 266–277). Berlin, Heidelberg: Springer-Verlag.

Wu, D., & Xia, X. (1995). Large-scale automatic extraction of an English-Chinese translation lexicon. *Machine Translation*, 9(3-4), 285–313. doi:10.1007/BF00980581

KEY TERMS AND DEFINITIONS

Ontology: An ontology is a data structure that describes the vocabulary in a certain domain, and that specifies the relation between the elements in that domain.

Ontology Learning from Text: Ontology learning from text is the process of identifying terms, concepts, relations and optionally, axioms from natural language text, and using them to construct and maintain an ontology.

Parallel Corpora: Parallel corpora are bilingual text collections consisting of the same content in two or more different languages.

Comparable Corpora: Comparable corpora contain texts that are not exact translations but closely related or taken from the same text domain in two or more different languages.

Parallel Sentences Extraction: Parallel sentence extraction is to extract parallel sentences from parallel corpora or from comparable corpora.

Bilingual Term Extraction: Bilingual term extraction is to extract parallel terms from bilingual domain-specific corpora.

Statistical Machine Translation (SMT): SMT is an approach to the automatic translation from one natural language into another one by using computers, which is characterized by the use of statistical and machine learning methods.

ENDNOTES

[1] Retrieved from http://www.collinslanguage.com/ on March 18, 2010.

[2] The data is available at http://www.wipo.int/ipstats/en/statistics/patents/csv/wipo_pat_appl_from_1883_list.csv (Please note that this data does not include utility models).

[3] http://www.statmt.org/moses

[4] http://www.sipo.gov.cn/

[5] http://www.cnipr.com/

[6] http://ictclas.org/

[7] http://projects.ldc.upenn.edu/Chinese/LDC_ch.htm

[8] http://www.keenage.com/html/e_index.html

Chapter 14
Cross–Language Ontology Learning

Hans Hjelm
alaTest.com, Sweden

Martin Volk
University of Zurich, Switzerland

ABSTRACT

A formal ontology does not contain lexical knowledge; it is by nature language-independent. Mappings can be added between the ontology and, arbitrarily, many lexica in any number of languages. The result of this operation is what is here referred to as a cross-language ontology. A cross-language ontology can be a useful resource for machine translation or cross-language information retrieval. This chapter focuses on ways of automatically building an ontology by exploiting cross-language information from parallel corpora. The goal is to improve the automatic learning results compared to learning an ontology from resources in a single language. The authors present a framework for cross-language ontology learning, providing a setting in which cross-language evidence (data) can be integrated and quantified. The aim is to investigate the following question: Can cross-language data teach us more than data from a single language for the ontology learning task?

INTRODUCTION

To indicate why we think integrating information from different languages is a good idea, we turn to the field of *lexical typology*. It is concerned with the ways in which different languages "dissect" semantics, or meaning, and form it into words

DOI: 10.4018/978-1-60960-625-1.ch014

(Koch, 2001). E.g., where English has 'sibling' as a unifying word for 'brother' and 'sister', French only has 'frère' and 'sœur' but no unifying word; how kinship relations are expressed varies greatly in the languages of the world (Koch, 2001). Another example is that English 'go' corresponds to both German 'gehen' (go by foot) and 'fahren' (go by some means of transportation) (Goddard, 2001). Figure 1 also depicts how a particular se-

mantic field is subject to different categorizations in different languages. We believe that this type of diversity will prove an asset in an ontology learning system, providing different "views" that each contributes useful information. We describe how such differences influence features in our machine learning experiments later in the chapter.

EXPLOITING CROSS-LANGUAGE DATA

Our major hypothesis is that combining information from different languages will improve the results of the ontology learning task, which is traditionally approached in a single language framework. We describe the process of going from a domain-specific parallel or comparable corpus and language-specific terms to a hierarchical is-a ordering of cross-language term sets.

Regarding cross-language data, especially data taken from a parallel corpus, there are two extreme standpoints possible. One could argue that, by adding texts translated into another language, we are in fact doubling the amount of data, basing the argument on crude numbers such as bytes used

for storage or the like. The other extreme would be to say that we do not add anything at all, but are merely repeating the exact same information, just using a different "encoding". We show that the use of an additional language reveals certain pieces of information that were hidden in the initial language.

According to Sager (1994), the notion of *equivalence* is central to the field of translation. Equivalence relations, in turn, have the properties of being reflexive (any word is a translation of itself), symmetrical (if A is a translation of B, then B is a translation of A) and transitive (if A is a translation of B, and B of C, then A is also a translation of C) (Boolos & Jeffrey, 1989). In practice, the notion of equivalence could be modified to a notion of relative equivalence (see Figure 1), just as the synonymy relation is commonly relativized.

In addition to lexico-typological aspects, there are other sources of discrepancy, when dealing with translations. For a given word in the source language, it is not always possible to come up with a single translation to that word. This can have different causes, apart from the typological differences already discussed:

Figure 1. Words related to trees/wood in different languages. Ewe is a language in the Niger-Congo family and is spoken in Ghana, Togo and Benin. Note how English and French are closer to each other in this example than to Swedish, even though English and Swedish are both Germanic languages. (Figure from Mikael Parkvall, Stockholm University, personal communication)

Ewe	Swedish	English	French
àtí	träd	tree	arbre
	stam	trunk	tronc
	gren	branch	branche
nákè	virke	(construction wood) **wood**	bois
àvé	ved	(firewood)	
	skog	forest	forêt

- The source word is polysemic or homonymic and the different senses of the word give rise to different translations in the target language.
- The target language has more than one word with more or less the same meaning, used interchangeably as translations of the source word (the target language words are synonyms).

We expect cases as the ones mentioned to occur less frequently in domain-specific text than they would in general, non-technical texts. Though problematic at times, we actually expect that these discrepancies will be a source for added information when trying to learn an ontology over a domain, rather than pose a problem.

Probabilistic Approaches to Ontology Learning

We propose a method that can be desribed as a probabilistic approach to ontology learning. We therefore wish to point the reader to other work along those lines.

In an experiment in Caraballo (2001), the assumption is made that there exists a "true" hierarchy from which observed co-occurrence data was generated; the task then is to find the hierarchy which gives the highest probability to observed data. Accordingly they assume a process which generates a noun n with probability $P(n)$ and then a context word w with probability $P(w \mid n)$. Caraballo then suggests a backing-off version of this, where the superordinate (hyperonym) node c of n is taken into account: $P(w \mid n) = \lambda P(w \mid n) + (1 - \lambda)P(w \mid c)$, incorporating the hierarchical structure in the calculations.

Snow et al. (2006) describe a probabilistic approach to constructing an ontology based on two classifiers trained to recognize hyperonym/hyponym pairs and cohyponym pairs, respectively.

The ontology is built up stepwise, by at each step adding the relation that maximizes the probability of the ontology *as a whole*. This is done by calculating all new relations that will be created by adding a particular relation to the ontology, using the transitive closures of the hyponymy and cohyponymy relations. This is also the approach we follow in our experiments.

Translational Equivalence for Terms

Because we wish to model words or terms from different languages in our learned ontologies, it becomes important to know which of them mean the same thing, which ones are *translational equivalents* of each other. In the absence of a translation dictionary, it is still possible to work with cross-language ontology learning, using techniques from bilingual dictionary extraction.

Tiedemann (2003, p. 12) gives the following definition for the task of bilingual lexicon/dictionary extraction: "*Bilingual lexicon extraction aims at the identification of lexical word type links in parallel corpora*". The focus lies on *word types*, in contrast with the task of *word alignment*, where the focus is on *word tokens*. The bilingual dictionary extraction task is thus not concerned with which word(s) in a particular source language sentence correspond to which word(s) in a particular target language sentence; instead, the entire corpus is taken into consideration and a most probable translation of the source language word(s) is sought in this global perspective. The two contrasting views give rise to different evaluation schemes, something worth keeping in mind when reading articles in the area.

The cross-language approach to ontology learning advocated in this chapter depends on the existence of a bilingual dictionary, or a parallel or comparable corpus from which to extract such a dictionary. Resnik & Smith (2003) propose a way of remedying the absence of these resources, by describing how the Web can be mined for parallel texts.

We use data from a bilingual dictionary extraction system in our experiments. We will not describe the system in detail here, but like Tiedemann (2003), we combine results from an automatic word-alignment system with similarity measurements from a distributional similarity model (Hjelm, 2007).

Other Efforts Towards Exploiting Cross-Language Data

This section looks at other attempts of profiting from cross-language information in a variety of NLP settings related to the ontology learning field.

Aizawa & Kageura (2001) look at co-occurrences of English and Japanese keywords in scientific articles. The co-occurrences are used to form a graph where the edges are weighted by the number of co-occurrences. They perform a clustering by splitting up the graph using the *minimum edge cut*, a graph-theoretically motivated approach. They do not compare their cross-language results with single language results, so we do not know if the cross-language data gives a better clustering than the single language data. On the other hand, the resulting resource (cross-language term clusters) has added value, because it can be used in, e.g., a cross-language information retrieval setting.

Simard (1999) and Borin (2000) look at the effects of adding a third language for solving problems normally involving two languages: sentence and word alignment in parallel corpora. They both conclude that information from the third language increases the accuracy of the system, evaluated on cross-language alignment tasks. Simard also concludes that "the more languages, the merrier", implying that adding a fourth language would improve the results further. Borin also notes that adding a language from the same language family is more helpful than adding a language from a different language family.

Dyvik (2005) proposes to use *semantic mirrors* to perform both word sense discrimination and a hierarchical ordering of word senses using a word-aligned parallel corpus. A key concept is the so called *t-image* of a word W, which consists of all the words in the target language which have been word-aligned with W. The linking process is then reversed by taking the t-image of all the words in the first t-image, which gives us a set of words in the source language, called the *inversed t-image* of W. By going back and forth between languages (Dyvik also forms what he calls a *second t-image* by going back to the target language from the inversed t-image), one is able to form sets of words in either language that share at least one member (apart from W). These sets correspond to senses of W. Further, these sets can be used to produce a hierarchy by using a set inclusion analysis to form an upper semilattice. A disadvantage is that the semantic mirroring process depends on high quality (i.e., manually produced) word alignments, something which is hard to come by on a larger scale. Dyvik also reports that the method works better for adjectives than for nouns.

Plas & Tiedemann (2006) use a cross-language distributional similarity model for targeting the extraction of synonyms. The idea, not unlike Dyvik's, is that synonyms will "co-occur" with the same translations in a parallel corpus, whereas this would be less true for other lexical semantic relations such as antonymy or hyperonymy. Their system outperforms a traditional, single language, distributional similarity model on the task of identifying synonyms in the Dutch EuroWordNet.

We have provided an overview of different approaches for solving problems involved in ontology learning, or, specifically, cross-language ontology learning. Not all approaches were developed with this application in mind, but most of them have proven useful in various types of ontology learning systems.

A common trait of all the methods discussed in this section is that they all deal with meaning in one way or another, whether they aim at capturing similarity or at exploiting asymmetries. A large part of our task will be to find strategies for combining this wealth of information in ways that take advantage of the strengths and weaknesses of the different approaches. We present experiments to this end in the next section.

EXPERIMENTAL SETUP AND RESOURCES

As mentioned, our approach to ontology learning is based on the method described by Snow et al. (2006), with some alterations, and we add a cross-language perspective by using probabilities based on evidence from different languages. Using the translational equivalence relation for merging data across languages, we use the merged data when training support vector machine classifiers. The output of the classifiers is in turn used as input when constructing the ontology.

Resources

A few initiatives, some of them ongoing, have been taken in the ontology learning field to establish a standard document collection along with a corresponding domain ontology to be used for evaluation. The existence of such a standard would facilitate automated qualitative comparisons among ontology learning systems and approaches. To date, one of the most ambitious initiatives was taken for the *2nd Workshop on Ontology Learning and Population*, held in Sydney, Australia, 2006. Participants were encouraged to perform experiments on the *OLP2 dataset*,[1] a corpus, ontology and knowledge base in the soccer domain. This dataset is still freely available for research purposes, but it has not yet had the needed homogenizing impact on the community. Of course, an exaggerated homogeneity can also be harmful to a field, such as is arguably the case with the use of the Wall Street Journal part of the Penn Treebank (Marcus et al., 1993) in the *parsing* community. For the ontology learning field, the danger lies rather in slipping into the opposite ditch, where the lack of standards is preventing competitive develop-

ment. We choose to work with a different setup: a corpus and a terminological ontology dealing with European Union (EU) related issues. There are several reasons for this, the main reason being the massively parallel nature of the corpus (see below). Another reason is the availability of a rather large terminological ontology, where all terms have been translated into most of the EU languages (also described below). This combination of a parallel corpus and a cross-language terminological ontology is crucial to our experiments. *JRC-ACQUIS Multilingual Parallel Corpus*

This corpus consists of legal texts concerning matters involving the EU. The number of words per language varies between 6.5 million (Swedish) and 7.8 million (French) among the languages used in the experiments: German, French, English and Swedish.[2] This choice of languages is to a certain extent arbitrary; it is based on the existence of readily available, high quality pre-processing software, such as lemmatizers and compound splitters. The corpus is parallel and contains over 20 European languages in total (Steinberger et al., 2006). Note that there is a release 3.0 of this corpus, which is almost three times bigger than the one in our experiments (version 2.2).

The corpus is distributed with automatic alignment on the paragraph level. The paragraphs are very short and usually only contain one sentence or even one part of a sentence. There are two alignment versions available for download;[3] we have opted for the version produced by the Vanilla aligner.[4] Since the alignment process is automatic, we are of course introducing an error source here; unfortunately we are unaware of any figures concerning alignment accuracy for this corpus and the languages involved. However, we consider the effects of this error source small but non-negligible.

Below is a short exemplifying passage from the corpus (excerpt from document "jrc32005R0123-en.xml").

Commission Regulation (EC) No 466/2001 [2], sets maximum levels for certain contaminants in foodstuffs. (2) According to Regulation (EC) No 466/2001, the Commission shall review the provisions as regards ochratoxin A (OTA) in dried vine fruit and with a view to including a maximum level for OTA in green and roasted coffee and coffee products, wine, beer, grape juice, cocoa and cocoa products and spices taking into account the investigations undertaken and the prevention measures applied to reduce the presence of OTA in these products.

Eurovoc

Eurovoc V4.2[5] is a freely available multilingual thesaurus with entries in more than 20 languages, and it covers topics where the EU is active, e.g., law, politics, economics and science. The thesaurus contains 6,645 concepts, each of which is given a *descriptor*, or recommended term, in each language. Only the descriptors are taken into consideration throughout all our experiments, which means that we make a simplifying assumption that there is a one-to-one relationship between terms and concepts. The average depth of the Eurovoc hierarchy is 4.32 and the maximum depth is 8. An example of a small is-a hierarchy is displayed in Figure 2.

Apart from hierarchical (is-a) relations, also equivalence and associative relations are listed in Eurovoc, but only the hierarchical relations are considered in our experiments. Eurovoc is divided into 21 *fields*, each representing a domain of interest in the EU. E.g., we have the fields 'politics', 'finance' and 'education and communications' and examples of terms from these respective fields are 'composition of parliament', 'financial accounting' and 'educational administration'.

To be able to perform cross-validation in our machine learning experiments, we split the Eurovoc taxonomy into ten parts, approximately equal in size. We do this by exploiting the fact that Eurovoc is already segmented into 21 fields. We have nine partitions containing two fields each and a tenth partition containing three fields and we number the partitions 0–9.

A minority of the terms in the hierarchy have more than one super-ordinate term; this concerns mainly geographical entities, which have both part-of and is-a relations marked (though the marking itself does not discriminate between the

Figure 2. Excerpt from Eurovoc, terms involving petroleum products

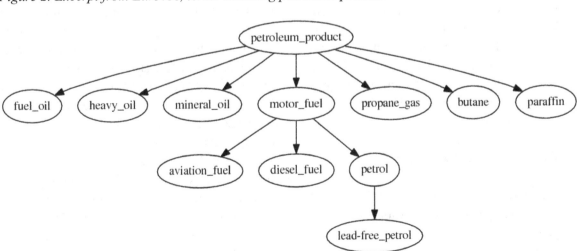

two relation types). E.g., 'Sweden' has 'Northern Europe' and 'EU member state' as super-ordinate terms, but only with the latter does it enter into an is-a relation. In such cases, we have processed the data to remove this type of polyhierarchy and only keep the is-a information (this is generally discernible using the ID numbers of the concepts, though this is only a heuristic). Some concepts have *only* part-of information listed, e.g., 'Skåne county' only has 'South Sweden' as parent in the hierarchy. These cases are not marked in the thesaurus, which means that we are not able to filter them out automatically, and in turn, that we end up with a small number of part-of relations in our gold standard. We estimate the number of such cases to make out no more than 2–3% of the total, which means that they will have a negligible effect on our evaluations.

Evaluation

Dellschaft & Staab (2006) point out that the existence of methodologies and datasets for evaluation in "batch mode" has played an important role in the success of fields like information retrieval and speech recognition (and this also holds for, e.g., text categorization and statistical machine translation). Also Maedche (2002) expresses the need for standardized datasets, especially cross-language ones, and evaluation measures to go with these datasets. Though there is ongoing work towards establishing benchmark datasets (see previous discussion) and evaluation metrics in ontology learning, there is still a great need for further understanding and refinement of today's measures. We briefly discuss the matter in the following section.

Evaluating Ontology Learning

We are interested in finding a metric for measuring the similarity between two ontologies. A first suggestion towards this goal within the ontology learning community was given in Maedche

(2002). The measures *taxonomic precision* (TP), *taxonomic recall* (TR) and TF (the harmonic mean of TP and TR) were introduced for this purpose. These measures make use of what Maedche calls *conceptual cotopy* or *semantic cotopy* (SC). The SC of a concept in a hierarchy consists of all its superconcepts, its subconcepts and the concept itself. To separate the evaluation of the overlap of the lexica of the two ontologies from the evaluation of the taxonomic structures, Dellschaft & Staab (2006) and Cimiano (2006) use *common semantic cotopy* (CSC), which disregards all concepts that are not found in *both* ontologies.

These measures have been applied in a number of different settings and are starting to establish themselves as the standard measures for evaluating an ontology learning system. We have argued in Hjelm (2009) that they are not applicable to all settings where such an evaluation measure is needed, and therefore use a new evaluation measure, based on Pearson's product-moment correlation coefficient (PMCC). We there show that the SC and CSC measures display an unwanted sensitivity to changes in the root node, which is not shared by the PMCC measure. The SC measure also has difficulties when the ontologies compared have different scales, e.g., when the reference ontology is much more extensive than the learned one. We also argue that the CSC measure is not applicable when evaluating certain learned ontologies, derived from hierarchical clustering. In a prototypical clustering, you will get mother nodes that have no labels of their own, but consist of a merge of two daughter nodes. Because of how the CSC measure is defined, it is not always capable of handling such cases – these are our main reasons for preferring the PMCC measure over the more established CSC or SC measures.

The PMCC measure uses two series of numbers, one series per ontology to be compared. The numbers in each list denote the distance, measured in number of steps, between each unordered pair of nodes in the ontologies. If the series are similar to each other, this means that nodes which are close in one ontology are also close in the other and that nodes far apart in the first are also far apart in the second. A PMCC measure of 1 means perfect similarity, 0 means that there is no correlation at all, and −1 means perfect negative correlation, somewhat simplified.

OUR ONTOLOGY LEARNING EXPERIMENTS

When constructing a hierarchy of terms, there are two relations which are more prominent than others. The first is the hyperonymy relation, that connects two terms in the vertical plane. The second is the cohyponymy relation, that instead connects two terms in the horizontal plane. Also Snow et al. (2006) and Ryu & Choi (2006) use these two relations as their basic building blocks. We look at a number of features which we think will be useful for recognizing either or both of two basic relations, which in turn will enable us to learn a terminological ontology. We use these features to train a support vector machine classifier, so the selection of some of the features is made with this type of classifier in mind.

Note that we do not necessarily expect any single feature *by itself* to be able to identify term pairs belonging to either of the two relations – rather we expect the collected evidence, when several features simultaneously point to the same result, to be the decisive factor. We use a total of 22 features per language in our experiments. We describe our features informally further on and there is a complete listing at the end; for a full account please see Hjelm (2009).

Merging Evidence across Languages

By using the translational equivalence relation for merging the data across languages, we achieve a positive effect when training support vector machine classifiers. We test two main approaches for performing the merging: one assumes that we have a domain-specific bilingual dictionary, the other assumes we do not. In the latter case we instead use the results of the automatic translation techniques mentioned earlier.

We were discussing how to view text in different languages previously – is it simply "more data" or are there special characteristics that should make us think of it differently? We will continue this discussion below and illustrate with examples from our corpora and ontologies.

We start with the scenario that we have access to a bilingual (or multilingual) domain-specific dictionary, and that we wish to learn a cross-language terminological ontology for the terms listed in it. We use the translation information that is encoded in the Eurovoc thesaurus for this purpose.

The English data forms our baseline for the experiments to follow. For each term pair in Eurovoc, where both terms occur at least once in the JRC-ACQUIS parallel corpus, we have 22 features, as described in the previous section. We next look up the translation of the two English terms in Swedish. If the two Swedish terms also occur at least once in the Swedish texts, we add the 22 Swedish features to the English, giving us a total of 44 features for the term pair. We repeat the same process for German and French, so that we in the end have 88 features per term pair (not all of which need to be instantiated in all languages for all term pairs). Term pairs where one or both terms do not occur at least once in the English texts are excluded from the experiments.

In the second approach, we envision that we have access to the output of an ideal term extraction system but that we do not have access to a translation dictionary. Instead of relying on the translation information in Eurovoc, we this time use the output of the automatic translation system as the basis for merging the evidence across languages. In order not to confuse the classifiers, we would like to merge the data only in cases where we are relatively sure that the translations are correct, so we use a filtering method where we use only the translations that give consistent results when compared across all language pairs. This means that the translations will be correct in about 98.4% of the cases, but that we are only merging data for about 36.5% of the terms. The effects of weighing precision against recall here is a parameter in our system we have yet to explore.

We contrast three different datasets in the following experiments. The first uses strictly English data and we will be referring to this set as "Mono". The second set uses the results from merging data across languages (English, Swedish, German and French), where we use Eurovoc for translating the terms – we will refer to this set as "All" (because "all" languages are included). The third set instead uses the output of the automated translation system for merging, and this set we refer to as "MT" (for "machine translation").[6]

We will continue by looking at how switching from one language to another can affect the features.

Distribution-Based Features

A large number of the features we are using to train the classifiers are based on the distribution of terms or the joint distribution of term pairs. Unless we have access to the perfect corpus, containing all relevant occurrences of our terms and no irrelevant occurrences, the distributional profile of a term will be fragmentary and contaminated by noise. However, switching languages, we are unlikely to have the *exact same* noise and fragmentation repeated; we can thus see the cross-language data as a way of abstracting away from such shortcomings, by giving the classifiers access to distributional data gathered from different languages. At the same time, we are of course introducing a new error source – new noise – by adding the cross-language data, but as we will show, the overall effect is positive.

We also expect differences in the distributional profile for a term in different languages, caused by the fact that homonymy and polysemy in a word or term rarely are kept intact when the word

is translated. This is likely to have an effect on features that use second order co-occurrences. Consider the following sentence from the JRC-ACQUIS corpus, given in English, German and French, respectively (terms are marked in bold):

- *The* **European Police College** *shall have its* seat *in Bramshill.*
- *Die* **Europäische Polizeiakademie** *hat ihren* Sitz *in Bramshill.*
- *Le* **Collège européen de police** *a son* siège *á Bramshill.*

The term/proper name 'European Police College' (or its translations) occurs in all three sentences, along with a number of context words. We have emphasized the word 'seat' and its translations in the example; we focus on this word not because of any remarkable traits that it possesses, but rather because its behavior is typical. We illustrate what happens when we translate the English 'seat' and the French 'siège' into German in Figure 3.

Both 'seat' and 'siège' share the translations 'Sitz' and 'Sitzplatz'; English has an additional four and French an additional five translations that are not shared.[7] This discrepancy will lead to 'seat' and 'siège' having different distributional patterns even in a parallel corpus, which will affect any feature making use of second order co-occurrences when measuring the similarity between terms – even though 'seat' itself is not a term. We believe that giving the classifiers access to cross-language distributional data allows them to abstract away from homonymy and polysemy in one language by weighing in information from the others.

Pattern-Based Features

Our only pattern-based features are the ones where we use Hearst-patterns (Hearst, 1992) to recognize our lexico-semantic relations of interest. We do not see the same theoretical motivation for the use-

Figure 3. Non-Transitivity of homonymy/polysemy

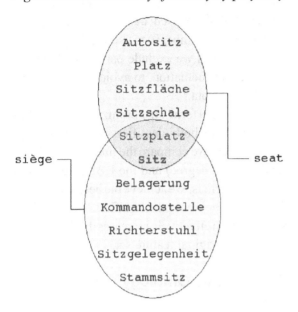

Head-Matching Features

We apply two head-matching features when training the classifiers: one for recognizing hyperonymy and one for cohyponymy. Both depend on the lexical head of a term explicitly marking the hierarchical semantic relation which it holds to its hyperonym – something which is rather an exception than a rule. We cannot expect the explicit expression of this relation to always occur for the same words in different languages. Whether it is expressed or not depends on different factors such as language-specific word formation rules and word-specific lexicalization factors. Table 1 contains example words from Eurovoc where the relation is not expressed in English but is expressed in at least one of the other languages.

Classification and Hierarchy Learning

We train two classifiers: one for recognizing hyperonymy relations and one for recognizing cohyponymy relations. We use the full set of 22 features for training the hyperonym classifier; for the cohyponym classifier, we use a subset of the features. We form the classifier data by taking all ordered pairs of terms within each partition of Eurovoc. When preparing data for the hyperonym classifier, we mark all term pairs (t, u) as positive examples where t is the direct parent of u in the Eurovoc thesaurus, and we do the same for siblings for the cohyponym classifier. All other term pairs are marked as negative examples, so the positive examples for one classifier are negative for the other.

We diverge from Cimiano (2006) and Snow et al. (2006) by not using the *transitive closure* of the dominance relation when collecting data for the hyperonym classifier. This is a deliberate choice, since we believe that the direct dominance relation gives more prototypical examples of hyperonyms than does the transitive closure of the relation.

fulness of cross-language data for pattern-based features as we do for distribution-based features. However, our patterns are rigid – if the text in one language happens to word an expression slightly differently from what we anticipated, our pattern matching component will miss it. Using more than one language then becomes a way of covering our bases – we get more chances of getting it right, working with more than one language. Below is an example from the JRC-ACQUIS corpus where the hyperonymy relation between 'vegetable oil' and 'olive oil' is captured in the German but not in the English, due to the use of ellipsis:

- *Für den Sektor Fette muß für die Bereitstellung von* **Olivenöl** *<und anderen>* **pflanzlichen Ölen** *eine zweckentsprechende Regelung getroffen werden.*
- *Whereas, in the oils and fats sector, appropriate rules and procedures should be laid down for mobilizing olive <and other>* **vegetable oils***;*

Terms are again marked in bold and the triggering Hearst-pattern is delimited with angle brackets.

There are many more term pairs within each partition of the ontology that are unrelated to each other than there are hyperonym or cohyponym pairs. We have a total of 1,078,480 examples, out of which 2,030 are positive hyperonym examples and 13,078 are positive cohyponym examples. This means that our data for training the classifiers is skewed (it contains many more negative examples than positive) and that we must find a strategy for dealing with this skewness – otherwise the classifiers might rationalize the problem by simply classifying every term pair as unrelated. We discuss this further below.

When evaluating the classifier results, we also have to take the data skewness into consideration. If we consider the overall accuracy of the classifier, we would get 99.8% correct for the hyperonym classifier and 98.8% correct for the cohyponym classifier, simply by classifying all examples as negative. Instead, the standard way of evaluating such datasets is to consider precision, recall and F-score of the positive class only and this is the evaluation method we employ in the following experiments.

To come to grips with the aforementioned problems with skewed data, we set aside one data partition (number 9) to use as a development set. This means we exclude partition 9 from all further experimentation, to avoid mixing testing and training data.[8]

We also perform an optimization, again on partition 9, for both classifiers for selecting the kernel, where we compare the linear, polynomial (2nd and 3rd degree) and the RBF (radial basis function) kernels. We achieve the best results with the RBF kernel for both classifiers – a non-linear kernel, which effectively increases the dimensionality of the original feature set.

Probabilistic Ontology Learning

We discussed previous efforts towards incorporating probability theory in ontology learning earlier. Our approach is based on the method described by Snow et al. (2006), with some alterations, and we add a cross-language perspective by using probabilities based on evidence from different languages. Snow et al. define two base relations

Table 1. Explicit expression of hyperonymy relations in different languages. The fifth column contains an approximate translation of the hyperonym, marked in bold in the non-English relevant cases.

English	German	French	Swedish	Hyperonym
jurisdiction	gerichtliche **Zuständigkeit**	**compétence** juridictionelle	domstolars be-**hörighet**	competence
concessionaire	Vertrags**händler**	concessionnaire	general**agent**	trader/agent
cohabitation	freie **Partnerschaft**	**union** libre	sambo	partnership
incorporation	Gesellschafts**gründung**	**constitution** de société	bolags**bildning**	formation
conglomerate	Misch**konzern**	conglomérat	konglomerat	concern
cannery	Konservenfabrik	conserverie	konserv**fabrik**	factory
assessment	Leistungs**kontrolle**	**contrôle** des connaissances	kunskaps**kontroll**	inspection
crustacean	Krebstier	crustacé	kräft**djur**	animal
devolution	Dekonzentration	déconcentration	begränsat själv-**styre**	government
delinquency	Straffälligkeit	délinquance	kriminellt be-**teende**	behavior

that are used to construct the hierarchy: hyponymy (and its inverse relation hyperonymy) and cohyponymy. The hierarchy is constructed by iteratively adding instances of either of the two relations, in such a way as to maximize the probability of the resulting hierarchy after each step. After a few terms have been added to the hierarchy, one is no longer free to add new relations at will, but the hierarchy constructed to that point imposes restrictions on any new relations to be added (e.g., term t and term u cannot be cohyponyms if t has already been specified as the hyperonym of u).

A new relation added to the ontology typically *implies* a further set of relations, because of the resulting new structure of the hierarchy. The probability of these implied relations is also taken into account when considering which instance of which of the two base relations to add next to the hierarchy. Snow et al. thus introduce a global perspective, considering the hierarchical structure in its entirety, into their ontology learning process; something which is absent in the (otherwise similar) approach suggested by Ryu & Choi (2006). As stated, this is also the method we follow in our experiments.

The algorithm we use is greedy for reasons of tractability; generating and testing every possible configuration for arranging the terms hierarchically would be much too expensive. We therefore try to find, in each step, the relation to add that will maximize the probability of the ontology at that given point. Assume we have an ontology O, evidence used to learn the ontology E (in our case the output of the SVM classifiers), two terms t and u and a relation R_{tu} between the two terms. We then calculate the multiplicative change in the overall probability of ontology O, caused by adding R_{tu}, like this:

$$\Delta_O(R_{tu}) = k\left(\frac{P(R_{tu} \in O \mid E_{tu}^R)}{1 - P(R_{tu} \in O \mid E_{tu}^R)}\right)$$

In the above equation, k is considered a constant, independent of O, t and u. Snow et al. (2006) use the same k for both base relations in their experiments; we investigate the effect of using different k values for the different base relations in our experiments.

Experimental Results

We report results on the three sets of data for all experiments, as described previously: "Mono", "All" and "MT". We compare the three resulting models by using them to build ontologies in our probabilistic ontology learning system. The learned ontologies are evaluated using the PMCC measure and the CSC measure, both discussed earlier. In order not to overestimate the similarities when testing with the CSC measure, we use a version of Eurovoc where the root concept has been changed to a neutral one (not occurring in the learned ontology).

Varying the Average Branching Factor

We can influence our ontology learning system towards building flatter or deeper trees, with higher or lower average branching factors, by using different values of k in Equation 1. We compare the results for different k values and all three models to the Eurovoc thesaurus. If we use k for the cohyponymy relation, we use $k' = 1 - (k - 1)$ for the hyperonymy relation – in other words, when the constant for one relation goes up, the constant for the other relation goes down, and vice versa. The results for the PMCC measure are given in Figure 4 and for the CSC measure in Figure 5. Remember from previous sections that values closer to 1 mean high similarity and values close to 0 mean little or no similarity between the compared ontologies.

We set the threshold to 1 for the multiplicative change (same as in Snow et al., 2006) for deciding when to stop adding new relations to the ontology in these experiments. This means, in our case, that we are on average adding about 80% of the terms scored by the classifiers to the ontology (same for all three models); for the rest, the evidence of them entering into any relation with the other terms is deemed too loose.

We see a sizable increase in the PMCC measure when using the "All" and the "MT" data, compared with using the "Mono" data. For the "All" data, the increase lies between 27% – 55%, depending on the k value, and for the "MT" data it lies between 20% – 70%. The results for the "MT" data lie almost flat across the different k values, the "All" data results peak at $k = 1.1$ and the "Mono" data shows an almost perfect linear increase. We stop investigating k values at 1.2, because beyond that, no or very few hierarchical relations are added, which defeats the purpose of our efforts. Using $k < 1$ would mean producing a tree with a branching factor less than two, and this is intuitively the wrong way to go.

Turning to the results for the CSC measure (Figure 5), the picture is different. We still see improved results for the "All" and "MT" data, but on a smaller scale: between 6% – 11% for the "All" data and 2% – 9% for the "MT" data. The

"All" data results peak at $k = 1.05$, otherwise the tendency is that the CSC measure decreases as k increases – practically the inverse situation to what we saw for the PMCC measure. This should not come as a big surprise; the CSC measure is "blind" to horizontal relations. As we increase the k value for the cohyponymy relation, fewer hyperonymy relations are added and the CSC score drops.

Choosing the appropriate k value for our purposes thus proves a less straightforward decision than we had hoped. We settle on using $k = 1.05$ for our future experiments strictly as a compromise between the results from the two evaluation measures. At $k = 1.05$, the CSC measure has not dropped too much from its state at $k = 1.0$, and the PMCC measure has had the chance to improve slightly. To some degree, setting $k = 1.05$ is an arbitrary decision, but the most important issue for the next experiment series is the *fixation* of k, rather than the value assigned.

Figure 4. Increasing values of k for cohyponymy, 9-fold cross validation, single and cross-language data, evaluated with the PMCC measure

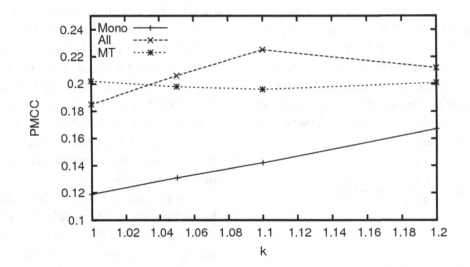

Varying the Probability Threshold

The experiments described here have the same basic setup as the ones in the preceding section, and once again we compare results using the three different datasets. We fix the value of $k = 1.05$ and instead measure what happens when we vary the threshold for when to stop adding new relations to the ontology. Snow et al. use a threshold of $t = 1$ in their system; here, we vary t in the range [0,2], starting at 0 and increasing it by steps of 0.5 for each run. We give the results for our PMCC measure in Figure 6 and for the CSC measure in Figure 7.

We see an increase in PMCC value using the "All" data over the "Mono" data of between 19% – 64%; for the "MT" data the same figures are 11% – 54%. The difference between using the "All" data and the "MT" data seems small here, with the "MT" data even giving slightly better results at $t = 0$. We see this as an effect of the hyperonym classifier working with higher precision when using the "MT" data; using a more conservative strategy, trading recall for precision,

is probably a good approach at this threshold level ($t = 0$).

For the CSC measure, the picture again is changed. The "All" data boosts the results with between 1%–15% but the "MT" data makes the result vary between -6%–4%. It seems that the conservative strategy that was useful for the PMCC evaluation here becomes a disadvantage. The high precision of the added hyperonymy relations cannot fully compensate for the loss in recall, when evaluating with the CSC measure (remember that cohyponymy relations are not considered by this measure).

Using a specific threshold, the number of concepts added to the ontology will vary slightly between our three datasets, depending on the distributions of the scores from the classifiers. Of course, it is easier to score high in these evaluations if one only adds relations for which the evidence is clear. In other words: the more concepts and relations added to the ontology, the harder the task, given that there is a sliding scale of certainty for the validity of the evidence. To verify that the differences in the evaluations in

Figure 5. Increasing values of k for cohyponymy, 9-fold cross validation, single and cross-language data, evaluated with the CSC measure

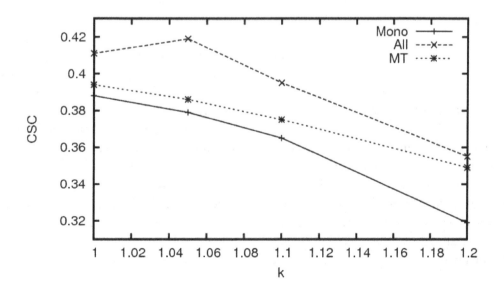

Figure 6. Increasing values of t, 9-fold cross validation, single and cross-language data, evaluated with the PMCC measure

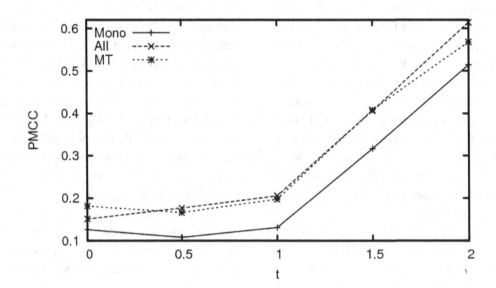

Figures 4–7 are not caused by such differences in lexical coverage, we also plot the percentage of concepts added against the different values of t for all three datasets in Figure 8.

There is obviously little or no difference between the three models in this aspect. Where they do differ, it is towards the "All" and "MT" data including more terms than the "Mono" data. Differences to the advantage of using the cross-language data shown in Figures 4–7 are thus *not* due to the system solving an easier problem in those cases; if anything, it solves a slightly harder problem, with a considerable increase in accuracy.

Example System Output

To give an idea of how the output of the system might look, we include part of the ontology for partition 3, learned using the "All" data, in Figure 9 (we have to exclude parts of the structure due to the restricted size of the page). We see that at the settings used to learn this ontology (using the non-tuned parameters $k = 1.0$, $t = 1.0$), a lot

of confidence is placed in the head-matching heuristic, both for hyperonymy and cohyponymy. But that is far from the whole story, especially for the cohyponymy relation; see, e.g., nodes 1, dealing with different kinds of cereals and grains, and 25, dealing with environmental issues. Also the hyperonymy relation shows some interesting departures from the head-matching heuristic, e.g., between the terms 'meat' → 'beef', 'sweetener' → 'honey', and 'natural_resource' → 'mineral_resource' (the last example actually goes against the head-matching heuristic for cohyponymy).

The numeric nodes in the learned ontology are produced when the ontology learning algorithm adds cohyponymy relations between terms not already in the ontology. By allowing the creation of these abstract nodes, we ensure that the relation maximizing the probability gets added in each iteration of the algorithm (otherwise we would only be allowed to add cohyponymy relations under an already specified hyperonym). It on the other hand means that the structure we produce is not a strict terminological ontology, but rather a structure which has characteristics both of a

Figure 7. Increasing values of t, 9-fold cross validation, single and cross-language data, evaluated with the CSC measure

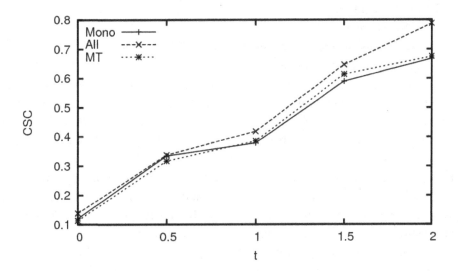

Figure 8. Increasing values of t, 9-fold cross validation, single and cross-language data, percent of concepts added

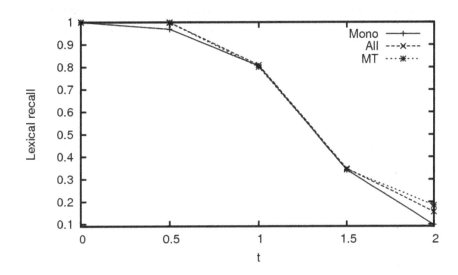

terminological and of a prototype-based ontology. We thus give precedence to producing the structure with the highest probability over producing a structure which adheres to the rules for terminological ontologies. This behavior could be changed easily, by disallowing the insertion of the numeric nodes.

Using SVM classifiers, especially with nonlinear kernels such as the RBF kernel in our experiments, it is not transparent which feature or combination of features lead to an item being classified as a positive or negative case. For the example with 'beef', it seems obvious that cross-language information has been useful, since all three other languages involved can use the head-matching heuristic. The translations are: 'Rindfleisch' (German), 'viande bovine' (French) and 'nötkött' (Swedish), where 'Fleisch', 'viande' and 'kött' all are translations of 'meat'. For the examples involving 'honey' and 'mineral_resource', the situation is less clear – there is no single feature to look to for an explanation. We simply have to regard the outcome as a result of all available information working together to produce the classification.

The average branching factor of the ontology in Figure 9 is much higher than two (two being the average branching factor of a *full binary tree*). We get a greater number of relations with high confidence values from the cohyponym classifier than we get from the hyperonym classifier, which in turn leads to more cohyponymy relations being added, even when using identical *k* values for both relations. If we want to create a system that is truly unbiased as to which of the two relation types it

prefers, such factors will have to be weighed in when setting the *k* values for the two relations.

DISCUSSION

Maedche (2002) presents an experiment for evaluating how closely two ontologies built by humans resemble each other. He uses an existing ontology from the tourist domain, constructed by knowledge engineering experts, as a gold standard. The ontology contains 310 concepts, in addition to some top level concepts defining the basic structure. Four undergraduate students in industrial and business engineering were given 310 terms, corresponding to the 310 concepts, and asked to arrange them in a hierarchy. Each student received a total of six hours of training in ontology building before starting the task. The students' results are compared to the gold standard, but Maedche also performed a mutual comparison of the results within the student group. The task

Figure 9. Excerpt of the ontology learned using the "All" data for partition 3, k = 1.0, t = 1.0

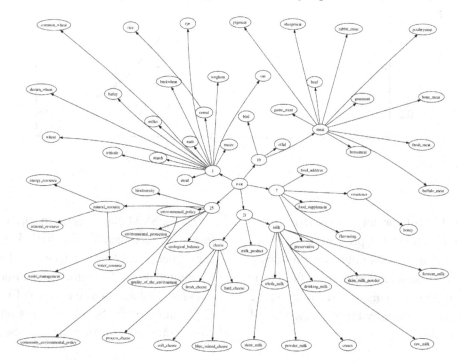

set for the students is similar to the one we have evaluated: given a set of terms, identify their relations when modeled in a hierarchical structure.

Maedche uses the semantic cotopy (SC) measure to compare the ontologies to one another. Because there are five ontologies to compare (four from the students plus the gold standard), we end up with a total of 20 comparisons. The SC values for these 20 comparisons range from 0.47 to 0.87, with an average value of 0.56 (the measure gives a value in the range [0,1]). Unfortunately we have not been able to perform any experiments with human subjects, so we are not sure what the corresponding figures under our conditions would be. It is reasonable to ascribe Maedche's figures some level of general applicability though; if our system manages to learn ontologies that give similarity figures that are in proximity of the ones in Maedche's study, we should take this as a favorable sign of the quality of the output of our system.

Here is where we run into problems with the SC measure. It is impossible to separate the values for lexical coverage from the values for precision and recall of the hierarchical relation (hyperonymy). Because we are using cross-validation in our experiments, we are only learning a small part of the ontology in each run, which means that all recall values will be very low using SC (typically below 0.01). Even if we disregard all other partitions of the ontology than the one we are using at the moment, we are only including a subset of the concepts (terms) within each partition in the learned ontology – namely those terms that occur at least once in the English texts (and the size of this subset will also vary with different values for the threshold t). Therefore, we cannot use the SC measure and expect meaningful results, in our case.

The common semantic cotopy (CSC) measure, however, provides exactly what we need: it calculates values of precision and recall taking *only* those concepts into consideration that occur in both ontologies. If we consider the CSC values at $t = 1.0$ (the standard threshold suggested in Snow et

al., 2006) in Figure 7, we get values in the range 0.38–0.42, depending on the dataset used for the experiment. So, the highest result (0.42) at this threshold is still lower than the lowest result (0.47) in the human–human comparison and another step away from the average human–human result (0.56). We should point out, though, that comparing evaluation results from the SC and CSC evaluation measures is not unproblematic.

We do not expect the ontology learning process to be *fully* automated for all applications – a domain expert can always be consulted for post editing the results, if necessary. In this light, the results measured in our experiments are positive, though there is still plenty of qualitative and methodological improvement that can and should be made, before the system can start performing on a human level, in terms of accuracy.

CONCLUSION

We have answered the questions we set out to investigate and indicated ways of improving ontology learning systems through the exploitation of cross-language data. Still, we have a long way to go before our ontology learning system performs on a human level. We end this chapter by discussing ideas for improving our system, and we also consider widening the scope of the problem towards including other kinds of semantic relations.

When considering the use of automatically generated term equivalence links, we mentioned that it would be possible to trade precision for recall when deciding which equivalents to merge and which not. In our current system, we are focusing on precision, but we cannot exclude the possibility that increasing the recall (at the cost of precision) would produce better results overall.

We discussed possible repercussions of not using the transitive closure of the hyperonymy relation, when creating the training examples for the hyperonym classifier. To see the rationale

Figure 10. Eurovoc excerpt, concepts dealing with animal products. 'Leather' and 'hide' have been added to the original Eurovoc structure

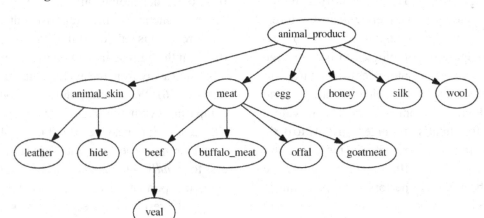

behind excluding the indirect relations, consider the Eurovoc excerpt in Figure 10. The relation between 'animal product' and 'beef' is different from the relation between 'meat' and 'beef'. In text, we would expect 'beef' to be compared to other kinds of 'meat', but rarely to other kinds of 'animal products' like 'silk' or 'wool'. This will affect tendencies of the two term pairs to appear in Hearst-patterns together, and also their distributional patterns in general. On the other hand, training separate classifiers for recognizing hyperonymy relations for each different number of intervening concepts will most likely mean throwing away many commonalities, and instead create a sparse data problem. One possible compromise would be to build one classifier for direct hyperonyms, and one for indirect ones, whatever the number of intervening concepts, or, to allow a number of intervening concepts up to a certain threshold. It is again difficult to predict what kind of effect this would have on the overall quality of the system output.

We described how we can steer the ontology learning system towards producing broader or narrower hierarchies (with larger or smaller average branching factors), by altering the value of a constant k. By setting the k value higher for either the hyperonymy or the cohyponymy relation, the system gets biased towards adding instances of one relation more frequently than the other. One could imagine finding an optimal k value for a particular dataset by generating ontologies using different parameterizations, and choosing the k value which generates the ontology with the highest probability. There is no guarantee that the most probable ontology (in this sense of 'probable') will also result in the best ontology by human standards, or by the standards of an ontology learning evaluation measure, but it is a possibility worth investigating.

We have made the simplifying assumption of a one-to-one correspondence between terms and concepts. Introducing the cross-language perspective, this assumption still holds, as long as we consider each language as an isolated system. If we were to add the synonymy relation to our two base relations hyperonymy and cohyponymy, we would have to abandon this simplification. Assume we allow the synonymy relation, and that we have currently learned the ontology in Figure 10. Assume further that we also have good evidence for the relations in Figure 11 (with an unspecified top node) and that we would like to add an instance of the synonymy relation between the terms 'animal skin' and 'skin'. Adding this instance means that a lot of implied relations will have to be considered,

Figure 11. Partially learned ontology dealing with animal products, unspecified top node

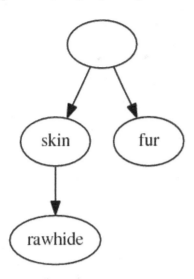

e.g., that 'animal product' will be a hyperonym of 'skin' and 'fur', and that 'skin' and 'fur' will be cohyponyms of 'meat', 'egg', 'honey', etc. But we should also consider whether 'fur' and 'rawhide' can be merged via synonymy with any of the terms in matching positions in the "main" ontology ('hide' and 'rawhide' would be good candidates for a merge in this example). This would result in the ontology in Figure 12, where alternative terms (synonyms) are separated by a |.

These further merges are not "implied" in the previous sense, but we would still like to consider their probabilities when deciding on the addition of a synonymy instance to the ontology. One approach would be to take positive evidence for further merges into account (such as for 'hide' and 'rawhide'), while the rest can be treated as terms in their own right (as for 'fur', which has no real candidates for merging). Adding a cross-language dimension to the discussion, we would have to consider synonymy relations for all languages involved, which would add further complexity (e.g., two English terms appear to be synonyms, but their German translations do not – how should this be handled?). Making synonymy a third base relation, in addition to hyperonymy and cohyponymy, would thus pose some interesting challenges, especially when wanting to fit all relations into the same framework.

The most obvious way of improving our system would be to make our 22 features produce more accurate results. 19 of our 22 features are based on distribution and frequencies, so they all most likely would benefit from using version 3.0 of the JRC-ACQUIS corpus, which is almost three times bigger than version 2.2 that we used in our work. The Hearst-pattern feature would probably also benefit from a bigger corpus, because related terms are more likely to appear in a Hearst-pattern, the more text we analyze. A cheap way of getting more co-occurrence data would be to use large general purpose corpora, in addition to our domain-specific ones. But this introduces problems with ambiguity, since we then can rely less on the "one sense per discourse" heuristic which we use for our domain-specific corpora.

It would be interesting to incorporate languages that are typologically further removed from the others in future experiments (e.g., to include Finnish or any of the Slavic languages from the JRC-ACQUIS corpus and Eurovoc in the experiments). One could argue that merging the data should be simpler, the more similar the involved languages are. On the other hand, dissimilar languages could be argued to introduce a higher degree of "orthogonality" in the data, meaning that they would express *new* information, where similar languages merely would repeat what is already known.

If we had access to a high quality coreference resolution system, this would be another factor in dealing with the sparse data problem, allowing us to exchange pronouns for the non-pronominal nouns or noun phrases they refer to, in the running text. Nilsson & Hjelm (2009) show the reverse side of this; how distributional similarity can be used for improving coreference resolution, which means that there is an opportunity for creating a bootstrapping effect between the two fields.

Figure 12. Ontology after merging (near) synonyms

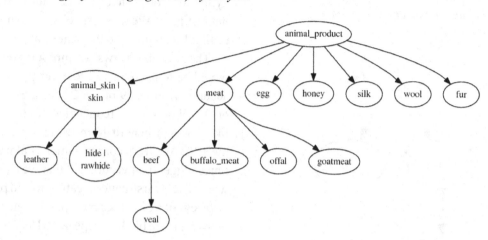

Another way of further improving our system such as it stands today, would be to perform more extensive feature weighting and parameter optimization for the support vector machine classifiers. Such optimizations are time consuming when performed on large enough datasets, which is why we had to settle for using standard parameterizations for certain parts of our system. It is also possible that we could improve our system further by a more sophisticated handling of missing feature values in our data, perhaps by reduplicating or interpolating data from other languages.

Finally, we feel that there is a lot of interesting work to be done in evaluating the effects of incorporating the semantic knowledge captured in a learned ontology in other NLP applications. We see some trends also in commercial settings towards incorporating ontological knowledge in information access-oriented companies such as Powerset,[9] Twine[10] and Hakia.[11] From a research perspective, it would of course be interesting to quantify the effects of incorporating ontological knowledge on the large scale (in terms of data and users) such commercializations allow. On a smaller scale, Nagypál (2007) has performed evaluations towards this end, that we feel would be worthwhile pursuing further.

To sum up, we have indicated many fields in NLP (machine translation is another such field of interest) where we suspect that ontology learning approaches have yet to demonstrate their full worth. In this we feel to be fully in line with dominating currents in NLP today, where, as noted in the introduction, more and more attention is given to handling semantics.

REFERENCES

Aizawa, A., & Kageura, K. (2001). A graph-based approach to the automatic generation of multilingual keyword clusters. In Bourigault, D. (Ed.), *Recent advances in computational terminology* (pp. 1–27). Philadelphia, PA: John Benjamins Publishing Company.

Boolos, G., & Jeffrey, R. (1989). *Computability and logic* (3 ed.). Cambridge, UK: Cambridge University Press.

Borin, L. (2000). You'll take the high road and I'll take the low road: Using a third language to improve bilingual word alignment. In *Proceedings of the 18th international Conference on computational linguistics* (Vol. 1, pp. 97–103).

Caraballo, S. A. (2001). *Automatic construction of a hypernym-labeled noun hierarchy from text.* Unpublished doctoral dissertation, Brown University, Providence, RI, USA.

Cimiano, P. (2006). *Ontology learning and population from text: Algorithms, evaluation and applications.* New York, NY: Springer-Verlag.

Dellschaft, K., & Staab, S. (2006). *On how to perform a gold standard based evaluation of ontology learning.* In 5th International Semantic Web Conference, Athens, GA, USA.

Dyvik, H. (2005). Translations as a semantic knowledge source. In *Proceedings of the second Baltic Conference on human language technologies.* Tallinn, Estonia.

Goddard, C. (2001). Universal units in the lexicon. In Haspelmath, M., König, E., Oesterreicher, W., & Raible, W. (Eds.), *Language typology and language universals* (*Vol. 2*, pp. 1178–1190). Berlin, Germany / New York, NY: Walter de Gruyter. doi:10.1515/9783110171549.2.11.1190

Hearst, M. (1992). Automatic acquisition of hyponyms from large text corpora. In *Proceedings of the 14th International Conference on computational linguistics.* Nantes, France.

Hjelm, H. (2007). Identifying cross language term equivalents using statistical machine translation and distributional association measures. In *Proceedings of NODALIDA 2007, the 16th Nordic Conference of computational linguistics.* Tartu, Estonia.

Hjelm, H. (2009). *Cross-language ontology learning: Incorporating and exploiting cross-language data in the ontology learning process* (vol. 1). Unpublished doctoral dissertation, Stockholm University, Stockholm, Sweden.

Koch, P. (2001). Lexical typology from a cognitive and linguistic point of view. In Haspelmath, M., König, E., Oesterreicher, W., & Raible, W. (Eds.), *Language typology and language universals* (*Vol. 2*, pp. 1142–1178). Berlin, Germany / New York, NY: Walter de Gruyter. doi:10.1515/978311017 1549.2.11.1142

Maedche, A. (2002). *Ontology learning for the Semantic Web.* Norwell, MA: Kluwer Academic Publishers.

Marcus, M. P., Marcinkiewicz, M. A., & Santorini, B. (1993). Building a large annotated corpus of English: The Penn treebank. *Computational Linguistics, 19*(2), 313–330.

Nagypál, G. (2007). *Possibly imperfect ontologies for effective information retrieval.* Unpublished doctoral dissertation, Universität Karlsruhe (TH), Karlsruhe, Germany.

Nilsson, K., & Hjelm, H. (2009). Using semantic features derived from word-space models for Swedish coreference resolution. In *Proceedings of the 17th Nordic Conference of computational linguistics NODALIDA 2009* (pp. 134–141). Northern European Association for Language Technology (NEALT).

Nirenburg, S., & Raskin, V. (2004). *Ontological semantics.* Cambridge, MA: The MIT Press.

Resnik, P., & Smith, N. A. (2003). The Web as a parallel corpus. *Computational Linguistics, 29*(3), 349–380. doi:10.1162/089120103322711578

Ryu, P. M., & Choi, K. S. (2006). Taxonomy learning using term specificity and similarity. In *Proceedings from the Workshop on ontology learning and population: Bridging the gap between text and knowledge (with COLING/ACL 2006)* (pp. 41 – 48). Sydney, Australia.

Sager, J. (1994). *Language engineering and translation: Consequences of automation.* Amsterdam, The Netherlands: John Benjamins Publishing Company.

Simard, M. (1999). Text-translation alignment: Three languages are better than two. In *Proceedings of the 1999 Joint SIGDAT Conference on empirical methods in natural language processing and very large corpora* (pp. 2–11).

Snow, R., Jurafsky, D., & Ng, A. Y. (2006). Semantic taxonomy induction from heterogeneous evidence. In *Proceedings of COLING/ACL 2006.* Sydney, Australia.

Steinberger, R., Pouliquen, B., Widiger, A., Ignat, C., Erjavec, T., & Tufis, D. (2006). The JRC-Acquis: A multilingual aligned parallel corpus with 20+ languages. In *Proceedings of the 5th international Conference on language resources and evaluation (LREC'2006).* Genoa, Italy.

Tiedemann, J. (2003). *Recycling translations: Extraction of lexical data from parallel corpora and their application in natural language processing.* Unpublished doctoral dissertation, Uppsala University, Uppsala, Sweden.

van der Plas, L., & Tiedemann, J. (2006). Finding synonyms using automatic word alignment and measures of distributional similarity. In *Proceedings of COLING/ACL 2006.* Sydney, Australia.

Volk, M., & Buitelaar, P. (2002). A systematic evaluation of concept-based cross-language information retrieval in the medical domain. In *Proc. of 3rd Dutch-Belgian information retrieval Workshop.* Leuven, Holland.

ADDITIONAL READING

Biemann, C. (2005). Ontology Learning from Text – a Survey of Methods. *LDV-Forum, 20*(2), 75–93.

Bloehdorn, S., Cimiano, C., Duke, A., Haase, P., Heizmann, J., Thurlow, I., & Völker, J. (2007). Ontology-based question answering for digital libraries. In *Proceedings of the 11th European Conference on Research and Advanced Technology for Digital Libraries (ECDL)*, pages 14–25, Budapest, Hungary.

Brown, P. F., Della Pietra, S. A., Della Pietra, V. J., & Mercer, R. L. (1993). The Mathematics of Statistical Machine Translation: Parameter Estimation. *Computational Linguistics, 19*(2), 263–311.

Deerwester, S., Dumais, S., Landauer, T., Furnas, G., & Harshman, R. (1990). Indexing by Latent Semantic Analysis. *Journal of the American Society for Information Science American Society for Information Science, 41*(6), 391–407. doi:10.1002/(SICI)1097-4571(199009)41:6<391::AID-ASI1>3.0.CO;2-9

Grefenstette, G. (1994). *Explorations in Automatic Thesaurus Discovery.* Boston, MA, USA: Kluwer Academic Publishers.

Harris, Z. Distributional Structure. *Word*, 10(2–3):775–793.

Hendrickx, I., Hoste, V., & Daelemans, W. (2008). Semantic and Syntactic features for Anaphora Resolution for Dutch. In *Proceedings of the CICLing-2008 conference*, Volume 4919 of *Lecture Notes in Computer Science*, pages 351–361. Springer Verlag, Berlin, Germany.

Kanerva, P., Kristoferson, J., & Holst, A. (2000). Random Indexing of Text Samples for Latent Semantic Analysis. In *Proceedings of the 22nd Annual Conference of the Cognitive Science Society*.

Koehn, P. (2010). *Statistical Machine Translation.* Cambridge, England: Cambridge University Press.

Lin, D. (1998). Automatic Retrieval and Clustering of Similar Words. In *COLING-ACL98*, Montreal, QC, Canada.

Liu, Z., & Chu, W. W. (2007). Knowledge-based Query Expansion to Support Scenario-specific Retrieval of Medical Free Text. *Information Retrieval, 10*(2), 173–202. doi:10.1007/s10791-006-9020-6

Maedche, A., & Staab, S. (2002). Measuring Similarity between Ontologies. In *Proceedings of the European Conference on Knowledge Acquisition and Management.*

Manning, C. D., Raghavan, P., & Schütze, H. (2008). *Introduction to Information Retrieval.* Cambridge, England: Cambridge University Press.

Matsumoto, Y. (2003). *Lexical Knowledge Aquisition. The Oxford Handbook of Computational Linguistics.* Oxford, England: Oxford University Press.

Melamed, D. (2000). Models of Translational Equivalence among Words. *Computational Linguistics, 26*(2), 221–249. doi:10.1162/089120100561683

Och, F. J., & Ney, H. (2003). A Systematic Comparison of Various Statistical Alignment Models. *Computational Linguistics, 29*(1), 19–51. doi:10.1162/089120103321337421

Sahlgren, M. (2006). *The Word-Space Model: Using Distributional Analysis to Represent Syntagmatic and Paradigmatic Relations between Words in High-Dimensional Vector Spaces.* PhD Thesis, Stockholm University, Stockholm, Sweden.

Schütze, H. (1992). Dimensions of Meaning. In [Los Alamitos, CA, USA.]. *Proceedings of Supercomputing, 92*, 787–796. doi:10.1109/SUPERC.1992.236684

Tai, K. (1979). The Tree-to-Tree Correction Problem. *Journal of the Association for Computing Machinery, 26*(3), 422–433.

Weeds, J., Downdall, J., Schneider, G., & Weir, D. (2005). Using Distributional Similarity to Organise Biomedical Terminology. *Terminology, 11*(1), 107–141. doi:10.1075/term.11.1.06wee

Widdows, D. (2004). *Geometry and Meaning.* Stanford, CA, USA: CSLI Publications.

KEY TERMS AND DEFINITIONS

Cross-Language Ontology Learning: is an approach to Ontology Learning which uses evidence from parallel corpora. The assumption is that translated texts provide more clues than monolingual texts for the automatic derivation of semantic relations between terms.

Distributional Similarity: model relies on the idea that words with a similar meaning occur in similar contexts. Based on this idea it is possible to compute semantic relations when given large text corpora.

Machine Learning: is a method to derive rules and preferences from past events in order to classify new instances. Machine Learning algorithms use certain properties of the past events. These properties are called features and their selection and weighting constitutes the core challenge in using Machine Learning.

Multilingual Thesaurus: is a lexical resource where terms in two or more languages are ordered based on synonym and antonym relations. Eurovoc is a Multilingual Thesaurus compiled by the European Union.

Parallel Corpus: is a text collection in one language together with its translation in another language.

Semantic Cotopy: of a concept in a hierarchy consists of all its superconcepts, its subconcepts and the concept itself. Semantic Cotopy is used in evaluating automatically learned ontologies.

Semantic Relation: describe the meaning relations between terms. Basic relations are synonymy (terms have similar meaning), antonymy (terms have opposite meaning), hyponymy (term A is hyponym to term B if A is a subclass of B), hyperonymy (term A is hyponym to term B if A is a superclass of B) and cohyponymy (term A is a cohyponym to term B if A and B have the same superclass C).

Support Vector Machines: are a family of Machine Learning algorithms which have proven to be useful for many Language Technology applications.

ENDNOTES

1   Available at http://www.dfki.de/sw-lt/olp2_dataset/

2   The differences are due to the idiosyncratic ways of the different languages of, e.g., forming compounds.

3   http://wt.jrc.it/lt/Acquis/

4   http://nl.ijs.si/telri/Vanilla/doc/ljubljana/

5   http://europa.eu/eurovoc/

6   Note that "machine translation" here does not refer to an entire machine translation system. Rather, it should be considered shorthand for "the word alignment part of a machine translation system".

7   The translations are taken from http://leo.dict.org.

8   Because of this, we are performing 9-fold cross validation in all experiments instead of the standard 10-fold.

9   www.powerset.com

10   www.twine.com

11   www.hakia.com

APPENDIX

Feature Listing

Table 2. Listing of all features used for identifying hyperonymy and cohyponymy. Each feature is represented by an index (running id number), an identifier (name) and a short description

Index	Identifier	Description
1	Subsumption-1st	The subsumption measure, using first order co-occurrence
2	Subsumption-2nd-3	The subsumption measure, using second order co-occurrence and window size 3
3	Subsumption-2nd-50	The subsumption measure, using second order co-occurrence and window size 50
4	Subsumption-2nd-500	The subsumption measure, using second order co-occurrence and window size 500
5	Similarity-1st	Distributional similarity, using first order co-occurrence and a non-reduced matrix
6	Similarity-2nd-3	Distributional similarity, using second order co-occurrence, window size 3 and a non-reduced matrix
7	Similarity-2nd-50	Distributional similarity, using second order co-occurrence, window size 50 and a non-reduced matrix
8	Similarity-2nd-500	Distributional similarity, using second order co-occurrence, window size 500 and a non-reduced matrix
9	SVD-1st	Distributional similarity, using first order co-occurrence and an SVD matrix
10	SVD-2nd-3	Distributional similarity, using second order co-occurrence, window size 3 and an SVD matrix
11	SVD-2nd-50	Distributional similarity, using second order co-occurrence, window size 50 and an SVD matrix
12	SVD-2nd-500	Distributional similarity, using second order co-occurrence, window size 500 and an SVD matrix
13	Hearst	Measure based on Hearst-patterns
14	Head-hyperonym	Head-matching heuristic for hyperonymy
15	Head-cohyponym	Head-matching heuristic for cohyponymy
16	Frequency-diff	Difference in absolute frequency
17	Entropy-diff-1st	Difference in distributional entropy, using first order co-occurrence
18	Entropy-diff-2nd-3	Difference in distributional entropy, using second order co-occurrence and window size 3
19	Entropy-diff-2nd-50	Difference in distributional entropy, using second order co-occurrence and window size 50
20	Entropy-diff-2nd-500	Difference in distributional entropy, using second order co-occurrence and window size 500
21	Frequency-1	Absolute frequency of the first term in the term pair
22	Frequency-2	Absolute frequency of the second term in the term pair

Compilation of References

Abney, S. P. (1991). Parsing by chunks. In S. P. Abney R. C. Berwick & C. Tenny (Eds.), *Principle-based parsing: Computation and psycholinguistics*, (pp. 257–278). Dordrecht, The Netherlands: Kluwer.

Aggarwal, C., Hinneburg, A., & Keim, D. (2001). On the surprising behavior of distance metrics in high dimensional space. In *Proceedings of the 8th International Conference Database Theory* (pp. 420-434).

Aizawa, A., & Kageura, K. (2001). A graph-based approach to the automatic generation of multilingual keyword clusters. In Bourigault, D. (Ed.), *Recent advances in computational terminology* (pp. 1–27). Philadelphia, PA: John Benjamins Publishing Company.

Alani, H. (2006). Position paper: Ontology construction from online ontologies. In L. Carr, D. D. Roure, A. Iyengar, C. A. Goble, & M. Dahlin (Eds.), *Proceedings of the 15th International Conference on World Wide Web (WWW 2006)* (pp. 491–495). Edinburgh, Scotland, UK: ACM.

Aleksovski, Z., ten Kate, W., & van Harmelen, F. (2006). Ontology matching using comprehensive ontology as background knowledge. In P. Shvaiko et al. (Eds.), *Proceedings of the International Workshop on Ontology Matching at ISWC 2006* (pp. 13–24). Athens, GA, USA: CEUR.

Altaf-Ul-Amin, M., Shinbo, Y., Mihara, K., Kurokawa, K., & Kanaya, S. (2006). Development and implementation of an algorithm for detection of protein complexes in large interaction networks. *BMC Bioinformatics*, 7, 207. doi:10.1186/1471-2105-7-207

Altschul, S. F., Madden, T. L., Schäffer, A. A., Zhang, J., Zhang, Z., Miller, W., & Lipman, D. J. (1997). Gapped BLAST and PSI-BLAST: A new generation of protein database search programs. *Nucleic Acids Research*, 25(17), 3389–3402. doi:10.1093/nar/25.17.3389

Ananiadou, S., Friedman, C., & Tsujii, J. (2004). Introduction: Named entity recognition in biomedicine. *Journal of Biomedical Informatics*, 37(6), 393–395. doi:10.1016/j.jbi.2004.08.011

Anaya-Sánchez, H., Pons-Porrata, A., & Berlanga-Llavori, R. (2008). A new document clustering algorithm for topic discovering and labeling. In *Ciarp '08: Proceedings of the 13th Ibero-American Congress on pattern recognition* (pp. 161–168). Berlin/Heidelberg, Germany: Springer-Verlag.

Andrieu, C., de Freitas, N., Doucet, A., & Jordan, M. I. (2003). An introduction to mcmc for machine learning. *Machine Learning*, 50(1-2), 5–43. doi:10.1023/A:1020281327116

Angeletou, S., Sabou, M., Specia, L., & Motta, E. (2007). *Bridging the gap between folksonomies and the Semantic Web: An experience report* (vol. 2).

Angjeli, A., Isaac, A., Cloarec, T., Martin, F., van der Meij, L., Matthezing, H., & Schlobach, S. (2009). Semantic Web and vocabulary interoperability: An experiment with illumination collections. *International Cataloguing and Bibliographic Control*, 38(2), 25–29.

Ankolekar, A., Krötzsch, M., Tran, D. T., & Vrandecic, D. (2008). The two cultures: Mashing up Web 2.0 and the Semantic Web. *Journal of Web Semantics*, 6(1), 70–75.

Artz, D., & Gil, Y. (2007). A survey of trust in computer science and the Semantic Web. *Journal of Web Semantics: Science. Services and Agents on the World Wide Web, 5*, 58–71. doi:10.1016/j.websem.2007.03.002

Ashburner, M., Ball, C. A., Blake, J. A., Botstein, D., Butler, H., Cherry, J. M., & Davis, A. P. (2000). Gene ontology: Tool for the unification of biology. The gene ontology consortium. *Nature Genetics, 25*(1), 25–29. doi:10.1038/75556

Asthana, S., King, O. D., & Gibbons, F. D. (2004). Predicting protein complex membership using probabilistic network reliability. *Genome Research, 14*(6), 1170–1175. doi:10.1101/gr.2203804

Babych, B., & Hartley, A. (2003). Improving machine translation quality with automatic named entity recognition. *Proceedings of EAMT/EACL Workshop on MT, Budapest.*

Bader, G. D., Betel, D., & Hogue, C. W. (2003). BIND: The biomolecular interaction network database. *Nucleic Acids Research, 31*(1), 248–250. doi:10.1093/nar/gkg056

Bader, J. S., Chaudhuri, A., Rothberg, J. M., & Chant, J. (2004). Gaining confidence in high throughput protein interaction networks. *Nature Biotechnology, 22*(1), 78–85. doi:10.1038/nbt924

Baeza-Yates, R. A., & Ribeiro-Neto, B. A. (1999). *Modern information retrieval.* ACM Press / Addison-Wesley.

Baker, C. F., Fillmore, C. J., & Lowe, J. B. (1998). The Berkeley FrameNet project. In *Proceedings of the COLING-ACL*, Montreal, Canada

Banko, M., Cafarella, M. J., Soderland, S., Broadhead, M., & Etzioni, O. (2007). Open information extraction from the Web. In [ACM.]. *Proceedings of IJCAI, 2007*, 68–74.

Barabasi, A. L., & Oltvai, Z. N. (2004). Network biology: Understanding the cell's functional organization. *Nature Reviews. Genetics, 5*(2), 101–113. doi:10.1038/nrg1272

Barker, K., Agashe, B., Chaw, S. Y., Fan, J., Glass, M., & Hobbs, J. … Yeh, P. (2007). Learning by reading: A prototype system, performance baseline and lessons learned. In *Proceedings of Twenty-Second National Conference on Artificial Intelligence*, (pp. 280-286). AAAI Press.

Barrell, D., Dimmer, E., Huntley, R. P., Binns, D., O'Donovan, C., & Apweiler, R. (2009). The GOA database in 2009–an integrated gene ontology annotation resource. *Nucleic Acids Research, 37*(1), D396–D403. doi:10.1093/nar/gkn803

Barutcuoglu, Z., Schapire, R. E., & Troyanskaya, O. G. (2006). Hierarchical multi-label prediction of gene function. *Bioinformatics (Oxford, England), 22*(7), 830–836. doi:10.1093/bioinformatics/btk048

Basili, R., Pazienza, M. T., & Vindigni, M. (2000). Corpus-driven learning of event recognition rules. In *Proceedings of Workshop on Machine Learning for Information Extraction held in conjunction with the 14th European Conference on Artificial Intelligence (ECAI-00)*, Berlin, Germany, 2000.

Becker, C., & Bizer, C. (2008). DBpedia mobile: A location-aware Semantic Web client. *Proceedings of the Semantic Web Challenge.*

Bederson, B. B., Shneiderman, B., & Wattenberg, M. (2002). Ordered and quantum treemaps: Making effective use of 2d space to display hierarchies. *ACM Transactions on Graphics, 21*(4), 833–854. Retrieved from http://hcil.cs.umd.edu/trs/2001-18/2001-18.pdf. doi:10.1145/571647.571649

Bender, E. M., Sag, I. A., & Wasow, T. (2003). *Syntactic theory: A formal introduction, 2nd edition, instructor's manual.* CSLI Publications. Retrieved July 23rd, 2010, from http://hpsg.stanford.edu/book/slides/index.html

Ben-Hur, A., & Noble, W. S. (2005). Kernel methods for predicting protein-protein interactions. *Bioinformatics (Oxford, England), 21*(1), i38–i46. doi:10.1093/bioinformatics/bti1016

Benjamins, V. R., Contreras, J., Blázquez, M., Dodero, J. M., García, A., & Navas, E. … Wert, C. (2004). Cultural heritage and the Semantic Web. In C. Bussler, J. Davies, D. Fensel, & R. Studer (Eds.), *The Semantic Web: Research and applications: First European Semantic Web Symposium, ESWS 2004, Heraklion, Crete, Greece, May 10-12, 2004: Proceedings* (LNCS 3053), (pp.433–444). Berlin, Germany: Springer-Verlag.

Berners-Lee, T., Hendler, J., & Lassila, O. (2001). The Semantic Web. *Scientific American, 284*(5), 34–43. doi:10.1038/scientificamerican0501-34

Berry, M. W., Dumais, S., O'Brien, G., Berry, M. W., & Dumais, S. T., & Gavin. (1995). Using linear algebra for intelligent information retrieval. *SIAM Review, 37,* 573–595. doi:10.1137/1037127

Berry, M. W., & Castellanos, M. (Eds.). (2008). *Survey of text mining II: Clustering, classification and retrieval.* Springer-Verlag.

Berry, M. W., Dumais, S. T., & O'Brien, G. W. (1995). Using linear algebra for intelligent information retrieval. *SIAM Review, 37,* 573–595. doi:10.1137/1037127

Bhagdev, R., Chakravarthy, A., Chapman, S., Ciravegna, F., & Lanfranchi, V. (2008). Creating and using organisational Semantic Webs in large networked organisations. In *ISWC '08: Proc., 7th International Conference on The Semantic Web* (pp. 723–736). Springer-Verlag.

Biemann, C. (2005). Ontology learning from text: A survey of methods. *LDV Forum, 20*(2), 75–93.

BioBLP/JNLPBA. (2004). *BioNLP/JNLPBA shared task on biomedical entity recognition.*

Biskri, I., Meunier, J. G., & Joyal, S. (2004). L'extraction des termes complexes: Une approche modulaire semiautomatique. In Purnelle, G., Fairon, C., & Dister, A. (Eds.), *Presses universitaires de louvain* (*Vol. 1*, pp. 192–201).

Bizer, C., Lehmann, J., Kobilarov, G., Auer, S., Becker, C., & Cyganiak, R. (2009). DBpedia - a crystallization point for the Web of data. *Journal of Web Semantics: Science. Services and Agents on the World Wide Web, 7*(3), 154–165. doi:10.1016/j.websem.2009.07.002

Blei, D., Griffiths, T., Jordan, M., & Tenenbaum, J. (2004). Hierarchical topic models and the nested Chinese restaurant process. *Advances in Neural Information Processing Systems, 16,* 106.

Blei, D. M., Ng, A. Y., Jordan, M. I., & Lafferty, J. (2003). Latent dirichlet allocation. *Journal of Machine Learning Research, 3,* 2003. doi:10.1162/jmlr.2003.3.4-5.993

Blei, D., Ng, A. Y., & Jordan, M. I. (2003). Latent dirichlet allocation. *Journal of Machine Learning Research, 3,* 993–1022. doi:10.1162/jmlr.2003.3.4-5.993

Blei, D. M., Ng, A. Y., & Jordan, M. I. (2003). Latent dirichlet allocation. *Journal of Machine Learning Research, 3,* 993–1022. doi:10.1162/jmlr.2003.3.4-5.993

Blei, D., & Lafferty, J. (2006). Dynamic topic models. In *Proceedings of the 23rd International Conference on Machine Learning* (p. 120).

Bloehdorn, S., & Hotho, A. (2004). Boosting for text classification with semantic features. In *Proceedings of the Workshop on Mining for and from the Semantic Web at the 10th ACM SIGKDD Conference on Knowledge Discovery and Data Mining* (pp. 70-87).

Bock, J. R., & Gough, D. A. (2001). Predicting protein - protein interactions from primary structure. *Bioinformatics (Oxford, England), 17*(5), 455–460. doi:10.1093/bioinformatics/17.5.455

Boeckmann, B., & Bairoch, A. (2003). The SWISS-PROT protein knowledgebase and its supplement TrEMBL in 2003. *Nucleic Acids Research, 31*(1), 365–370. doi:10.1093/nar/gkg095

Bonifacio, M., Bouquet, P., & Cuel, R. (2002). Knowledge nodes: The building blocks of a distributed approach to knowledge management. *Journal for Universal Computer Science, 8*(6), 652–661.

Boolos, G., & Jeffrey, R. (1989). *Computability and logic* (3 ed.). Cambridge, UK: Cambridge University Press.

Borin, L. (2000). You'll take the high road and I'll take the low road: Using a third language to improve bilingual word alignment. In *Proceedings of the 18th international Conference on computational linguistics* (Vol. 1, pp. 97–103).

Boyd-Graber, J., Chang, J., Gerrish, S., Wang, C., & Blei, D. (2009). Reading tea leaves: How humans interpret topic models. [NIPS]. *Advances in Neural Information Processing Systems, 31.*

Breslin, J. G., Passant, A., & Decker, S. (2010). *The social Semantic Web.* Springer-Verlag.

Brewster, C., Ciravegna, F., & Wilks, Y. (2003). Background and foreground knowledge in dynamic ontology construction: viewing text as knowledge maintenance. In *Proceedings of Conference Semantic Web Workshop, SIGIR03*: Association of Computing Machinery.

Brewster, C., Iria, J., Zhang, Z., Ciravegna, F., Guthrie, L., & Wilks, Y. (2007). Dynamic iterative ontology learning. In *RANLP '07: Proc., the Recent Advances in Natural Language Processing Conference.*

Brin, S., & Page, L. (1998). The anatomy of a large-scale hypertextual Web search engine. *Computer Networks and ISDN Systems, 30*(1–7), 107–117.

Briscoe, E., & Carroll, J. (2006). Evaluating the accuracy of an unlexicalized statistical parser on the PARC DepBank. In *Proceedings of the COLING/ACL 2006 Main Conference Poster Sessions*, Sydney, Australia. (pp. 41-48).

Brooks, R. A. (1991). Intelligence without representation. *Artificial Intelligence, 47*, 139–159. doi:10.1016/0004-3702(91)90053-M

Brown, P. F., Cocke, J., Pietra, S. A. D., Pietra, V. J. D., Jelinek, F., & Lafferty, J. D. (1990). A statistical approach to machine translation. *Computational Linguistics, 16*(2), 79–85.

Brown, P. F., Pietra, S. A. D., Pietra, V. J. D., & Mercer, R. L. (1993). Mathematics of statistical machine translation: Parameter estimation. *Computational Linguistics, 19*(2), 263–311.

Brown, P. F., Lai, J. C., & Mercer, R. L. (1991). Aligning sentences in parallel corpora. In *Proceedings of the Annual Meeting of the Association of Computational Linguistics (ACL)*. (pp. 169-176).

Brun, C., Chevenet, F., Martin, D., Wojcik, J., Guenoche, A., & Jacq, B. (2003). Functional classification of proteins for the prediction of cellular function from a protein–protein interaction network. *Genome Biology, 5*(1), R6. doi:10.1186/gb-2003-5-1-r6

Buckner, C., Niepert, M., & Allen, C. (2010). From encyclopedia to ontology: Toward dynamic representation of the discipline of philosophy. *Synthese*.

Budanitsky, A., & Hirst, G. (2006). Evaluating word-net-based measures of lexical semantic relatedness. *Computational Linguistics, 32*(1), 13–47. doi:10.1162/coli.2006.32.1.13

Buitelaar, P., & Cimiano, P. (Eds.). (2008). *Ontology learning and population: Bridging the gap between text and knowledge. Frontiers in Artificial Intelligence and Applications Series* (*Vol. 167*). IOS Press.

Buitelaar, P., Cimiano, P., & Magnini, B. (2005). Ontology learning from text: An overview. In Buitelaar, P., Cimiano, P., & Magnini, B. (Eds.), *Ontology learning from text: Methods, applications and evaluation* (pp. 3–12). IOS Press.

Bunescu, R., & Pasca, M. (2006). *Using encyclopedic knowledge for named entity disambiguation. ECAL-06*. The Association for Computer Linguistics.

Bunescu, R., & Mooney, R. (2005). A shortest path dependency kernel for relation extraction. In *Proceedings of the Human Language Technology Conference and Conference on Empirical Methods in Natural Language Processing*, (pp. 724–731). ACL.

Butters, J., & Ciravegna, F. (2008). Using similarity metrics for terminology recognition. *Proceedings in the sixth Language Resource Evaluation Conference*. European Language Resources Association (ELRA)

Byrne, K. (2007). Nested named entity recognition in historical archive text. *Proceedings of the International Conference on Semantic Computing*. (pp. 589-896). IEEE Computer Society

Caraballo, S. A. (2001). *Automatic construction of a hypernym-labeled noun hierarchy from text*. Unpublished doctoral dissertation, Brown University, Providence, RI, USA.

Carvalho, R., Chapman, S., & Ciravegna, F. (2008). Extracting semantic meaning from photographic annotations using a hybrid approach. *MMIU'08: Proceedings of the 1st International Workshop on Metadata Mining for Image Understanding*.

Castro, A. G., Rocca-Serra, P., Stevens, R., Taylor, C., Nashar, K., Ragan, M. A., & Sansone, S.-A. (2006). The use of concept maps during knowledge elicitation in ontology development processes - the nutrigenomics use case. *BMC Bioinformatics, 7*(267).

Chang, C. C., & Lin, C. J. (2010). *LIBSVM: A library for support vector machines*. Retrieved from http://www.csie.ntu.edu.tw/cjlin/libsvm

Chen, J. C., & Yuan, B. (2006). Detecting functional modules in the yeast protein–protein interaction network. *Bioinformatics (Oxford, England), 22*(18), 2283–2290. doi:10.1093/bioinformatics/btl370

Chen, P. (2008). Predicting and validating protein interactions using network structure. *PLoS Computational Biology, 4*(7), e1000118. doi:10.1371/journal.pcbi.1000118

Chen, Y., & Xu, D. (2004). Global protein function annotation through mining genome-scale data in yeast Saccharomyces cerevisiae. *Nucleic Acids Research, 32*(21), 6414–6424. doi:10.1093/nar/gkh978

Chen, S. F. (1993). Aligning sentences in bilingual corpora using lexical information. In *Proceedings of the Annual Meeting of the Association of Computational Linguistics (ACL)*. (pp. 9-16). Columbus, OH.

Chen, S., Wang, H., & Zhou, S. (2009). *Concept clustering of evolving data*. In IEEE International Conference on Data Engineering (pp. 1327–1330).

Cheng, J., Cline, M., Martin, J., Finkelstein, D., Awad, T., & Kulp, D. (2004). A knowledge-based clustering algorithm driven by gene ontology. *Journal of Biopharmaceutical Statistics, 14*(3), 687–700. doi:10.1081/BIP-200025659

Chiang, D. (2007). Hierarchical phrase-based translation. *Computational Linguistics, 33*(2), 201–228. doi:10.1162/coli.2007.33.2.201

Chiang, D. (2005). A hierarchical phrase-based model for statistical machine translation. In *Proceedings of the Association for Computational Linguistics (ACL)*. (pp. 263-270).

Chiang, D., Wang, W., & Knight, K. (2009). 11,001 new features for statistical machine translation. In *Proceedings of NAACL-HLT*, (pp. 218–226).

Chien, C., Bartel, P., Sternglanz, R., & Fields, S. (1991). The two-hybrid system: A method to identify and clone genes for proteins that interact with a protein of interest. *Proceedings of the National Academy of Sciences of the United States of America, 88*(21), 9578–9582. doi:10.1073/pnas.88.21.9578

Chinchor, N. (1998). Overview of MUC-7/MET-2. *Proceedings of the Seventh Message Understanding Conference MUC-7*.

Chou, K. C., & Cai, Y. D. (2006). Predicting protein–protein interactions from sequences in a hybridization space. *Journal of Proteome Research, 5*(2), 316–322. doi:10.1021/pr050331g

Chua, H. N., Sung, W. K., & Wong, L. (2006). Exploiting indirect neighbours and topological weight to predict protein function from protein–protein interactions. *Bioinformatics (Oxford, England), 22*(13), 1623–1630. doi:10.1093/bioinformatics/btl145

Chua, H. N., Sung, W. K., & Wong, L. (2007). An efficient strategy for extensive integration of diverse biological data for protein function prediction. *Bioinformatics (Oxford, England), 23*(24), 3364–3373. doi:10.1093/bioinformatics/btm520

Church, K. W., & Hanks, P. (1990). Word association norms, mutual information and lexicography. In *Proceedings of the 27th Annual Conference of the Association of Computational Linguistics*, (pp. 22-29). MIT Press.

Cimiano, P. (2006). *Ontology learning and population from text: Algorithms, evaluation and applications*. Springer.

Cimiano, P., & Völker, J. (2005). Text2Onto. *NLDB, 2005*, 227–238.

Cimiano, P. (2006). *Ontology learning and population from text: Algorithms, evaluation and applications*. Secaucus, NJ: Springer-Verlag New York, Inc.

Cimiano, P., Pivk, A., Schmidt-Thieme, L., & Staab, S. (2005). Learning taxonomic relations from heterogeneous sources of evidence. In *Ontology learning from text: Methods, evaluation and applications* (pp. 59–73). IOS Press.

Cimiano, P., & Staab, S. (2004). Learning by Googling. *SIGKDD Explorations, 6*(2), 24–33. doi:10.1145/1046456.1046460

Cimiano, P., Völker, J., & Studer, R. (2006). Ontologies on demand? - A description of the state-of-the-art, applications, challenges and trends for ontology learning from text. *Information. Wissenschaft und Praxis, 57*(6-7), 315–320.

Cimiano, P. (2006). *Ontology learning and population from text: Algorithms, evaluation and applications*. New York, NY: Springer-Verlag.

Cimiano, P., Pivk, A., Schmidt-Thieme, L., & Staab, S. (2005). Learning taxonomic relations from heterogeneous sources of evidence. In Buitelaar, P., Cimiano, P., & Magnini, B. (Eds.), *Ontology learning from text: Methods, evaluation and applications* (pp. 59–73). IOS Press.

Cimiano, P., & Völker, J. (2005). Text2onto. In *Natural language processing and information systems* (pp. 227-238).

Cimiano, P., Haase, P., & Heizmann, J. (2007). Porting natural language interfaces between domains – a case study with the ORAKEL system. In *Proceedings of the International Conference on Intelligent User Interfaces* (IUI), (pp. 180–189).

Cimiano, P., Völker, J., & Studer, R. (2006). Ontologies on demand? A description of the state-of-the-art, applications, challenges and trends for ontology learning from text information. *Information, Wissenschaft und Praxis, 57*(6-7), 315-320. Retrieved from http://www.aifb.uni-karlsruhe.de/Publikationen/showPublikation?publ id=1282

Ciravegna, F., Greengrass, M., Hitchcock, T., Chapman, S., McLaughlin, J., & Bhagdev, R. (2008). Finding needles in haystacks: Data-mining in historical datasets. In Greengrass, M., & Hughes, L. (Eds.), *The virtual representation of the past* (pp. 65–79). Farnham, UK: Ashgate.

Ciravegna, F., & Staab, S. (2005). *Large scale cross-media knowledge acquisition, sharing and reuse in X-Media*. In EWIMT 2005: The 2nd European Workshop on the Integration of Knowledge, Semantics and Digital Media Technology (pp. 407–408).

Ciravegna, F., Dingli, A., Petrelli, D., & Wilks, Y. (2002). *Timely and non-intrusive active document annotation via adaptive information extraction*. In Semantic Authoring, Annotation & Knowledge Markup (SAAKM 2002), ECAI 2002 Workshop, (pp. 7-13)

Ciula, A., Spence, P., & Vieira, J. M. (2008). Expressing complex associations in medieval historical documents: The Henry III Fine Rolls project. *Literary and Linguistic Computing, 23*(3), 311–325. doi:10.1093/llc/fqn018

Cleuziou, G. (2007). Okm: Une extension des k-moyennes pour la recherche de classes recouvrantes. In M. Noirhomme-Fraiture & G. Venturini (Eds.), *Egc* (Vol. RNTI-E-9, p. 691-702). Cépaduès-Éditions. Retrieved from http://dblp.uni-trier.de/db/conf/f-egc/egc2007.html#Cleuziou07

Cleuziou, G. (2009). Okmed et wokm: Deux variantes de okm pour la classification recouvrante. In J. G. Ganascia & P. Gancarski (Eds.), *Egc* (vol. RNTI-E-15, p. 31-42). Cépaduès-Éditions. Retrieved from http://dblp.uni-trier.de/db/conf/f-egc/egc2009.html#Cleuziou09

Consortium, T. U. (2009). The universal protein resource (uniprot) 2009. *Nucleic Acids Research, 37*(1), D169–D174. doi:10.1093/nar/gkn664

Corcho, O. (2006). Ontology based document annotation: Trends and open research problems. *IJMSO, 1*(1), 47–57. doi:10.1504/IJMSO.2006.008769

Couto, F. M., Silva, M. J., & Coutinho, P. M. (2007). Measuring semantic similarity between gene ontology terms. *Data & Knowledge Engineering, 61*(1), 137–152. doi:10.1016/j.datak.2006.05.003

Crane, G., Seales, B., & Terras, M. (2009). Cyberinfrastructure for classical philology. *Digital Humanities Quarterly, 3*(1). Retrieved March 10, 2010, from http://www.digitalhumanities.org/dhq/vol/3/1/000023.html

Crestani, F. (1997). Application of spreading activation techniques in information retrieval. *Artificial Intelligence Review, 11*, 453–482. doi:10.1023/A:1006569829653

Cucerzan, S. (2007). Large-scale named entity disambiguation based on Wikipedia data. *Proceedings of the 2007 Joint Conference on Empirical Methods in Natural Language Processing and Computational Natural Language Learning* (pp. 708-716)

Cunningham, H. (2005). *Information extraction, automatic* (2nd ed.). Encyclopedia of Language and Linguistics.

Curran, J. R. (2002). Ensemble methods for automatic thesaurus extraction. In *Proceedings of ACL* (pp. 222–229).

D'Agostini, G. (2003). Bayesian inference in processing experimental data: Principles and basic applications. *Reports on Progress in Physics, 66*(9), 1383–1419. doi:10.1088/0034-4885/66/9/201

d'Aquin, M., Motta, E., Sabou, M., Angeletou, S., Gridinoc, L., & Lopez, V. (2008). Toward a new generation of Semantic Web applications. *IEEE Intelligent Systems, 23*(3), 20–28. doi:10.1109/MIS.2008.54

d'Aquin, M., Sabou, M., Motta, E., Angeletou, S., Gridinoc, L., & Lopez, V. (2008). What can be done with the Semantic Web? An overview of Watson-based applications. In A. Gangemi, J. Keizer, V. Presutti, & H. Stoermer (Eds.), *Proceedings of the 5th workshop on Semantic Web applications and perspectives (swap2008)* (Vol. 426). Rome, Italy: CEUR-WS.org.

Dadzie, A.-S., Lanfranchi, V., & Petrelli, D. (2009). Seeing is believing: Linking data with knowledge. *Information Visualization*, *8*(3), 197–211. doi:10.1057/ivs.2009.11

Dadzie, A.-S., Iria, J., Petrelli, D., & Xia, L. (2009). The XMediaBox: Sensemaking through the use of knowledge lenses. In L. Aroyo, et al. (Eds.), *ESWC 2009: The Semantic Web: Research and Applications, Proc., 6th European Semantic Web Conference* (pp. 811–815).

Dahlquist, K. D., Salomonis, N., Vranizan, K., Lawlor, S. C., & Conklin, B. R. (2002). GenMAPP, a new tool for viewing and analyzing microarray data on biological pathways. *Nature Genetics*, *31*(1), 19–20. doi:10.1038/ng0502-19

Daille, B., Gaussier, É., & Langé, J. M. (1994). Towards automatic extraction of monolingual and bilingual terminology. In *Proceedings of the 15th Conference on Computational Linguistics*.

de Boer, V., van Someren, M., & Wielinga, B. (2006). Extracting instances of relations from Web documents using redundancy. In Y. Sure & J. Domingue (Eds.), *The Semantic Web: Research and applications: 3rd European Semantic Web Conference, ESWC 2006 Budva, Montenegro, June 11-14, 2006, Proceedings* (LNCS 4011), (pp. 245-258). Berlin, Germany: Springer-Verlag.

De Marneffe, M.-C., MacCartney, B., & Manning, C. D. (2006). Generating typed dependency parses from phrase structure parses. In *Proceedings of LREC*, (pp. 449-454). ELRA.

Deerwester, S. C., Dumais, S. T., Landauer, T. K., Furnas, G. W., & Harshman, R. A. (1990). Indexing by latent semantic analysis. *JASIS*, *41*(6), 391–407. doi:10.1002/(SICI)1097-4571(199009)41:6<391::AID-ASI1>3.0.CO;2-9

Dellschaft, K., & Staab, S. (2006). *On how to perform a gold standard based evaluation of ontology learning*. International Semantic Web Conference, (pp. 228-241).

Deng, M., Zhang, K., Mehta, S., Chen, T., & Sun, F. (2003). Prediction of protein function using protein–protein interaction data. *Journal of Computational Biology*, *10*(6), 947–960. doi:10.1089/106652703322756168

Dias, G., Guilloré, S., & Lopes, J. G. P. (2000). Extraction automatique d'associations textuelles à partir de corpora non traités. In M. Rajman & JC. Chapelier (Eds.), *Journées Internationales d'Analyse Statistique de Données Textuelles, 2*, 213-220. Lausanne, France: Ecole Polytechnique Fédérale de Lausanne.

Dickinger, A., Scharl, A., Stern, H., Weichselbraun, A., & Wöber, K. (2008). Applying optimal stopping for optimizing queries to external Semantic Web resources. In P. O'Connor, H. Wolfram, & G. Ulrike (Eds.), *Information and communication technologies in tourism 2008, Proceedings of the International Conference in Innsbruck, Austria, 2008* (pp. 545–555). Vienna, Austria/New York, NY: Springer.

Diederich, J., & Balke, W. T. (2007). The semantic growbag algorithm: Automatically deriving categorization systems. In *European Conference on research and advanced technology for digital libraries* (pp. 1-13).

Doddington, G., Mitchell, A., Przybocki, M., Ramshaw, L., Strassel, S., & Weischedel, R. (2004). The Automatic Content Extraction (ACE) program – tasks, data, and evaluation. *Proceedings of the fourth Conference on Language Resources and Evaluation (LREC)* (pp. 837-840). European Language Resources Association (ELRA).

Doerr, M. (2003). The CIDOC CRM: An ontological approach to semantic interoperability of metadata. *AI Magazine*, *24*(3), 75–92.

Downey, D., Broadhead, M., & Etzioni, O. (2007). Locating complex named entities in Web text. *Proceedings of the 20th International Joint Conference on Artifical intelligence* (pp. 2733-2739). Morgan Kaufmann Publishers Inc.

Du, P., Feng, G., Flatow, J., Song, J., Holko, M., Kibbe, W. A., & Lin, S. M. (2009). From disease ontology to disease-ontology lite: Statistical methods to adapt a general-purpose ontology for the test of gene-ontology associations. *Bioinformatics (Oxford, England)*, *25*(12), i63–i68. doi:10.1093/bioinformatics/btp193

Du, Z., Li, L., Chen, C. F., Yu, P. S., & Wang, J. Z. (2009). G-sesame: Web tools for go-term-based gene similarity analysis and knowledge discovery. *Nucleic Acids Research*, *37*(2), W345–349.

Dunn, J. C. (1973). A fuzzy relative of the iso-data process and its use in detecting compact well-separated clusters. *Journal of Systems and Cybernetics*, *3*(3), 32–57. Retrieved from http://www.informaworld.com/10.1080/01969727308546046. doi:10.1080/01969727308546046

Dyvik, H. (2005). Translations as a semantic knowledge source. In *Proceedings of the second Baltic Conference on human language technologies*. Tallinn, Estonia.

Eckert, K., Pfeffer, M., & Stuckenschmidt, H. (2008). Assessing thesaurus-based annotations for semantic search applications. *International Journal on Metadata. Semantics and Ontologies*, *3*(1), 53–67. doi:10.1504/IJMSO.2008.021205

Eckert, K., Stuckenschmidt, H., & Pfeffer, M. (2007). Interactive thesaurus assessment for automatic document annotation. In *Proceedings of the Fourth International Conference on knowledge capture (k-cap 2007)*, Whistler, Canada.

Eisenberg, D., Marcotte, E. M., Xenarios, I., & Yeates, T. O. (2000). Protein function in the postgenomic era. *Nature*, *405*(6788), 823–826. doi:10.1038/35015694

English, J., & Nirenburg, S. (2007). Ontology learning from text using automatic ontological-semantic text annotation and the Web as the corpus. *Proceedings of the AAAI 2007 Spring Symposium Series on Machine Reading*. Retrieved from http://www.aaai.org/Papers/Symposia/Spring/2007/SS-07-06/SS07-06-008.pdf

Erdmann, M., Nakayama, K., Hara, T., & Nishio, S. (2009). Improving the extraction of Bilingual terminology from Wikipedia. *ACM Transactions on Multimedia Computing. Communications and Applications*, *5*(4), 1–17.

Ernst, N. A., & Storey, M.-A. (2003). *A preliminary analysis of visualization requirements in knowledge engineering tools. (Tech. Rep.)*. CHISEL, University of Victoria.

Estruch, V., Orallo, J., & Quintana, M. (2008). *Bridging the gap between distance and generalisation: Symbolic learning in metric spaces*. Unpublished doctoral dissertation, Universitat Politècnica de València.

Etzioni, O., Banko, M., Soderland, S., & Weld, D. S. (2008). Open information extraction from the Web. *Communications of the ACM*, *51*(12), 68–74. doi:10.1145/1409360.1409378

Etzioni, O., Cafarella, M. J., Downey, D., Kok, S., Popescu, A., & Shaked, T. … Yates, A. (2004). Web-scale information extraction in Knowitall: Preliminary results. In *Proceedings of WWW* (pp. 100-110).

Evans, R. (2003). A framework for named entity recognition in the open domain. In *Proceedings of Recent Advances in Natural Language Processing 2003*.

Fellbaum, C. (1998). *WordNet: An electronic lexical database*. Cambridge, MA: The MIT Press.

Ferrández, S., Toral, A., Ferrández, Í., & Ferrández, A. (2009). Exploiting Wikipedia and EuroWordNet to solve cross-lingual question answering. [Elsevier Science Inc.]. *Information Sciences: An International Journal*, *179*(20), 3473–3488.

Finn, R. D., Tate, J., Mistry, J., Coggill, P. C., Sammut, S. J., & Hotz, H. R. (2008). The pfam protein families database. *Nucleic Acids Research*, *36*(1), D281–D288.

Fisher, D. H. (1987). Knowledge acquisition via incremental conceptual clustering. *Machine Learning*, *2*(2), 139–172. doi:10.1007/BF00114265

Fontana, P., Cestaro, A., Velasco, R., Formentin, E., & Toppo, S. (2009). Rapid annotation of anonymous sequences from genome projects using semantic similarities and a weighting scheme in gene ontology. *PLoS ONE*, *4*(2), e4619. doi:10.1371/journal.pone.0004619

Frank, E., Paynter, G. W., Witten, I. H., Gutwin, C., & Nevill-Manning, C. G. (1999). Domain-specific keyphrase extraction. In *IJCAI* (p. 668-673). Morgan Kaufmann.

Frantzi, K. T., & Ananiadou, S. (1999). The C-Value/NC-Value domain independent method for multi-word term extraction. *Journal of Natural Language Processing*, *6*(3), 145–179.

Frantzi, K. T., & Ananiadou, S. (1997). Automatic term recognition using contextual cues. In *Proceedings of the IJCAI Workshop on Multilinguality in Software Industry: the AI Contribution*, Japan.

Friedl, J. E. F. (2002). *Mastering regular expressions* (2nd ed.). Sebastopol, CA: O'Reilly Media.

Friedrich, C., Revillion, T., Hofmann, M., & Fluck, J. (2006). Biomedical and chemical named entity recognition with conditional random fields: The advantage of dictionary features. *Proceedings of the Second International Symposium on Semantic Mining in Biomedicine.*

Fujii, A., Utiyama, M., Yamamoto, M., & Utsuro, T. (2008). Overview of the patent translation task at the NTCIR-7 workshop. In *Proceedings of the 7th NTCIR Workshop Meeting on Evaluation of Information Access Technologies (NTCIR).* (pp. 389-400). Tokyo, Japan.

Fullam, K., & Barber, S. (2006). *Learning trust strategies in reputation exchange networks.* AAMAS'06, May 8-12, 2006, Hakodate, Hokkaido, Japan

Gabrilovich, E., Broder, A., Fontoura, M., Joshi, A., Josifovski, V., Riedel, L., & Zhang, T. (2009). Classifying search queries using the Web as a source of knowledge. *ACM Transactions on the Web, 3*(2), 1–28. doi:10.1145/1513876.1513877

Gabrilovich, E., & Markovitch, S. (2006). Overcoming the brittleness bottleneck using Wikipedia: Enhancing text categorization with encyclopedic knowledge. *Proceedings of the 21st National Conference on Artificial intelligence, vol. 2* (pp. 1301-1306). AAAI Press

Gabrilovich, E., & Markovitch, S. (2007). Computing semantic relatedness using Wikipedia-based explicit semantic analysis. *Proceedings of the 20th International Joint Conference on Artifical intelligence.* (pp. 1606-1611). Morgan Kaufmann Publishers Inc.

Gale, W. A., & Church, K. W. (1991). A program for aligning sentences in bilingual corpora. In *Proceedings of the Annual Meeting of the Association of Computational Linguistics (ACL).* (pp. 79-85).

Ganti, V., Konig, A., & Vernica, R. (2008). Entity categorization over large document collections. *Proceeding of the 14th ACM SIGKDD International Conference on Knowledge discovery and data mining.* (pp. 274-282). Association for Computing Machinery

Gavin, A. C., Aloy, P., Grandi, P., Krause, R., Boesche, M., Marzioch, M., & Rau, C. (2006). Proteome survey reveals modularity of the yeast cell machinery. *Nature, 440*(7084), 631–636. doi:10.1038/nature04532

Gavin, A. C., Bösche, M., Krause, R., Grandi, P., Marzioch, M., Bauer, A., & Schultz, J. (2002). Functional organization of the yeast proteome by systematic analysis of protein complexes. *Nature, 415*(6868), 141–147. doi:10.1038/415141a

Geleijnse, G., & Korst, J. (2007). Creating a dead poets society: Extracting a social network of historical persons from the Web. In K. Aberer, P. Cudré-Mauroux, K. Choi, N. Noy, D. Allemang, K. Lee, … G. Schreiber (Eds.), *Proceedings of the 6th International Semantic Web and 2nd Asian Conference on Asian Semantic Web Conference (Busan, Korea, November 11 - 15, 2007)* (LNCS 4825), (pp. 156-168). Berlin, Germany: Springer-Verlag.

Gennari, J. H., Musen, M. A., Fergerson, R. W., Grosso, W. E., Crubézy, M., & Eriksson, H. (2003). The evolution of Protégé: An environment for knowledge-based systems development. *International Journal of Human-Computer Studies, 58*(1), 89–123. doi:10.1016/S1071-5819(02)00127-1

Geraci, F., Pellegrini, M., Maggini, M., & Sebastiani, F. (2006). *Cluster generation and cluster labelling for Web snippets: A fast and accurate hierarchical solution* (pp. 25–36). Retrieved from http://dx.doi.org/10.1007/11880561\3

Gildea, D., & Jurafsky, D. (2002). Automatic labeling of semantic roles. *Computational Linguistics, 28*(3), 245–288. doi:10.1162/089120102760275983

Giles, J. (2005). Internet encyclopedias go head to head. *Nature, 438*, 900–901. doi:10.1038/438900a

Gill, T. (2004). Building semantic bridges between museums, libraries and archives: The CIDOC Conceptual Reference Model. *First Monday, 9*(5). Retrieved March 10, 2010, from http://firstmonday.org/htbin/cgiwrap/bin/ojs/index.php/fm/article/view/1145/1065

Gillam, L., Tariq, M., & Ahmad, K. (2005). Terminology and the construction of ontology. *Terminology, 11*, 55–81. doi:10.1075/term.11.1.04gil

Giot, L., Bader, J. S., Brouwer, C., Chaudhuri, A., Kuang, B., Li, Y., & Hao, Y. L. (2003). A protein interaction map of Drosophila melanogaster. *Science, 302*(5651), 1727–1736. doi:10.1126/science.1090289

Giovannetti, E., Marchi, S., Montemagni, S., & Bartolini, R. (2008). Ontology learning and semantic annotation: A necessary symbiosis. In *LREC '08: Proc., 6th International Conference on Language Resources and Evaluation* (pp. 2079–2085).

Girju, R., Badulescu, A., & Moldovan, D. (2006). Automatic discovery of part-whole relations. *Computational Linguistics, 32*(1), 83–135.

Giuglea, A., & Moschitti, A. (2006). Shallow semantic parsing based on FrameNet, VerbNet and PropBank. In *Proceedings of 17th European Conference on Artificial intelligence*, (pp. 563-567). IOS Press.

Giuliano, C., Lavelli, A., & Romano, L. (2007). Relation extraction and the influence of automatic named-entity recognition. *ACM Transactions on Speech and Language Processing, 5*(1), 1–26. doi:10.1145/1322391.1322393

Giuliano, C. (2009). Fine-grained classification of named entities exploiting latent semantic kernels. In [Morristown, NJ: Association for Computational Linguistics]. *Proceedings of CoNLL, 09*, 201–209. doi:10.3115/1596374.1596406

Giuliano, C., Lavelli, A., & Romano, L. (2006). Exploiting shallow linguistic information for relation extraction from biomedical literature. In *Proceedings of the 11th Conference of the European Chapter of the Association for Computational Linguistics*.

Giullano, C., & Gliozzo, A. (2008). Instance-based ontology population exploiting named-entity substitution. In *Proceedings of the 22nd International Conference on Computational Linguistics,* vol. 1 (pp. 265-272). Association for Computational Linguistics

Goddard, C. (2001). Universal units in the lexicon. In Haspelmath, M., König, E., Oesterreicher, W., & Raible, W. (Eds.), *Language typology and language universals* (*Vol. 2*, pp. 1178–1190). Berlin, Germany / New York, NY: Walter de Gruyter. doi:10.1515/9783110171549.2.11.1190

Godoy, D., & Amandi, A. (2006). Modeling user interests by conceptual clustering. *Information Systems, 31*(4-5), 247–265. doi:10.1016/j.is.2005.02.008

Golder, S. A., & Huberman, B. A. (2006). Usage patterns of collaborative tagging systems. *Journal of Information Science, 32*, 198–208. doi:10.1177/0165551506062337

Goldschmidt, D., & Krishnamoorthy, M. (2008). Comparing keyword search to semantic search: A case study in solving crossword puzzles using the Google™ API. [John Wiley & Sons Inc.]. *Software, Practice & Experience, 38*(4), 417–445. doi:10.1002/spe.840

Google Press Center online. (2006). *Google to acquire YouTube for $1.65 billion in stock*. Retrieved from http://www.google.com/press/pressrel/google_youtube.html

Gracia, J., Trillo, R., Espinoza, M., & Mena, E. (2006). Querying the Web: A multiontology disambiguation method. In D. Wolber, N. Calder, C. Brooks, & A. Ginige (Eds.), *Proceedings of the 6th International Conference on Web Engineering (ICWE 2006)* (pp. 241–248). Palo Alto, CA, USA: ACM.

Grau, B. C., Parsia, B., Sirin, E., & Kalyanpur, A. (2006). Modularity and Web ontologies. In P. Doherty, J. Mylopoulos, & C. A. Welty (Eds.), *KR2006: Proc., 10th International Conference on Principles of Knowledge Representation and Reasoning* (pp. 198–209).

Greengrass, M. (2007). *Ontologies and semantic interoperability for humanities data*. Paper presented at Ontologies and Semantic Interoperability for Humanities Data workshop, Edinburgh. Retrieved March 10, 2010, from http://www.nesc.ac.uk/action/esi/download.cfm?index=3524

Greenwood, M. A., Stevenson, M., Guo, Y., Harkema, H., & Roberts, A. (2005). Automatically acquiring a linguistically motivated genic interaction extraction system. In *Proceedings of the 4th Learning Language in Logic workshop* (LLL05), Bonn, Germany.

Grefenstette, G. (1994). *Explorations in automatic thesaurus discovery*. Heidelberg, Germany: Springer.

Grefenstette, G., & Hearst, M. A. (1992). A method for refining automatically-discovered lexical relations: Combining weak techniques for stronger results. In *AAAI Workshop on statistically-based natural language programming techniques* (pp. 64–72). Menlo Park, CA: AAAI Press.

Griffiths, T. (2002). *Gibbs sampling in the generative model of latent dirichlet allocation. (Tech. Rep.)*. Stanford University.

Griffiths, T. L., & Steyvers, M. (2004, April). Finding scientific topics. *Proceedings of the National Academy of Sciences of the United States of America*, *101*(1), 5228–5235. doi:10.1073/pnas.0307752101

Griffiths, T., & Steyvers, M. (2002). A probabilistic approach to semantic representation. In *Proceedings of the 24th annual Conference of the cognitive science society.*

Grishman, R., & Sundheim, B. (1996). Message understanding conference - 6: A brief history. *Proceedings of the 16ᵗʰ International Conference on Computational Linguistics,* vol. 1 (pp.466-471). Association for Computational Linguistics.

Gruber, T. R. (1995). Toward principles for the design of ontologies used for knowledge sharing? *International Journal of Human-Computer Studies*, *43*(5-6), 907–928. doi:10.1006/ijhc.1995.1081

Gruber, T. (1993). A translation approach to portable ontology specifications. *Knowledge Acquisition*, *5*(2), 199–220. doi:10.1006/knac.1993.1008

Gruber, T. (2008). Collective knowledge systems: Where the social web meets the Semantic Web. *Journal of Web Semantics*, *6*(1), 4–13.

Gruber, T. R. (2003). A translation approach to portable ontology specifications. *Knowledge Acquisition*, *5*(2), 199–220. doi:10.1006/knac.1993.1008

Gruber, T. (2007). Ontology of Folksonomy: A mash-up of apples and oranges. *International Journal on Semantic Web and Information Systems*, *3*(2).

Guarino, N. (1998). *Formal ontology in Information Systems*. IOS Press.

Gulla, J., Borch, H., & Ingvaldsen, J. (2007). Ontology learning for search applications. In Meersman, R., & Tari, Z. (Eds.), *OTM 2007, part I, (LNCS 4803)* (pp. 1050–1062).

Guo, X., Liu, R., Shriver, C. D., Hu, H., & Liebman, M. N. (2006). Assessing semantic similarity measures for the characterization of human regulatory pathways. *Bioinformatics (Oxford, England)*, *22*(8), 967–973. doi:10.1093/bioinformatics/btl042

Ha, L. A., Fernandez, G., Mitkov, R., & Corpas, G. (2008). Mutual bilingual terminology extraction. In *Proceedings of the Sixth International Language Resources and Evaluation (LREC).* (pp. 1818-1824).

Haase, P., & Völker, J. (2008). Ontology learning and reasoning - dealing with uncertainty and inconsistency. In *Proceedings of the Workshop on Uncertainty Reasoning for the Semantic Web*, (pp. 366-384). Berlin / Heidelberg, Germany: Springer.

Halliday, M. A. K., & Hasan, R. (1976). *Cohesion in English*. Longman Pub Group.

Hammouda, K. M., Matute, D. N., & Kamel, M. S. (2005). Corephrase: Keyphrase extraction for document clustering. *MLDM*, *2005*, 265–274.

Han, J. D., & Bertin, N. (2004). Evidence for dynamically organized modularity in the yeast protein-protein interaction network. *Nature*, *430*(6995), 88–93. doi:10.1038/nature02555

Han, J. D., Dupuy, D., Bertin, N., Cusick, M. E., & Vidal, M. (2005). Effect of sampling on topology predictions of protein-protein interaction networks. *Nature Biotechnology*, *23*(7), 839–844. doi:10.1038/nbt1116

Han, H., & Elmasri, R. (2003). *Ontology extraction and conceptual modeling for Web information. Information modeling for Internet applications* (pp. 174–188). Hershey, PA: IGI Global.

Harabagiu, S. (1999). From lexical cohesion to textual coherence: A data driven perspective. *Journal of Pattern Recognition and Artificial Intelligence*, *13*, 247–265. doi:10.1142/S0218001499000148

Harris, Z. (1968). *Mathematical structures of language*. John Wiley & Sons.

Hart, G. T., Lee, I., & Marcotte, E. R. (2007). A high-accuracy consensus map of yeast protein complexes reveals modular nature of gene essentiality. *BMC Bioinformatics*, *8*, 236. doi:10.1186/1471-2105-8-236

Hart, G. T., Ramani, A. K., & Marcotte, E. M. (2006). How complete are current yeast and human protein-interaction networks? *Genome Biology*, *7*(11), 120. doi:10.1186/gb-2006-7-11-120

Hassan, S., & Mihalcea, R. (2009). Cross-lingual semantic relatedness using encyclopedic knowledge. *Proceedings of the 2009 Conference on Empirical Methods in Natural Language Processing* (pp.1192-1201). Association for Computational Linguisticts

Hayes, P., Eskridge, T. C., Saavedra, R., Reichherzer, T., Mehrotra, M., & Bobrovnikoff, D. (2005). Collaborative knowledge capture in ontologies. In *K-CAP '05: Proc., 3rd International Conference on Knowledge Capture* (pp. 99–106). ACM.

Hearst, M. (1992). Automatic acquisition of hyponyms from large text corpora. *Proceedings of the 14th Conference on Computational linguistics*, vol. 2 (pp. 539-545). Association for Computational Linguistics.

Heath, T., Motta, E., & Petre, M. (2007). Computing word-of-mouth trust relationships in social networks from Semantic Web and Web 2.0 data sources. In *Proceedings of the Workshop on bridging the gap between Semantic Web and Web 2.0.*

Hermjakob, H., & Monetcchi-Palazzi, L. (2004). IntAct: An open source molecular interaction database. *Nucleic Acids Research*, *32*, D452–D455. doi:10.1093/nar/gkh052

Heymann, P., & Garcia-Molina, H. (2006, April). *Collaborative creation of communal hierarchical taxonomies in social tagging systems* (Technical Report No. 2006-10). Computer Science Department.

Hishigaki, H., Nakai, K., Ono, T., Tanigami, A., & Takagi, T. (2001). Assessment of prediction accuracy of protein function from protein–protein interaction data. *Yeast (Chichester, England)*, *18*(6), 523–531. doi:10.1002/yea.706

Hjelm, H. (2007). Identifying cross language term equivalents using statistical machine translation and distributional association measures. In *Proceedings of NODALIDA 2007, the 16th Nordic Conference of computational linguistics.* Tartu, Estonia.

Hjelm, H. (2009). *Cross-language ontology learning: Incorporating and exploiting cross-language data in the ontology learning process.* Unpublished doctoral dissertation, Stockholm University, Sweden.

Hoffman, R. R., Shadbolt, N. R., Burton, A. M., & Klein, G. (1995). Eliciting knowledge from experts: A methodological analysis. *Organizational Behavior and Human Decision Processes*, *62*(2), 129–158. doi:10.1006/obhd.1995.1039

Hofmann, T. (2001). Unsupervised learning by probabilistic latent semantic analysis. *Machine Learning*, *42*(1/2), 177–196. doi:10.1023/A:1007617005950

Holloway, T., Bozicevic, M., & Börner, K. (2007). Analyzing and visualizing the semantic coverage of Wikipedia and its authors. *Journal of Complexity, Special issue on Understanding Complex Systems, 12*(3), 30-40.

Horton, R., Morrissey, R., Olsen, M., Roe, G., & Voyer, R. (2009). Mining eighteenth century ontologies: Machine learning and knowledge classification in the Encyclopédie. *DHQ: Digital Humanities Quarterly, 3*(2). Retrieved March 10, 2010 from http://digitalhumanities.org/dhq/vol/3/2/000044.html

Hotho, A., Staab, S., & Stumme, G. (2003). Wordnet improves text document clustering. In *Proceedings of Semantic Web Workshop, the 26th annual International ACM SIGIR Conference* (pp. 541-544).

Hu, P., Bader, G., Wigle, D. A., & Emili, A. (2007). Computational prediction of cancer gene function. *Nature Reviews. Cancer, 7*(1), 23–34. doi:10.1038/nrc2036

Hu, P., Jiang, H., & Emili, A. (2010). Predicting protein functions by relaxation labelling protein interaction network. *BMC Bioinformatics, 11*(1), S64. doi:10.1186/1471-2105-11-S1-S64

Hu, J., Fang, L., Cao, Y., Zeng, H., Li, H., Yang, Q., & Chen, Z. (2008). Enhancing text clustering by leveraging Wikipedia semantics. In *Proceedings of the 31st Annual international ACM SIGIR Conference on Research and Development in information Retrieval* (pp. 179-186).

Hubmann-Haidvogel, A., Scharl, A., & Weichselbraun, A. (2009). Multiple coordinated views for searching and navigating Web content repositories. *Information Sciences, 179*(12), 1813–1821. doi:10.1016/j.ins.2009.01.030

Huynen, M., Snel, B., Lathe, W. III, & Bork, P. (2000). Predicting protein function by genomic context: Quantitative evaluation and qualitative inferences. *Genome Research, 10*(8), 1204–1210. doi:10.1101/gr.10.8.1204

Hyvönen, E., Mäkelä, E., Kauppinen, T., Alm, O., Kurki, J., & Ruotsalo, T. … Nyberg, K. (2009). CultureSampo - a national publication system of cultural heritage on the Semantic Web 2.0. In L. Aroyo, P. Traverso, F. Ciravegna, P. Cimiano, T. Heath, E. Hyvönen, … E. Simperl (Eds.) *The Semantic Web: Research and applications: ESWC 2009 Heraklion, Crete, Greece, May 31–June 4, 2009 Proceedings* (LNCS 5554) (pp. 851-856). Berlin, Germany: Springer-Verlag.

Iria, J. (2009). Automating knowledge capture in the aerospace domain. *Proceedings of the fifth International Conference on Knowledge capture* (pp. 97-104). Association for Computing Machinery.

Isaac, A., Wang, S., Zinn, C., Matthezing, H., van der Meij, L., & Schlobach, S. (2009). Evaluating thesaurus alignments for semantic interoperability in the library domain. *IEEE Intelligent Systems, 24*(2), 76–86. doi:10.1109/MIS.2009.26

Ito, T., Chiba, T., Ozawa, R., Yoshida, M., Hattori, M., & Sakaki, Y. (2001). A comprehensive two hybrid analysis to explore the yeast protein interactome. *Proceedings of the National Academy of Sciences of the United States of America, 98*(8), 4569–4574. doi:10.1073/pnas.061034498

Itti, L., & Baldi, P. (2006). Bayesian surprise attracts human attention. [Cambridge, MA: MIT Press.]. *Advances in Neural Information Processing Systems, 19*, 547–554.

Jain, A. K., Murty, M. N., & Flynn, P. J. (1999). Data clustering: A review. *ACM Computing Surveys, 31*(3), 264–323. doi:10.1145/331499.331504

Jansen, R., & Gerstein, M. (2004). Analyzing protein function on a genomic scale: The importance of gold-standard positives and negatives for network prediction. *Current Opinion in Microbiology, 7*(5), 535–545. doi:10.1016/j.mib.2004.08.012

Jansen, R., Yu, H., Greenbaum, D., Kluger, Y., Krogan, N. J., & Chung, S. (2003). A Bayesian networks approach for predicting protein–protein interactions from genomic data. *Science, 302*(5644), 449–453. doi:10.1126/science.1087361

Jeffrey, S., Richards, J., Ciravegna, F., Chapman, S., & Zhang, Z. (2009). *The Archaeotools project: Faceted classification and natural language processing in an archaeological context. Special Theme Issues of the Philosophical Transactions of the Royal Society A, Crossing Boundaries: Computational Science.* E-Science and Global E-Infrastructures.

Jiang, X., Nariai, N., Steffen, M., Kasif, S., & Kolaczyk, E. D. (2008). Integration of relational and hierarchical network information for protein function prediction. *BMC Bioinformatics, 9*, 350. doi:10.1186/1471-2105-9-350

Jiang, J. J., & Conrath, D. W. (1997). *Semantic similarity based on corpus statistics and lexical taxonomy.* In International Conference Research on Computational Linguistics.

Jimeno, A., Ruiz, E., Lee, V., Gaudan, S., Berlanga, R., & Schuhmann, D. (2007). Assessment of disease named entity recognition on a corpus of annotated sentences. *Proceedings of the Second International Symposium on Languages in Biology and Medicine (LBM).* BMC Bioinformatics

Joho, H., Sanderson, M., & Beaulieu, M. (2004). A study of user interaction with a concept-based interactive query expansion support tool. In S. McDonald & J. Tait (Eds.), *Advances in information retrieval, 26th European Conference on IR research (ECIR 2004)* (Vol. 2997, p. 42-56). Sunderland, UK: Springer.

Jurafsky, D., & James, H. M. (2009). *Speech and language processing: An introduction to natural language processing, speech recognition, and computational linguistics* (2nd ed.). Prentice-Hall.

Kageura, K., & Umino, B. (1996). Methods of automatic term recognition: A review. *Terminology*, *3*(2), 259–289. doi:10.1075/term.3.2.03kag

Kageura, K., Tsuji, K., & Aizawa, A. N. (2000). Automatic thesaurus generation through multiple filtering. In *Proceedings Coling* (pp. 397–403).

Kaji, N., & Kitsuregawa, M. (2008). Using hidden Markov random fields to combine distributional and pattern-based word clustering. In *Proceedings of Coling* (pp. 401–408).

Kalfoglou, Y., & Schorlemmer, M. (2003). Ontology mapping: The state of the art. *The Knowledge Engineering Review*, *18*(1), 1–31. doi:10.1017/S0269888903000651

Kamp, H., & Reyle, U. (1993). From discourse to logic. In *Model-theoretic semantics of natural language, formal logic and discourse representation theory, studies in linguistics and philosophy*.

Kanehisa, M., Goto, S., Kawashima, S., Okuno, Y., & Hattori, M. (2004). The KEGG resource for deciphering the genome. *Nucleic Acids Research*, *32*, D277–D280. doi:10.1093/nar/gkh063

Katia Lida Kermanidis, M M., Thanopoulos, A., & Fakotakis, N. (2008). Eksairesis: A domain-adaptable system for ontology building from unstructured text. In *Proceedings of LREC*.

Katifori, A., Halatsis, C., Lepouras, G., Vassilakis, C., & Giannopoulou, E. (2007). Ontology visualization methods—a survey. *ACM Computing Surveys*, *39*(4), 10. doi:10.1145/1287620.1287621

Kauppinen, T., & Hyvönen, E. (2007). Modeling and reasoning about changes in ontology time series. In Kishore, R., Ramesh, R., & Sharman, R. (Eds.), *Ontologies: A handbook of principles, concepts and applications in Information Systems* (pp. 319–338). Berlin, Germany: Springer-Verlag.

Kazama, J., & Torisawa, K. (2007). Exploiting Wikipedia as external knowledge for named entity recognition. *Proceedings of the 2007 Joint Conference on Empirical Methods in Natural Language Processing and Computational Natural Language Learning (EMNLP-CoNLL)*. (pp. 698-707). Association for Computational Linguistics.

Kazama, J., & Torisawa, K. (2008). Inducing gazetteers for named entity recognition by large-scale clustering of dependency relations. In *Proceedings of ACL-08: HLT.* (pp. 407-415). Association for Computational Linguistics.

Kietz, J., Maedche, A., & Volz, R. (2000). *A method for semi-automatic ontology acquisition from a corporate intranet*. EKAW-2000 Workshop âœOntologies and Textâ, Juan-Les-Pins, France, October 2000.

Kim, D., Barker, K., & Porter, B. (2009). Knowledge integration across multiple texts. In *Proceedings of the Fifth International Conference on Knowledge Capture (KCAP2009)*, (pp. 49-56). ACM.

Kim, J., Ohta, T., Tsuruoka, Y., Tateisi, Y., & Collier, N. (2004). Introduction to the bio-entity recognition task at JNLPBA. *Proceedings of the International Joint Workshop on Natural Language Processing in Biomedicine and its Applications (JNLPBA'04)* (pp. 70-75). Association for Computational Linguistics.

Kiryakov, A., Popov, B., Terziev, I., Manov, D., & Ognyanoff, D. (2004). Semantic annotation, indexing, and retrieval. *Journal of Web Semantics*, *2*(1), 49–79. doi:10.1016/j.websem.2004.07.005

Kislinger, T., Cox, T. B., Kannan, A., Chung, C., Hu, P., & Ignatchenko, A. (2006). Global survey of organ and organelle protein expression in mouse: Combined proteomic and transcriptomic profiling. *Cell*, *125*(1), 173–186. doi:10.1016/j.cell.2006.01.044

Klein, D., & Manning, C. D. (2003). Accurate unlexicalized parsing. *Proceedings of the 41st Meeting of the Association for Computational Linguistics*, (pp. 423-430).

Kliegr, T., Chandramouli, K., Nemrava, J., Svatek, V., & Izquierdo, E. (2008). Combining image captions and visual analysis for image concept classification. *Proceedings of the 9th International Workshop on Multimedia Data Mining: held in conjunction with the ACM SIGKDD 2008* (pp. 8-17). Association for Computing Machinary.

Klinger, R., Friedrich, C., Fluck, J., & Hofmann-Apitius, M. (2007). Named entity recognition with combinations of conditional random fields. *Proceedings of the Second BioCreative Challenge Evaluation Workshop*.

Kobilarov, G., Scott, T., Raimond, Y., Oliver, S., Sizemore, C., & Smethurst, M. … Lee, R. (2009). Media meets Semantic Web – how the BBC uses DBpedia and linked data to make connections. *Proceedings of the 6th European Semantic Web Conference on The Semantic Web: Research and Applications* (pp. 723-737). Springer-Verlag.

Koch, P. (2001). Lexical typology from a cognitive and linguistic point of view. In Haspelmath, M., König, E., Oesterreicher, W., & Raible, W. (Eds.), *Language typology and language universals* (*Vol. 2*, pp. 1142–1178). Berlin, Germany / New York, NY: Walter de Gruyter. doi:10.15 15/9783110171549.2.11.1142

Koehn, P. (2004). Pharaoh: A beam search decoder for phrase-based statistical machine translation models. In *Proceedings of the Conference of the Association for Machine Translation in the Americas (AMTA)*.

Koehn, P. (2005). Europarl: A parallel corpus for statistical machine translation. In *Proceedings of MT Summit X*.

Koehn, P., Hoang, H., Birch, A., Callison-Burch, C., Federico, M., & Bertoldi, N. … Herbst, E. (2007). Moses: Open source toolkit for statistical machine translation. In *Proceedings of the Annual Meeting of the Association of Computational Linguistics (ACL) Demo Session.* (pp. 177-180).

Kotis, K., Vouros, G., & Stergiou, K. (2006). Towards automatic merging of domain ontologies: The HCONE-merge approach. [JWS]. *Journal of Web Semantics*, *4*(1), 60–79. doi:10.1016/j.websem.2005.09.004

Kotis, K., & Papasalouros, A. (2010). *Learning useful kick-off ontologies from query logs: HCOME revised.* 4th International Conference on Complex, Intelligent and Software Intensive Systems (CISIS-2010).

Krizhanovsky, A., & Lin, F. (2009). Related terms search based on WordNet / Wiktionary and its application in ontology matching. *Proceedings of the 11th Russian Conference on Digital Libraries RCDL*.

Krogan, N. J., & Cagney, G. (2006). Global landscape of protein complexes in the yeast Saccharomyces cerevisiae. *Nature*, *440*(7084), 637–643. doi:10.1038/nature04670

Kübler, S., McDonald, R. T., & Nivre, J. (2009). *Dependency parsing*. Morgan & Claypool Publishers.

Kupiec, J. (1993). An algorithm for finding noun phrase correspondences in bilingual corpora. In *Proceedings of the 31st Annual Meeting of the Association for Computational Linguistics* (ACL).

Lafferty, D. (2006). Correlated topic models. In *Advances in neural information processing systems 18: Proceedings of the 2005 conference* (p. 147).

Lanckriet, G. R., De Bie, T., Cristianini, N., Jordan, M. I., & Nobel, W. S. (2004). A statistical framework for genomic data fusion. *Bioinformatics (Oxford, England)*, *20*(16), 2626–2635. doi:10.1093/bioinformatics/bth294

Landauer, T., & Dumais, S. (1997). A solution to Plato's problem: The latent semantic analysis theory of acquisition, induction and representation of knowledge. *Psychological Review*, *104*(2), 211–240. doi:10.1037/0033-295X.104.2.211

Larsen, B., & Aone, C. (1999). Fast and effective text mining using linear-time document clustering. In *Proceedings of the fifth ACM SIGKDD International Conference on Knowledge discovery and data mining* (pp. 16-22).

Larsson, N. J. (1998). *Notes on suffix sorting*. (LU-CS-TR:98-199, LUNDFD6/(NFCS-3130)/1–43/(1998)).

Lau, R., Li, Y., & Xu, Y. (2007). *Mining fuzzy domain ontology from textual databases*. IEEE/WIC/ACM International Conference on Web Intelligence, 2007.

Lee, H., Tu, Z., Deng, M., Sun, F., & Chen, T. (2006). Diffusion kernel-based logistic regression models for protein function prediction. *OMICS: J Integr Biol*, *10*(1), 40–55. doi:10.1089/omi.2006.10.40

Lemaire, B., & Denhière, G. (2006). Effects of high-order co-occurrences on word semantic similarities. *Current Psychology Letters, 18*(1).

Lesk, M. (1986). Automatic sense disambiguation using machine readable dictionaries: How to tell a pine cone from an ice cream cone. In *Sigdoc '86: Proceedings of the 5th annual international conference on systems documentation* (pp. 24–26). New York, NY: ACM.

Letovsky, S., & Kasif, S. (2003). Predicting protein function from protein-protein interaction data: a probabilistic approach. *Bioinformatics (Oxford, England)*, *19*(1), i197–i204. doi:10.1093/bioinformatics/btg1026

Li, X., & Roth, D. (2001). Exploring evidence for shallow parsing. In *Proceedings of the 2001 Workshop on Computational Natural Language Learning - Volume 7. Annual Meeting of the ACL*, (pp.1-7). ACL.

Lin, D., Zhao, S., Qin, L., & Zhou, M. (2003). Identifying synonyms among distributionally similar words. In. *Proceedings of, IJCAI-03*, 1492–1493.

Lin, D. (1998). *An information-theoretic definition of similarity*. In International Conference on Machine Learning (pp. 296–304).

Lin, D. (2008). *An information-theoretic definition of similarity, semantic similarity based on corpus statistics and lexical taxonomy*. Fifteenth International Conference on Machine Learning. (pp. 296–304).

Lin, D., & Pantel, P. (2001). Induction of semantic classes from natural language text. In *Proceedings of ACM Conference on Knowledge Discovery and Data Mining*, (pp. 317-322). ACM.

Liu, W., Weichselbraun, A., Scharl, A., & Chang, E. (2005). Semi-automatic ontology extension using spreading activation. *Journal of Universal Knowledge Management*, *1*, 50–58.

Liu, Y., Lü, Y., & Liu, Q. (2009). Improving tree-to-tree translation with packed forests. In *Proceedings of ACL/IJCNLP*, (pp. 558-566).

Lopez, A. (2008). Statistical machine translation. *ACM Computing Surveys*, *40*(3), 1–49. doi:10.1145/1380584.1380586

Lord, P. W., Stevens, R. D., Brass, A., & Goble, C. A. (2003). Investigating semantic similarity measures across the gene ontology: The relationship between sequence and annotation. *Bioinformation*, *19*(10), 1275–1283. doi:10.1093/bioinformatics/btg153

Lu, B., & Tsou, B. K. Y. (2009). Towards bilingual term extraction in comparable patents. In *Proceedings of the 23rd Pacific Asia Conference on Language, Information and Computation (PACLIC)*. (pp. 755-762). Hong Kong. December, 2009.

Lu, B., Tsou, B. K. Y., Zhu, J., Jiang, T., & Kwong, O. Y. (2009). The construction of a Chinese-English patent parallel corpus. In *Proceedings of MT Summit XII 3rd Workshop on Patent Translation*. Ottawa, Canada.

Lubovac, Z., Gamalielsson, J., & Olsson, B. (2006). Combining functional and topological properties to identify core modules in protein interaction networks. *Proteins*, *64*(4), 948–959. doi:10.1002/prot.21071

Ma, X. (2006). Champollion: A robust parallel text sentence aligner. In *Proceedings of the 5th International Conference on Language Resources and Evaluation (LREC)*. Genova, Italy.

MacKay, D. J. (2003). *Information theory, inference, and learning algorithms*. Cambridge University Press.

MacQueen, J. (1967). Some methods for classification and analysis of multivariate observations. In *Proceedings of the 5th Berkeley Symposium on Mathematical Statistics and Probability - vol 1, Statistics*.

Macqueen, J. B. (1967). Some methods of classification and analysis of multivariate observations. In *Proceedings of the fifth Berkeley Symposium on mathematical statistics and probability* (pp. 281–297).

Maedche, A., & Staab, S. (2001). Ontology learning for the Semantic Web. *IEEE Intelligent Systems*, *16*(2), 72–79. doi:10.1109/5254.920602

Maedche, A. (2002). *Ontology learning for the Semantic Web*. Norwell, MA: Kluwer Academic Publishers.

Maedche, A., Pekar, V., & Staab, S. (2002). Ontology learning part one-on discovering taxonomic relations from the Web. In Zhong, N., Liu, J., & Yao, Y. (Eds.), *Web intelligence* (pp. 301–322). Springer.

Maedche, A., & Volz, R. (2001). The ontology extraction maintenance framework Text-To-Onto. In *Proceedings of the Workshop on Integrating Data Mining and Knowledge Management*.

Maedche, A., Pekar, V., & Staab, S. (2002). Ontology learning part one - on discovering taxonomic relations from the Web. *Web Intelligence*, 301–322.

Manber, U., & Myers, G. (1990). Suffix arrays: A new method for on-line string searches. In *Proceedings of the first annual ACM-SIAM Symposium on discrete algorithms* (pp. 319–327).

Manning, C. D., & Schuetze, H. (1999). *Foundations of statistical natural language processing*. MIT Press.

Manning, C. D., Raghavan, P., & Schôtze, H. (2008). *Introduction to information retrieval*. Cambridge University Press.

Marcus, M. P., Marcinkiewicz, M. A., & Santorini, B. (1993). Building a large annotated corpus of English: The Penn treebank. *Computational Linguistics, 19*(2), 313–330.

Massey, L. (2005). Real-world text clustering with adaptive resonance theory neural networks. In *Proceedings of 2005 International Joint Conference on Neural Networks*.

Massjouni, N., Rivera, C. G., & Murali, T. M. (2006). VIRGO: Computational prediction of gene functions. *Nucleic Acids Research, 34*, W340–4. doi:10.1093/nar/gkl225

Mateos, A., Dopazo, J., Jansen, R., Tu, Y., Gerstein, M., & Stolovitzky, G. (2002). Systematic learning of gene functional classes from DNA array expression data by using multilayer perceptrons. *Genome Research, 12*(11), 1703–1715. doi:10.1101/gr.192502

Matsuo, Y., Sakaki, T., Uchiyama, K., & Ishizuka, M. (2006). Graph-based word clustering using a Web search engine. In *Proceedings of EMNLP* (pp. 542–550).

Mayfield, J., McNamee, P., & Piatko, C. (2003). Named entity recognition using hundreds of thousands of features. *Proceedings of the seventh conference on Natural language learning at HLT-NAACL 2003*, vol. 4 (pp. 184-187). Association for Computational Linguistics.

McDermott, J., Bumgarner, R., & Samudrala, R. (2005). Functional annotation from predicted protein interaction networks. *Bioinformatics (Oxford, England), 21*(15), 3217–3226. doi:10.1093/bioinformatics/bti514

McDowell, L., & Cafarella, M. J. (2008). Ontology-driven, unsupervised instance population. *Journal of Web Semantics, 6*(3), 218–236. doi:10.1016/j.websem.2008.04.002

McShane, M., Nirenburg, S., Beale, S., & O'Hara, T. (2005). Semantically rich human-aided machine annotation. In *CorpusAnno '05: Proc., Workshop on Frontiers in Corpus Annotations II* (pp. 68–75).

Mei, Q., Shen, X., & Zhai, C. (2007). Automatic labeling of multinomial topic models. In *Proceedings of the 13th ACM SIGKDD International Conference on knowledge discovery and data mining* (p. 499).

Mewes, H. W. (2002). MIPS: A database for genomes and protein sequences. *Nucleic Acids Research, 30*(1), 31–34. doi:10.1093/nar/30.1.31

Michalsky, R., & Stepp, R. (1983). Learning from observation: Conceptual clustering. In In, R., Michalski, J. G. C., & Mitchell, T. M. (Eds.), *Machine learning: An artificial intelligence approach* (pp. 331–363). Morgan Kauffmann.

Mihalcea, R., Chklovski, T., & Kilgarriff, A. (2004). The Senseval-3 English Lexical Sample Task, in Proc. of Senseval-3, pp. 25--28, Spain.

Mika, P. (2007). Ontologies are us: A unified model of social networks and semantics. *Journal of Web Semantics, 5*(1), 5–15. doi:10.1016/j.websem.2006.11.002

Mika, P. (2007). Ontologies are us: A unified model of social networks and semantics. *Journal of Web Semantics, 5*, 5–15. doi:10.1016/j.websem.2006.11.002

Miller, G. A. (1956). The magical number seven, plus or minus two: Some limits on our capacity for processing information. *Psychological Review, 63*, 81–97. doi:10.1037/h0043158

Miller, S., Guinness, J., & Zamanian, A. (2004). Name tagging with word clusters and discriminative training. [Association for Computational Linguistics.]. *Proceedings of, HLT-04*, 337–342.

Milne, D. N., Witten, I. H., & Nichols, D. M. (2007). A knowledge-based search engine powered by Wikipedia. In *Proceedings of the Sixteenth ACM Conference on Conference on information and Knowledge Management* (pp. 445-454).

Mirzaee, V., Iverson, L., & Hamidzadeh, B. (2005). Computational representation of semantics in historical documents. In *Humanities, Computers and Cultural Heritage: Proceedings of the XVI International Conference of the Association for History and Computing, 14-17 September 2005* (pp. 199-206). Amsterdam, The Netherlands: Royal Netherlands Academy of Arts and Sciences.

Mistry, M., & Pavlidis, P. (2008). Gene ontology term overlap as a measure of gene functional similarity. *BMC Bioinformatics, 9*(1), 327. doi:10.1186/1471-2105-9-327

Mödritscher, F. (2009). Semantic lifecycles: Modelling, application, authoring, mining, and evaluation of meaningful data. *International Journal of Knowledge and Web Intelligence*, *1*(1/2), 110–124. doi:10.1504/IJKWI.2009.027928

Mohit, B., & Hwa, R. (2005). Syntax-based semi-supervised named entity tagging. *Proceedings of ACL '05* (pp. 57-60). Association for Computational Linguistics.

Mollá, O., Zaanen, M., & Smith, D. (2006). Named entity recognition for question answering. *Proceedings of the 2006 Australasian Language Technology Workshop (ALTW2006)*.

Moore, R. C. (2002). Fast and accurate sentence alignment of bilingual corpora. In *Proceedings of AMTA.* (pp. 135-144).

Mostafavi, S., & Morris, Q. (2009). Using the gene ontology hierarchy when predicting gene function. In *Proceedings of the Twenty-Fifth Conference on Uncertainty in Artificial Intelligence (UAI-09)* (pp. 419-427). Oregon: AUAI Press.

Mularz, D., & Lyell, M. (2004). Integrating concept mapping and Semantic Web technologies for knowledge management. In *DEXA2004: Proc., 15th International Workshop on Database and Expert Systems Applications* (pp. 449–453).

Müller, C., & Gurevych, I. (2009). Using Wikipedia and Wiktionary in domain-specific information retrieval. In *Evaluating Systems for Multilingual and Multimodal Information Access* (pp. 219–226). Berlin / Heidelberg, Germany: Springer. doi:10.1007/978-3-642-04447-2_28

Munday, J. (2001). *Introducing translation studies: Theories and applications*. Oxon, UK: Routledge.

Munteanu, D. S., & Marcu, D. (2005). Improving machine translation performance by exploiting non-parallel corpora. *Computational Linguistics*, *31*(4), 477–504. doi:10.1162/089120105775299168

Murali, T. M., Wu, C. J., & Kasif, S. (2006). The art of gene function prediction. *Nature Biotechnology*, *24*(12), 1474–1475. doi:10.1038/nbt1206-1474

Murphy, T., McIntosh, T., & Curran, J. (2006). *Named entity recognition for astronomy literature*. In Australasian Language Technology Workshop.

Mutton, P., & Golbeck, J. (2003). Visualization of semantic metadata and ontologies. In *INFOVIS 2003: Proc., 7th International Conference on information visualization* (pp. 300–305).

Myers, C. L., & Troyanskaya, O. G. (2007). Context-sensitive data integration and prediction of biological networks. *Bioinformatics (Oxford, England)*, *23*(17), 2322–2330. doi:10.1093/bioinformatics/btm332

Nabieva, E., Jim, K., Agarwal, A., Chazelle, B., & Singh, M. (2005). Whole proteome prediction of protein function via graph-theoretic analysis of interaction maps. *Bioinformatics (Oxford, England)*, *21*(1), i302–i310. doi:10.1093/bioinformatics/bti1054

Nadeau, D. (2007). *Semi-supervised named entity recognition: Learning to recognize 100 entity types with little supervision*. Unpublished PhD thesis.

Nagar, A., & Al-Mubaid, H. (2008). *A new path length measure based on GO for gene similarity with evaluation using sgd pathways*. In IEEE International Symposium on Computer-Based Medical Systems (pp. 590–595).

Nagypál, G., Deswarte, R., & Oosthoek, J. (2005). Applying the Semantic Web: The VICODI experience in creating visual contextualization for history. *Literary and Linguistic Computing*, *20*(3), 327–349. doi:10.1093/llc/fqi037

Nagypál, G. (2005). History ontology building: The technical view. In *Humanities, Computers and Cultural Heritage: Proceedings of the XVI International Conference of the Association for History and Computing, 14-17 September 2005* (pp. 207-214). Amsterdam, The Netherlands: Royal Netherlands Academy of Arts and Sciences.

Nagypál, G. (2007). *Possibly imperfect ontologies for effective information retrieval*. Unpublished doctoral dissertation, Universität Karlsruhe (TH), Karlsruhe, Germany.

Nakagawa, H., & Mori, T. (2002). A simple but powerful automatic term extraction method. In *Proceedings of the International Conference on Computational Linguistics (COLING)*.

Nanas, N., Uren, V., & de Roeck, A. (2003). *A comparative study of term weighting methods for information filtering*. KMi, (Technical report no. KMI-TR-128).

Navarro, B., Marcos, R., & Abad, P. (2005). *Semantic annotation and inter-annotators agreement in Cast3LB corpus*. In TLT 2005: 4th Workshop on Treebanks and Linguistic Theories.

Navarro, E., Sajous, F., Gaume, B., Prévot, L., Shu Kai, H., & Tzu-Yi, K. … Chu-Ren, H. (2009). Wiktionary and NLP: Improving synonymy networks. *Proceedings of the Workshop on the People's Web Meets NLP, ACL-IJCNLP*.

Nguyen, D. P. T., Matsuo, Y., & Ishizuka, M. (2007). *Exploiting syntactic and semantic information for relation extraction from Wikipedia*. In IJCAI07-TextlinkWS. Retrieved from http://citeseerx.ist.psu.edu/viewdoc/download?doi=10.1.1.73.9398&rep=rep1&type=pdf

Niepert, M., Buckner, C., & Allen, C. (2007). A dynamic ontology for a dynamic reference work. In *JCDL '07: Proceedings of the 7th ACM/IEEE-CS Joint Conference on digital libraries* (pp. 288–297). New York, NY: ACM.

Niepert, M., Buckner, C., & Allen, C. (2008). Answer set programming on expert feedback to populate and extend dynamic ontologies. In *Proceedings of the twenty-first international Florida artificial intelligence research society Conference, May 15-17, 2008, Coconut Grove, Florida, USA* (pp. 500-505).

Niepert, M., Buckner, C., & Allen, C. (2009). Working the crowd: Design principles and early lessons from the social- Semantic Web. In *Proceedings of the Workshop on Web 3.0: Merging Semantic Web and social Web at ACM Hypertext*.

Nikolov, A., Uren, V., Motta, E., & de Roeck, A. (2008). Integration of semantically annotated data by the KnoFuss architecture. In *EKAW 2008: Proc., 16th International Conference on Knowledge Engineering: Practice and Patterns* (pp. 265–274).

Nilsson, K., & Hjelm, H. (2009). Using semantic features derived from word-space models for Swedish coreference resolution. In *Proceedings of the 17th Nordic Conference of computational linguistics NODALIDA 2009* (pp. 134–141). Northern European Association for Language Technology (NEALT).

Nirenburg, S., & Raskin, V. (2004). *Ontological semantics*. Cambridge, MA: The MIT Press.

Nivre, J. (2005). *Dependency grammar and dependency parsing*. Last retrieved from http://stp.ling.uu.se/~nivre/docs/05133.pdf

Nothman, J., Curran, J., & Murphy, T. (2008). *Transforming Wikipedia into named entity training data*. In ALTA-08.

O'Hara, K., Alani, H., Kalfoglou, Y., & Shadbolt, N. (2004). Trust strategies for the Semantic Web. In *Proceedings of Workshop on Trust, Security, and Reputation on the Semantic Web, 3rd International Semantic Web Conference*, 2004.

Och, F. J., & Ney, H. (2003). A systematic comparison of various statistical alignment models. *Computational Linguistics, 29*(1), 19–51. doi:10.1162/089120103321337421

Och, F. J., & Ney, H. (2004). The alignment template approach to machine translation. *Computational Linguistics, 30*(4), 417–449. doi:10.1162/0891201042544884

Ohta, T., Tateisi, Y., Kim, J., Mima, H., & Tsuji, J. (2002). The GENIA corpus: An annotated research abstract corpus in molecular biology domain. *Proceedings of the Second International Conference on Human Language Technology Research* (pp. 82-86). Morgan Kaufmann Publishers Inc.

Olsson, F. (2008). Bootstrapping named entity annotation by means of active machine learning: A method for creating corpora. Unpublished PhD thesis.

Ore, C., & Eide, Ø. (2009). TEI and cultural heritage ontologies: Exchange of information? *Literary and Linguistic Computing, 24*(2), 161–172. doi:10.1093/llc/fqp010

Osborne, J. D., & Flatow, J. (2009). Annotating the human genome with disease ontology. *BMC Genomics, 10*(1), S6. doi:10.1186/1471-2164-10-S1-S6

Osinski, S. (2003). *An algorithm for clustering of Web search results*. Unpublished Master's thesis, Poznań University of Technology, Poland.

Othman, R., Deris, S., & Illias, R. (2008). A genetic similarity algorithm for searching the gene ontology terms and annotating anonymous protein sequences. *Journal of Biomedical Informatics, 41*(1), 65–81. doi:10.1016/j.jbi.2007.05.010

Prˇzulj, N., Wigle, D., & Jurisica, I. (2004). Functional topology in a network of protein interactions. *Bioinformatics (Oxford, England)*, *20*(3), 340–348. doi:10.1093/bioinformatics/btg415

Palla, G., Der'enyi, I., Farkas, I. J., & Vicsek, T. (2005). Uncovering the overlapping modular structure of protein interaction networks. *Nature*, *435*(7043), 814–818. doi:10.1038/nature03607

Palma, R., Haase, P., Corcho, O., Gómez-Pérez, A., & Ji, Q. (2008). An editorial workflow approach for collaborative ontology development. In *ASWC 2008: Proc., 3rd Asian Semantic Web Conference* (pp. 227–241).

Pantel, P., & Pennacchiotti, M. (2008). Automatically harvesting and ontologizing semantic relations. In Buitelaar, P., & Cimiano, P. (Eds.), *Ontology learning and population: Bridging the gap between text and knowledge* (pp. 171–195). IOS Press.

Pantel, P., & Lin, D. (2002). Discovering word senses from text. In *Proceedings of ACM SIGKDD Conference on Knowledge Discovery and Data Mining, 2002* (pp. 613-619). Edmonton, Canada.

Pantel, P., & Ravichandran, D. (2004). Automatically labeling semantic classes. In *Proceedings of Human Language Technology- North American Association for Computational Linguistics*, (pp. 321-328). ACL.

Park, Y., Byrd, R., & Boguraev, B. (2003). Towards ontologies on demand. *Proceedings of Workshop on Semantic Web Technologies for Scientific Search and Information Retrieval, In Conjunction with the 2nd International Semantic Web Conference.*

Parsons, L., Haque, E., & Liu, H. (2004). Subspace clustering for high dimensional data: A review. *ACM SIGKDD Explorations Newsletter*, *6*(1), 90–105. doi:10.1145/1007730.1007731

Pease, A., Niles, I., & Li, J. (2002). *The suggested upper merged ontology: A large ontology for the Semantic Web and its applications*. In Working Notes of the AAAI-2002 Workshop on Ontologies and the Semantic Web, (pp. 7-10). AAAI Press.

Peri, S., & Navarro, J. D. (2003). Development of human protein reference database as an initial platform for approaching systems biology in humans. *Genome Research*, *13*(10), 2363–2371. doi:10.1101/gr.1680803

Pesquita, C., Faria, D., Bastos, H., Ferreira, A. E., Falcão, A. O., & Couto, F. M. (2008). Metrics for GO based protein semantic similarity: A systematic evaluation. *BMC Bioinformatics*, *9*(5). doi:10.1186/1471-2105-9-S5-S4

Pesquita, C., Faria, D., Falcão, A. O., Lord, P., & Couto, F. M. (2009). Semantic similarity in biomedical ontologies. *PLoS Computational Biology*, *5*(7), e1000443. doi:10.1371/journal.pcbi.1000443

Petrelli, D., Dadzie, A. S., & Lanfranchi, V. (2009). Mediating between AI and highly specialized users. *AI Magazine*, *30*(4), 95–102.

Piperidis, S., & Harlas, I. (2006). Mining bilingual lexical equivalences out of parallel corpora. *Lecture Notes in Computer Science, Advances in Artificial Intelligence.*

Polikar, R. (2006). Ensemble based systems in decision making. *IEEE Circuits and Systems Magazine*, *6*(3), 21–45. doi:10.1109/MCAS.2006.1688199

Pollach, I., Scharl, A., & Weichselbraun, A. (2009). Web content mining for comparing corporate and third party online reporting: A case study on solid waste management. *Business Strategy and the Environment*, *18*(3), 137–148. doi:10.1002/bse.549

Porter, M. F. (1980). An algorithm for suffix stripping. *Program*, *14*(3), 130–137. Retrieved from http://dx.doi.org/10.1007/11880561\ 3

Power, D., et al. (2007). *The lands of the Normans in England (1204–1244): Technical background*. Retrieved August 6th, 2010, from http://www.hrionline.ac.uk/normans/technical.shtml

Qi, G., Haase, P., Huang, Z., Ji, Q., Pan, J. Z., & Völker, J. (2008). A kernel revision operator for terminologies - algorithms and evaluation. In *Proceedings of the International Semantic Web Conference*, (pp. 419-434). Springer-Verlag.

Rajagopala, S. V., & Titz, B. (2007). The protein network of bacterial motility. *Molecular Systems Biology*, *3*, 128. doi:10.1038/msb4100166

Ravasz, E., Somera, A. L., Mongru, D. A., Oltvai, Z. N., & Barabási, A. L. (2002). Hierarchical organization of modularity in metabolic networks. *Science, 297*(5586), 1551–1555. doi:10.1126/science.1073374

Resnik, P. (1999). Semantic similarity in a taxonomy: An information-based measure and its application to problems of ambiguity in natural language. *Journal of Artificial Intelligence Research, 11*(2), 95–130.

Resnik, P., & Smith, N. A. (2003). The Web as a parallel corpus. *Computational Linguistics, 29*(3), 349–380. doi:10.1162/089120103322711578

Resnik, P. (1995). Using information content to evaluate semantic similarity in a taxonomy. In *Proceedings of the 14th International joint Conference on artificial intelligence (ijcai-95)*. Retrieved from http://arxiv.org/pdf/cmp-lg/9511007

Riley, M., & Abe, T. (2006). Escherichia coli K-12: A cooperatively developed annotation snapshot–2005. *Nucleic Acids Research, 34*(1), 1–9. doi:10.1093/nar/gkj405

Riloff, E., & Jones, R. (1999). Learning dictionaries for information extraction by multi-level bootstrapping. *Proceedings of the sixteenth National Conference on Artificial intelligence and the eleventh Innovative applications of artificial intelligence conference innovative applications of artificial intelligence* (pp. 474-479). American Association for Artificial Intelligence.

Riva, P., Doerr, M., & Žumer, M. (2009). FRBRoo: Enabling a common view of information from cultural heritage institutions. *International Cataloguing and Bibliographic Control, 38*(2), 30–34.

Rives, A. W., & Galitski, T. (2003). Modular organization of cellular networks. *Proceedings of the National Academy of Sciences of the United States of America, 100*(3), 1128–1133. doi:10.1073/pnas.0237338100

Rizoiu, M. A., Velcin, J., & Chauchat, J. H. (2010). *Regrouper les donnèes textuelles et nommer les groupes à l'aide des classes recouvrantes*. In 10ème Conférence extraction et gestion des connaissances (egc 2010), hammamet, tunisie (Vol. E-19, p. 561-572).

Roberts, A., Gaizauskas, R., Hepple, M., & Guo, Y. (2008). Combining terminology resources and statistical methods for entity recognition: An evaluation. In *Proceedings of the Sixth International Conference on Language Resources and Evaluation (LREC 2008)*. European Language Resources Association (ELRA).

Roche, M. (2004). *Intégration de la construction de la terminologie de domaines spécialisés dans un processus global de fouille de textes*. Unpublished doctoral dissertation, Université de Paris 11. Thèse de Doctorat Université de Paris 11.

Rodrìguez, C. (2005). The ABC of model selection: AIC, BIC and the New CIC. *Bayesian Inference and Maximum Entropy Methods in Science and Engineering, 803*, 80–87.

Romanello, M., Berti, M., Boschetti, F., Babeu, A., & Crane, G. (2009). Rethinking critical editions of fragmentary texts by ontologies. In S. Mornati & T. Hedlund (Eds.), *Rethinking Electronic Publishing: Innovation in Communication Paradigms and Technologies: Proceedings of 13th International Conference on Electronic Publishing* (pp. 155-174). Milan, Italy: CILEA.

Ryu, P. M., & Choi, K. S. (2006). Taxonomy learning using term specificity and similarity. In *Proceedings from the Workshop on ontology learning and population: Bridging the gap between text and knowledge (with COLING/ACL 2006)* (pp. 41 – 48). Sydney, Australia.

Sag, I., Wasow, T., & Bender, E. (2003). *Syntactic theory: A formal introduction* (2nd ed.). CSLI.

Sager, J. (1994). *Language engineering and translation: Consequences of automation*. Amsterdam, The Netherlands: John Benjamins Publishing Company.

Saha, S., Sarkar, S., & Mitra, P. (2009). Feature selection techniques for maximum entropy based biomedical named entity recognition. *Journal of Biomedical Informatics, 42*(5), 905–911. doi:10.1016/j.jbi.2008.12.012

Salton, G., Wong, A., & Yang, C. S. (1975). A vector space model for information retrieval. *Communications of the ACM, 18*(11), 613–620. doi:10.1145/361219.361220

Salton, G., & Buckley, C. (1988). Term-weighting approaches in automatic text retrieval. *Information Processing & Management, 24*(5), 515–523. doi:10.1016/0306-4573(88)90021-0

Salton, G., Wong, A., & Yang, C. S. (1975). A vector space model for automatic indexing. *Communications of the ACM, 18*(11), 613–620. Retrieved from http://dx.doi.org/10.1145/361219.361220. doi:10.1145/361219.361220

Salton, G., & Lesk, M. E. (1968). Computer evaluation of indexing and text processing. *Journal of the ACM, 15*(1), 8–36. doi:10.1145/321439.321441

Sánchez-Alonso, S., & García, E. (2006). Making use of upper ontologies to foster interoperability between SKOS concept schemes. *Online Information Review, 30*(3), 263–277. doi:10.1108/14684520610675799

Sanderson, M., & Croft, W. B. (1999). *Deriving concept hierarchies from text* (pp. 206–213). In SIGIR.

Sanderson, M., & Croft, W. B. (1999). Deriving concept hierarchies from text. In *22nd Annual International ACM Sigir Conference on research and development in information retrieval* (pp. 206–213). Berkeley, CA.

Sarmento, L., Jijkoun, V., Rijke, M., & Oliveira, E. (2007). More like these: Growing entity classes from seeds. In *Proceedings of the sixteenth ACM Conference on information and knowledge management* (CIKM'07)

Schlicker, A., Domingues, F. S., Rahnenfuhrer, J., & Lengauer, T. (2006). A new measure for functional similarity of gene products based on gene ontology. *BMC Bioinformatics, 7*, 302. doi:10.1186/1471-2105-7-302

Schmitz, P. (2006). *Inducing ontology from flickr tags*. In Collaborative Web tagging workshop at WWW 2006. Edinburgh, Scotland.

Schreiber, G., Amin, A., Aroyo, L., van Assem, M., de Boer, V., & Hardman, L. (2008). Semantic annotation and search of cultural-heritage collections: The MultimediaN e-culture demonstrator. *Journal of Web Semantics, 6*(4), 243–249. doi:10.1016/j.websem.2008.08.001

Schwikowski, B., Uetz, P., & Fields, S. (2000). A network of protein–protein interactions in yeast. *Nature Biotechnology, 18*(12), 1257–1261. doi:10.1038/82360

Scott, S., & Matwin, S. (1999). Feature engineering for text classification. In *Proceedings of the 16th International Conference on Machine Learning* (pp. 379-388).

Sebastiani, F. (2002). Machine learning in automated text categorization. *ACM Computing Surveys, 34*(1), 1–47. doi:10.1145/505282.505283

Seco, N., Veale, T., & Hayes, J. (2004). An intrinsic information content metric for semantic similarity in wordnet. In *Proceedings of the 16th European Conference on artificial intelligence* (pp. 1089-1090). Valencia, Spain. Retrieved from http://eden.dei.uc.pt/~nseco/ecai2004b.pdf

Segal, E., Yelensky, R., & Koller, D. (2003). Genome-wide discovery of transcriptional modules from DNA sequence and gene expression. *Bioinformatics (Oxford, England), 19*(1), 1273–1282. doi:10.1093/bioinformatics/btg1038

Sekine, A., & Suzuki, H. (2007). *Acquiring ontological knowledge from query logs*. WWW 2007, May 8-12, 2007, Banf, Canada.

Sevilla, J. L., Segura, V., Podhorski, A., Guruceaga, E., Mato, J. M., & Martinez-Cruz, L. A. (2005). Correlation between gene expression and GO semantic similarity. *IEEE/ACM Transactions on Computational Biology and Bioinformatics, 2*(4), 330–338. doi:10.1109/TCBB.2005.50

Sheehan, B., Quigley, A., Gaudin, B., & Dobson, S. (2008). A relation based measure of semantic similarity for gene ontology annotations. *BMC Bioinformatics, 9*(1), 468. doi:10.1186/1471-2105-9-468

Shen, J., Zhang, J., Luo, X., Zhu, W., Yu, K., & Chen, K. … Jiang, H. (2007). Predicting protein-protein interactions based only on sequences information. *Proceedings of the National Academy of Sciences USA, 104*(11), 4337–41.

Shneiderman, B. (1992). Tree visualization with treemaps: 2-d space-filling approach. *ACM Transactions on Graphics, 11*(1), 92–99. doi:10.1145/102377.115768

Shneiderman, B., & Wattenberg, M. (2001, 06). *Ordered treemap layouts*. Retrieved on February 19, 2007, from ftp://ftp.cs.umd.edu/pub/hcil/Reports-Abstracts-Bibliography/2001-06html/2001-06.htm

Silva, J. da, Dias, G., Guilloré, S., & Pereira. (1999). Using localmaxs algorithm for the extraction of contiguous and non-contiguous multiword lexical units. *Progress in Artificial Intelligence, 849*. Retrieved from http://dx.doi.org/10.1007/3-540-48159-1\ 9

Simard, M., & Plamondon, P. (1998). Bilingual sentence alignment: Balancing robustness and accuracy. *Machine Translation, 13*(1), 59–80. doi:10.1023/A:1008010319408

Simard, M. (1999). Text-translation alignment: Three languages are better than two. In *Proceedings of the 1999 Joint SIGDAT Conference on empirical methods in natural language processing and very large corpora* (pp. 2–11).

Smadja, F. A. (1991). From n-grams to collocations: An evaluation of xtract. In *Proceedings of the 29th Annual Meeting on association for computational linguistics* (pp. 279–284). Morristown, NJ: Association for Computational Linguistics.

Snow, R., Jurafsky, D., & Ng, A. Y. (2004). Learning syntactic patterns for automatic hypernym discovery. *Advances in Neural Information Processing Systems, 17*, 1297–1304.

Snow, R., Jurafsky, D., & Ng, A. Y. (2006). Semantic taxonomy induction from heterogeneous evidence. In *Proceedings of COLING/ACL 2006.* Sydney, Australia.

Spärck Jones, K. (1972). A statistical interpretation of term specificity and its application in retrieval. *The Journal of Documentation, 28*(1), 11–21. doi:10.1108/eb026526

Specia, L., & Motta, E. (2007). *Integrating folksonomies with the Semantic Web.* In The Semantic Web: Research and applications, 4th European Semantic Web Conference (eswc-2007) (Vol. 4519, p. 624-639). Berlin, Germany: Springer.

Spiliopoulos, V., Kotis, K., & Vouros, G. A. (2008). Semantic retrieval and ranking of SW documents using free-form queries. *International Journal of Metadata. Semantics and Ontologies, 3*(2), 95–108. doi:10.1504/IJMSO.2008.021888

Srihari, R., & Peterson, E. (2008). Named entity recognition for improving retrieval and translation of Chinese documents. In *Proceedings of the 11th International Conference on Asian Digital Libraries: Universal and Ubiquitous Access to Information* (pp. 404-405). Springer-Verlag.

Staab, S., Studer, R., Schnurr, H.-P., & Sure, Y. (2001). Knowledge processes and ontologies. *IEEE Intelligent Systems, 16*(1), 26–34. doi:10.1109/5254.912382

Steedman, M. (2001). *The syntactic process.* MIT Press.

Steinbach, M., Karypis, G., & Kumar, V. (2000). *A comparison of document clustering techniques.*

Steinberger, R., Pouliquen, B., Widiger, A., Ignat, C., Erjavec, T., & Tufis, D. (2006). The JRC-Acquis: A multilingual aligned parallel corpus with 20+ languages. In *Proceedings of the 5th international Conference on language resources and evaluation (LREC'2006).* Genoa, Italy.

Stevenson, M., & Greenwood, M. A. (2009). Dependency pattern models for information extraction. [Springer]. *Journal of Research on Language & Computation, 7*(1), 13–39. doi:10.1007/s11168-009-9061-2

Steyvers, M., & Griffiths, T. (2005). Probabilistic topic models. In T. Landauer, D. Mcnamara, S. Dennis, & W. Kintsch (Eds.), *Latent semantic analysis: A road to meaning.* Laurence Erlbaum.

Strube, M., & Ponzetto, S. (2006). WikiRelate! Computing semantic relatedness using Wikipedia. *Proceedings of the 21st National Conference on Artificial intelligence,* vol. 2 (pp. 1419-1424). AAAI Press.

Studer, R. R., Benjamins, R., & Fensel, D. (1998). Knowledge engineering: Principles and methods. *Data & Knowledge Engineering, 25*(1-2), 161–197. doi:10.1016/S0169-023X(97)00056-6

Sudo, K., Sekine, S., & Grishman, R. (2001). Automatic pattern acquisition for Japanese information extraction. In *Proceedings of the Human Language Technology,* (pp. 1-7). ACL.

Sudo, K., Sekine, S., & Grishman, R. (2003). An improved extraction pattern representation model for automatic IE pattern acquisition. In *Proceedings of the 41st Annual Meeting of the Association for Computational Linguistics (ACL-03),* Sapporo, Japan, (pp. 224–231).

Sun, Y. (2003). Determinants of foreign patents in China. *World Patent Information, 25*, 27–37. doi:10.1016/S0172-2190(02)00086-8

Tanay, A., Sharan, R., Kupiec, M., & Shamir, R. (2004). Revealing modularity and organization in the yeast molecular network by integrated analysis of highly heterogeneous genomewide data. *Proceedings of the National Academy of Sciences of the United States of America, 101*(9), 2981–2986. doi:10.1073/pnas.0308661100

Tang, J., Leung, H. F., Luo, Q., Chen, D., & Gong, J. (2009). Towards ontology learning from folksonomies. In *Ijcai'09: Proceedings of the 21st International Joint Conference on Artifical Intelligence* (pp. 2089–2094). San Francisco, CA, USA: Morgan Kaufmann Publishers Inc.

Tao, Y., Sam, L., Li, J., Friedman, C., & Lussier, Y. A. (2007). Information theory applied to the sparse gene ontology annotation network to predict novel gene function. *Bioinformatics (Oxford, England), 23*(13), i529–i538. doi:10.1093/bioinformatics/btm195

Tempich, C., Pinto, H. S., & Staab, S. (2006). Ontology engineering revisited: An iterative case study. In Y. Sure & J. Domingue (Eds.), *ESWC 2006: The Semantic Web: Research and Applications, Proc., 3rd European Semantic Web Conference* (pp. 110–124).

Thanopoulos, A. N., Fakotakis, N., & Kokkinakis, G. (2002). Comparative evaluation of collocation extraction metrics. In *Proceedings of the 3rd language resources evaluation Conference* (pp. 620–625).

Tho, Q. T., Hui, S. C., Fong, A. C. M., & Tru Hoang, C. (2006). Automatic fuzzy ontology generation for Semantic Web. *IEEE Transactions on Knowledge and Data Engineering, 18*(6), 842–856. doi:10.1109/TKDE.2006.87

Tiedemann, J. (2003). *Recycling translations: Extraction of lexical data from parallel corpora and their application in natural language processing*. Unpublished doctoral dissertation, Uppsala University, Uppsala, Sweden.

Toral, A., & Muñoz, R. (2006). A proposal to automatically build and maintain gazetteers for named entity recognition by using Wikipedia. *In Proceedings of the Workshop on NEW TEXT Wikis and blogs and other dynamic text sources in the 11th EACL.*

Toutanova, K., Klein, D., Manning, C., & Singer, Y. (2003). Feature-rich part-of-speech tagging with a cyclic dependency network. In. *Proceedings of HLT-NAACL, 2003*, 252–259.

Toutanova, K., & Manning, C. D. (2000). Enriching the knowledge sources used in a maximum entropy part-of-speech tagger. In *Proceedings of the Joint SIGDAT Conference on Empirical Methods in Natural Language Processing and Very Large Corpora (EMNLP/VLC-2000)*, (pp. 63-70).

Troyanskaya, O. G., Dolinski, K., Owen, A. B., Altman, R. B., & Botstein, D. (2003). A Bayesian framework for combining heterogeneous data sources for gene function prediction in Saccharomyces cerevisiae. *Proceedings of the National Academy of Sciences of the United States of America, 100*(14), 8348–8353. doi:10.1073/pnas.0832373100

Tsuda, K., Shin, H., & Schölkopf, B. (2005). Fast protein classification with multiple networks. *Bioinformatics (Oxford, England), 21*(2), ii59–ii65. doi:10.1093/bioinformatics/bti1110

Turcato, D., Popowich, F., Toole, J., Fass, D., Nicholson, D., & Tisher, G. (2000). Adapting a synonym database to specific domains. In *Proceedings of the ACL-2000 Workshop on recent advances in natural language processing and information retrieval* (pp. 1–11). Morristown, NJ: Association for Computational Linguistics.

Turdakov, D., & Velikhov, P. (2008). *Semantic relatedness metric for Wikipedia concepts based on link analysis and its application to word sense disambiguation*. In Colloquium on Databases and Information Systems (SYRCoDIS).

Turney, P. D. (2001). Mining the Web for synonyms: Pmi-ir versus lsa on toefl. In *Proceedings of EMCL* (pp. 491–502).

Utiyama, M., & Isahara, H. (2003). Reliable measures for aligning Japanese-English news articles and sentences. In *Proceedings of the Annual Meeting of the Association of Computational Linguistics (ACL)*. (pp. 72–79).

Utiyama, M., & Isahara, H. (2007). A Japanese-English patent parallel corpus. In *Proceeding of MT Summit XI*. (pp. 475–482).

van der Plas, L., & Tiedemann, J. (2006). Finding synonyms using automatic word alignment and measures of distributional similarity. In *Proceedings of Coling* (pp. 866–873).

van der Plas, L., & Tiedemann, J. (2006). Finding synonyms using automatic word alignment and measures of distributional similarity. In *Proceedings of COLING/ACL 2006*. Sydney, Australia.

VanRijsbergen, C. J. (1979). *Information retrieval*. London, UK: Butterworths.

Varga, D., Halacsy, P., Kornai, A., Nagy, V., Nemeth, L., & Tron, V. (2005). Parallel corpora for medium density languages. In *Proceedings of RANLP 2005 Conference.*

Vazquez, A., Flammini, A., Maritan, A., & Vespignani, A. (2003). Global protein function prediction from protein–protein interaction networks. *Nature Biotechnology, 21*(6), 697–700. doi:10.1038/nbt825

Velardi, P., Cucchiarelli, A., & Petit, M. (2007). A taxonomy learning method and its application to characterize a scientific Web community. *IEEE Transactions on Knowledge and Data Engineering, 19*(2), 180–191. doi:10.1109/TKDE.2007.21

Velcin, J., & Ganascia, J. G. (2007). *Topic extraction with agape* (pp. 377–388). In ADMA.

Veltman, K. H. (2004). Towards a Semantic Web for culture. *JoDI: Journal of Digital Information, 4*(4). Retrieved March 10, 2010, from http://jodi.ecs.soton.ac.uk/Articles/v04/i04/Veltman/

Vervenne, D. (1999). Advanced document management through thesaurus-based indexing: The IKEM platform. *CWI Quarterly, 12*(2), 159–172.

Vieira, J. M., & Ciula, A. (2007). *Implementing an RDF/OWL ontology on Henry the III Fine Rolls.* Paper presented at OWLED 2007, Innsbruck, Austria. Retrieved March 10, 2010, from http://www.webont.org/owled/2007/PapersPDF/submission_6.pdf

Vintar, Š. (2001). *Using parallel corpora for translation-oriented term extraction. Babel Journal.* John Benjamins Publishing.

Volk, M., & Buitelaar, P. (2002). A systematic evaluation of concept-based cross-language information retrieval in the medical domain. In *Proc. of 3rd Dutch-Belgian information retrieval Workshop.* Leuven, Holland.

Von Mering, C., Huynen, M., Jaeggi, D., Schmidt, S., Bork, P., & Snel, B. (2003). STRING: A database of predicted functional associations between proteins. *Nucleic Acids Research, 31*(1), 258–261. doi:10.1093/nar/gkg034

Vouros, G., Kotis, K., Chalkiopoulos, C., & Lelli, N. (2007). *The HCOME-3O framework for supporting the collaborative engineering of evolving ontologies.* ESOE 2007 International Workshop on Emergent Semantics and Ontology Evolution, ISWC 2007.

Wan, X. (2008). Using bilingual knowledge and ensemble techniques for unsupervised Chinese sentiment analysis. In *Proceeding of EMNLP2008.* (pp. 553-561).

Wang, W., Barnaghi, P., & Bargiela, A. (2009). Probabilistic topic models for learning terminological ontologies. *IEEE Transactions on Knowledge and Data Engineering, 99.*

Wang, J. Z., Du, Z., Payattakool, R., Yu, P. S., & Chen, C. F. (2007). A new method to measure the semantic similarity of GO terms. *Bioinformatics (Oxford, England), 23*(10), 1274–1281. doi:10.1093/bioinformatics/btm087

Wang, J. Z., Du, Z., Payattakool, R., Yu, P. S., & Chen, C. F. (2007). A new method to measure the semantic similarity of GO terms. *Bioinformatics (Oxford, England), 23*(10), 1274–1281. doi:10.1093/bioinformatics/btm087

Wang, W., May, J., Knight, K., & Marcu, D. (2010). Restructuring, re-labeling, and re-aligning for syntax-based statistical machine translation. *Computational Linguistics, 36*(2). doi:10.1162/coli.2010.36.2.09054

Wang, C., & Blei, D. (2009). *Variational inference for the Nested Chinese Restaurant Process.*

Wang, C., Blei, D., & Heckerman, D. (2008). *Continuous time dynamic topic models.* In The 23rd Conference on uncertainty in artificial intelligence.

Wang, C., Collins, M., & Andkoehn, P. (2007). Chinese syntactic reordering for statistical machine translation. In *Proceedings of EMNLP-CoNLL.* (pp. 737-745).

Wang, X., McCallum, A., & Wei, X. (2007). Topical n-grams: Phrase and topic discovery, with an application to information retrieval. In *Proceedings of the 7th IEEE International Conference on data mining* (pp. 697–702).

Weale, T., Brew, C., & Fosler-Lussier, E. (2009). Using the Wiktionary graph structure for synonym detection. *Proceedings of the Workshop on the People's Web Meets NLP, ACL-IJCNLP.*

Weber, N., & Buitelaar, P. (2006). Web-based ontology learning with ISOLDE. In *Proceedings of the Workshop on Web Content Mining with Human Language, International Semantic Web Conference (ISWC).*

Weber, R., Schek, H., & Blott, S. (1998). A quantitative analysis and performance study for similarity-search methods in high-dimensional spaces. In *Proceedings of the 24rd international Conference on Very Large Databases* (pp.194-205).

Weichselbraun, A., Wohlgenannt, G., & Scharl, A. (2010). Refining non-taxonomic relation labels with external structured data to support ontology learning. *Data & Knowledge Engineering, 69*(8), 763–778. doi:10.1016/j.datak.2010.02.010

Weiner, J. M. (2005). Differences in indexing term vocabularies and agreement with subject specialists. *Electronic Journal of Academic and Special Librarianship, 6*(1-2). Retrieved from http://southernlibrarianship.icaap.org/content/v06n01/weiner j01.htm

Wenger, E. (2004). Knowledge management is a donut: Shaping your knowledge strategy with communities of practice. *Ivey Business Journal, 68*(3), 1–8.

Wilks, Y. (2008). The Semantic Web: Apotheosis of annotation, but what are its semantics? *IEEE Intelligent Systems, 23*(3), 41–49. doi:10.1109/MIS.2008.53

Wilks, Y., & Brewster, C. (2009). Natural language processing as a foundation of the Semantic Web. [Now Publishers Inc.]. *Foundations and Trends in Web Science, 1*(3-4), 199–327.

Witschel, H. F. (2005). Using decision trees and text mining techniques for extending taxonomies. In *Proceedings of the Workshop on learning and extending lexical ontologies by using machine learning methods.*

Wodak, S. J., & Mendez, R. (2004). Prediction of protein-protein interactions: The CAPRI experiment, its evaluation and implications. *Current Opinion in Structural Biology, 14*(2), 242–249. doi:10.1016/j.sbi.2004.02.003

Wong, W., Liu, W., & Bennamoun, M. (2007). Tree-traversing ant algorithm for term clustering based on featureless similarities. *Data Mining and Knowledge Discovery, 15*(3), 349–381. doi:10.1007/s10618-007-0073-y

Wong, W., Liu, W., & Bennamoun, M. (2008). *Determination of unithood and termhood for term recognition. Handbook of research on text and Web mining technologies.* Hershey, PA: IGI Global.

Wong, W., Liu, W., & Bennamoun, M. (2009). A probabilistic framework for automatic term recognition. *Intelligent Data Analysis, 13*(4), 499–539.

Wong, W., Liu, W., & Bennamoun, M. (2008). Determination of unithood and termhood for term recognition. In Song, M., & Wu, Y. (Eds.), *Handbook of research on text and Web mining technologies.* Hershey, PA: IGI Global. doi:10.4018/9781599049908.ch030

Wong, W. Y. (2009). *Learning lightweight ontologies from text across different domains using the Web as background knowledge.* Unpublished doctoral dissertation, University of Western Australia, Australia.

Wong, W., Liu, W., & Bennamoun, M. (2010). Constructing specialised corpora through domain representativeness analysis of websites. *Language Resources and Evaluation.*

Wu, X., Zhu, L., Guo, J., Zhang, D. Y., & Lin, K. (2006). Prediction of yeast protein-protein interaction network: Insights from the gene ontology and annotations. *Nucleic Acids Research, 34*(7), 2137–2150. doi:10.1093/nar/gkl219

Wu, D., & Fung, P. (2005). Inversion transduction grammar constraints for mining parallel sentences from quasi-comparable corpora. In *Proceedings of IJCNLP2005.*

Wu, D., & Xia, X. (1994). Learning an English-Chinese lexicon from a parallel corpus. In *Proceedings of the First Conference of the Association for Machine Translation in the Americas.*

Wu, H., & Zhou, M. (2003). Optimizing synonym extraction using monolingual and bilingual resources. In *Proceedings of the Second International Workshop on paraphrasing* (pp. 72–79).

Xenarios, I., Salwinski, L., Duan, X. J., Higney, P., Kim, S. M., & Eisenberg, D. (2002). DIP, the database of interacting proteins: A research tool for studying cellular networks of protein interactions. *Nucleic Acids Research, 30*(1), 303–305. doi:10.1093/nar/30.1.303

Xia, L., & Iria, J. (2008). An approach to modeling heterogeneous resources for information extraction. In *LREC'08: Proc., 6th International Conference on Language Resources and Evaluation* (pp. 2768–2772).

Xu, T., Du, L., & Zhou, Y. (2008). Evaluation of go-based functional similarity measures using s. cerevisiae protein interaction and expression profile data. *BMC Bioinformatics, 9*(1), 472. doi:10.1186/1471-2105-9-472

Yangarber, R. (2003). Counter-training in the discovery of semantic patterns. In *Proceedings of the 41st Annual Meeting of the Association for Computational Linguistics (ACL-03)*, (pp. 343–350). ACL.

Yates, F. (1934). Contingency table involving small numbers and the χ^2 test. *Supplement to the Journal of the Royal Statistical Society, 1*(2), 217–235. doi:10.2307/2983604

Yeh, J., & Yang, N. (2008). Ontology construction based on latent topic extraction in a digital library. *Digital Libraries: Universal and Ubiquitous Access to Information*, 93–103.

Yon Rhee, S., Wood, V., Dolinski, K., & Draghici, S. (2008). Use and misuse of the gene ontology annotations. *Nature Reviews. Genetics, 9*(7), 509–515. doi:10.1038/nrg2363

Yu, H., Braun, P., Yildirim, M. A., Lemmens, I., Venkatesan, K., & Sahalie, J. (2008). High-quality binary protein interaction map of the yeast interactome network. *Science, 322*(5898), 104–110. doi:10.1126/science.1158684

Yu, K., & Tsujii, J. (2009). Bilingual dictionary extraction from Wikipedia. In *Proceedings of Machine Learning Summit XII.*

Zablith, F., Sabou, M., d'Aquin, M., & Motta, E. (2008). *Using background knowledge for ontology evolution.* In International Workshop on Ontology Dynamics (IWOD) at the International Semantic Web Conference (ISWC 2008).

Zanzoni, A., Montecchi-Palazzi, L., Quondam, M., Ausiello, G., Helmer-Citterich, M., & Cesareni, G. (2002). MINT: a Molecular INTeraction database. *FEBS Letters, 513*(1), 135–140. doi:10.1016/S0014-5793(01)03293-8

Zavitsanos, E., Paliouras, G., Vouros, G. A., & Petridis, S. (2007). Discovering subsumption hierarchies of ontology concepts from text corpora. In *Wi '07: Proceedings of the IEEE/WIC/ACM International Conference on Web intelligence* (pp. 402–408). Washington, DC: IEEE Computer Society.

Zesch, T., & Gurevych, I. (2007). Analysis of the Wikipedia category graph for NLP applications. *Proceedings of the TextGraphs-2 Workshop (NAACL-HLT).*

Zesch, T., Müller, C., & Gurevych, I. (2008). Using Wiktionary for computing semantic relatedness. *Proceedings of the 23rd National Conference on Artificial intelligence* (pp. 861-866). AAAI Press.

Zhang, B., & Horvath, S. (2005). A general framework for weighted gene co-expression network analysis. *Statistical Applications in Genetics and Molecular Biology, 4*, 17. doi:10.2202/1544-6115.1128

Zhang, J., Xiong, M., & Yu, Y. (2006). *Mining query log to assist ontology learning from relational database. (LNCS 3841)* (pp. 437–448). Springer – Verlag.

Zhang, Z., & Iria, J. (2009). A novel approach to automatic gazetteer generation using Wikipedia. In *Proceedings of the ACL'09 Workshop on Collaboratively Constructed Semantic Resources*, Singapore, August 2009.

Zhang, Z., Iria, J., Brewster, C., & Ciravegna, F. (2008). A comparative evaluation of term recognition algorithms. *Proceedings of the Sixth International Language Resources and Evaluation*, (pp. 2108-2113). ELRA.

Zhang, Z., Xia, L., Greenwood, M. A., & Iria, J. (2009). Too many mammals: Improving the diversity of automatically recognized terms. In *RANLP '09: Proc., International Conference on Recent Advances in Natural Language Processing.*

Zhao, X. M., Chen, L. N., & Aihara, K. (2007). Gene function prediction with the shortest path in functional linkage graph. *Lect Notes Oper Res, 7*, 68–74.

Zhao, X. M., Wang, Y., Chen, L. N., & Aihara, K. (2008). Gene function prediction using labeled and unlabeled data. *BMC Bioinformatics, 9*, 57. doi:10.1186/1471-2105-9-57

Zhao, J., & Huang, C. N. (1999). The model for Chinese baseNP structure analysis. *Chinese Journal of Computer, 22*(2), 141–146.

Zhao, B., & Vogel, S. (2002). Adaptive parallel sentences mining from Web bilingual news collection. In *Proceedings of Second IEEE International Conference on Data Mining (ICDM'02).*

Zhao, T., Yang, M., Liu, F., Yao, J., & Yu, H. (2000). Statistics based hybrid approach to Chinese base phrase identification. In *Proceedings of the Second Workshop on Chinese Language Processing*. (pp. 73-77).

Zhou, X. J., Kao, M. C., Huang, H., Wong, A., Nunez-Iglesias, J., & Primig, M. (2005). Functional annotation and network reconstruction through cross-platform integration of microarray data. *Nature Biotechnology, 23*(2), 238–243. doi:10.1038/nbt1058

Zhou, L. (2007). Ontology learning: State of the art and open issues. *Information Technology Management, 8*, 241–252. doi:10.1007/s10799-007-0019-5

Zhou, L. (2007). Ontology learning: State of the art and open issues. *Information Technology Management, 8*(3), 241–252. doi:10.1007/s10799-007-0019-5

Zhu, Q., Inkpen, D., & Asudeh, A. (2007). Automatic extraction of translations from Web-based bilingual materials. *Machine Translation, 2*.

Zöllner-Weber, A. (2010). *Text encoding and ontology – enlarging an ontology by semi-automatic generated instances*. Paper presented at Digital Humanities 2010. Retrieved August 5, 2010, from http://dh2010.cch.kcl.ac.uk/academic-programme/abstracts/papers/pdf/ab-643.pdf

Zouaq, A., Gagnon, M., & Ozell, B. (2010). Semantic analysis using dependency-based grammars and upper-level ontologies. [Bahri Publications.]. *International Journal of Computational Linguistics and Applications, 1*(1-2), 85–101.

Zouaq, A., & Nkambou, R. (2009). Evaluating the generation of domain ontologies in the Knowledge Puzzle Project. *IEEE Transactions on Knowledge and Data Engineering, 21*(11), 1559–1572. doi:10.1109/TKDE.2009.25

Zouaq, A. (2008). *An ontological engineering approach for the acquisition and exploitation of knowledge in texts*. PhD Thesis, University of Montreal (in French).

Zunde, P., & Dexter, M. E. (1969). Indexing consistency and quality. *American Documentation, 20*(3), 259–267. doi:10.1002/asi.4630200313

About the Contributors

Wilson Wong is a Postdoctoral Research Associate at the University of Western Australia (UWA) working on the application of text mining and natural language processing across different domains such as healthcare. Wilson was an Endeavour IPRS Scholar for his PhD study at UWA. His doctoral dissertation investigates the use of Web data for automatically acquiring knowledge from natural language texts across different domains. Wilson also has a BIT (First Class Honours) (Data Communications) degree, and an MSc (Information and Communication Technology) by research degree in the field of natural language processing from Malaysia. Wilson has close to 30 publications in book chapters, reputable conferences (e.g. IJCNLP, IJCAI, PACLING), and high-impact journals (e.g. DMKD, IDA). His areas of interest include text mining, natural language processing, Web technologies, and health informatics.

Wei Liu is an Assistant Professor at the University of Western Australia, and currently the Lab Coordinator for Adaptive System Group. She obtained her PhD from the University of Newcastle on Multi-Agent Belief Revision, Australia in 2003. Her current research interest is on ontology learning to bootstrap agent knowledge base. Dr. Wei Liu's research strength lies in ontology learning and data-driven ontology change. She leads the work on developing automatic and semi-automatic ontology learning system from 2004, which addresses the cold-start issues (labour intensive and time consuming) of manual ontology engineering. The research contributes significantly to the investigation of emergent semantics through text mining. The first paper reporting the techniques and the system modules won one of the best papers in the conference and was invited for journal publication. The techniques developed including co-occurrence analysis to identify taxonomic and non-taxonomic relations, and spreading activation to identify the core, extended, and peripheral concepts. Information network analysis and clustering algorithms are also developed to measure the evolution of an ontology in both temporal and spatial scope.

Mohammed Bennamoun received his PhD from Queen's University, Canada/Queensland University of Technology (QUT), Australia in the area of Computer Vision. He has been a full Professor and the Head of the School of Computer Science and Software Engineering (CSSE) at the University of Western Australia (UWA) since 2007. Prior to this, he was an Associate Professor at CSSE, a Senior Lecturer at QUT, and a Lecturer at Queen's. He was an Erasmus Mundus Scholar at the University of Edinburgh in 2006. He was also a Visiting Professor at several other institutions including CNRS (Centre National de la Recherche Scientifique), Telecom Lille1, Helsinki University of Technology, University of Bourgogne and University of Paris 13. He is the co-author of the book "Object Recognition: Fundamentals and Case Studies" published by Springer-Verlag. He published over 140 journal and conference publications, and served as a guest editor for several special issues in international journals. His areas of interest include control theory, robotics, obstacle avoidance, object recognition, artificial neural networks, signal/image processing, and computer vision, and lately, in the development of tools for combining text and image analysis.

* * *

Marco Alvarez is a PhD Student in Computer Science at Utah State University. Previously, Mr. Alvarez earned a BSc degree in Computer Science at the Federal University of Mato Grosso do Sul, Brazil and a MSc Degree in Computer Science at the University of Sao Paulo, Brazil. From 1999 to 2004, Mr. Alvarez was a full-time professor at the Dom Bosco Catholic University, Brazil. His main research interests include machine learning, computer vision, bioinformatics, and computing education.

Andrzej Bargiela is Professor and Director of Computer Science at the University of Nottingham, Malaysia Campus. He is member of the Automated Scheduling and Planning research group in the School of Computer Science at the University of Nottingham. Since 1978, he has pursued research focused on processing of uncertainty in the context of modelling and simulation of various physical and engineering systems. His current research falls under the general heading of computational intelligence and involves mathematical modelling, information abstraction, parallel computing, artificial intelligence, fuzzy sets, and neurocomputing.

Payam Barnaghi is a researcher in the Centre for Communication Systems Research (CCSR) at the University of Surrey. He completed his PhD in Computer Science at the University of Malaya in September 2007. His current research interests include Semantic Web, ontologies, machine learning, semantic sensor networks, Semantic Web services, and information search and retrieval.

Toby Burrows is an Honorary Research Fellow in the School of Humanities at the University of Western Australia. Between 2005 and 2010, he was the Digital Services Director for the Australian Research Council's Network for Early European Research (NEER). He also manages the Scholars' Centre in the University of Western Australia Library. He has a PhD in medieval history and professional qualifications in library science, and has held visiting fellowships at University College London, Churchill College (University of Cambridge), and the Vrije Universiteit in Amsterdam. His research has been funded by the Australian Research Council, the Australian Academy of the Humanities, and the European Science Foundation.

Fabio Ciravegna is Full Professor of Language and Knowledge Technologies at the University of Sheffield where he coordinates the Organisations, Information and Knowledge (OAK) Group. His research field concerns methodologies and technologies for the Intelligent and Semantic Web, with focus on knowledge management applications. He has considerable engagement with industry and user communities with projects funded by Rolls Royce, Kodak Eastman, Lycos, and the Environment Agency. He is part of the editorial board of the International Journal on Web Semantics and of the International Journal of Human Computer Studies. He is director of research of K-Now, a spin-off company of the University of Sheffield focusing on supporting dynamic distributed communities in large organizations. He holds a PhD from the University of East Anglia and a doctorship from the University of Torino, Italy.

Aba-Sah Dadzie is a research associate working with the OAK (Organisations, Information and Knowledge) Group at the Department of Computer Science, the University of Sheffield. She does research in human-computer interaction and visual analytics, with a focus on applications for knowledge management using Semantic Web technology. She currently works on the SmartProducts project, before which she coordinated a major industrial use case in X-Media. She also worked on the IPAS and XS-PAN projects. She holds a PhD in Computer Science from Heriot-Watt University, Edinburgh, Scotland, where she applied information visualisation to data analysis in bioinformatics. She has also worked in management in the manufacturing industry and in a research laboratory in the banking sector.

Kai Eckert is a PhD student at the Mannheim University in the group of Heiner Stuckenschmidt. He holds two Master degrees from the University of Mannheim, one in computer science, one in business informatics. His research is focused on the semi-automatic construction and maintenance of concept hierarchies, like thesauri, and on the evaluation of thesauri in retrieval settings.

Andrew Emili is a Full Professor in the Banting and Best Department of Medical Research, the Donnelly Centre for Cellular and Biomolecular Research (CCBR), and the Department of Molecular Genetics at the University of Toronto. Dr. Emili is an expert in molecular biology, functional genomics, and proteomics. Before joining the University of Toronto in 2000, Dr. Emili pursued post-doctoral studies with Dr. Leland Hartwell, noted geneticist and Nobel laureate (2001) and Dr. John Yates III, a pioneer in protein mass spectrometry. His Toronto research group uses multi-disciplinary technologies to investigate the biological roles and global proprieties of proteins and genes in diverse model organisms such as yeast, E. coli, mouse, and in human cells. The goals are to understand how cells and tissues function at a system's level, and to translate this knowledge into novel diagnostics and therapeutics.

Hans Hjelm is working in the Language Technology field at Swedish Internet company alaTest. He has a PhD in Computational Linguistics from Stockholm University, on the topic of multilinguality and ontology learning. He has worked as a guest researcher at the German Research Center for Artificial Intelligence in Saarbrücken and is an alumnus in the Swedish Graduate School of Language Technology. He has worked as a consultant for several European Language Technology companies, and his current research interests lie in distributional semantics and record linkage.

Pingzhao Hu is a PhD candidate in Machine-Learning at York University. His education background is in statistics and computer science. Being an active molecular biostatistician, he has worked on different genomic data analysis projects for over six years. He collaborates extensively with Emili laboratory, and his current main research interest is in developing computational methods for integrating molecular interaction networks as a means for predicting gene function.

Hui Jiang received the BEng and MEng degrees from the University of Science and Technology of China, and his PhD degree from the University of Tokyo, Japan, all in electrical engineering. From 1999 to 2000, he was with the Department of Electrical and Computer Engineering, University of Waterloo, Canada, as a postdoctoral fellow. From 2000 to 2002, he worked at Lucent Technologies Inc., Murray Hill, New Jersey. He joined the Department of Computer Science and Engineering, York University, Toronto, Canada, as assistant professor in 2002 and was promoted to associate professor in 2007. His current research interests include speech/audio/language processing, bioinformatics, machine learning, and statistical data modeling. He is a Member of the IEEE and has served as an associate editor for IEEE Transactions on Audio, Speech, and Language Processing since 2009.

Tao Jiang received his ME in computer science from Northeastern University, P.R. China in 2007. He is currently a research assistant in ChiLin Star Corporation, Zhuhai, P.R. China. His research interests are in natural language processing, especially statistical machine translation.

Konstantinos Kotis was born in 1973 in Samos, Greece. He graduated from the Computation Department at the University of Manchester (UMIST), UK in 1995. He has obtained his PhD in Knowledge Management and Representation from the Department of Information and Communication Systems Eng. at the University of Aegean. He has worked as post-doc researcher at Ai-Lab, Dept. of Information and Communication Systems Eng. University of the Aegean (2005-2006), where he has also worked as a researcher since 2006. He is a member of the Hellenic Artificial Intelligence Society and reviewer in several international journals and conferences. He has authored more than 40 publications related to Semantic Web technologies, ontology engineering, Semantic Web services, and Grid.

Oiyee Kwong received her PhD from the Computer Laboratory of the University of Cambridge, with a doctoral thesis on automatic word sense disambiguation. She is currently an assistant professor in the Department of Chinese, Translation, and Linguistics of the City University of Hong Kong. Her research interests are in natural language processing and corpus linguistics, in particular word sense disambiguation, lexical semantics, computational lexicography, language resources, and Chinese language processing. Her current research projects focus on various areas, including a computational lexicon based on the intrinsic nature of word senses, personal name transliteration, and computational analysis of children's stories. In recent years, she has also been actively involved in the organisation of many international conferences in the field.

Bin Lu received an MS in Computer Science from Peking University in 2007. He is currently a PhD candidate at the Department of Chinese, Translation, and Linguistics, City University of Hong Kong. He has published more than 20 academic papers in the area of natural language processing and computational linguistics, and holds two China patents. His research focuses on statistical machine translation, especially in the patent domain, as well as sentiment analysis and opinion mining.

Louis Massey is an Assistant Professor in the department of Computer Science at the Royal Military College of Canada. Before joining academia, he was a software engineer and project manager for the Canadian Air Force. Dr. Massey's current research interests in adaptable and autonomous real-world textual information management systems.

Robert Meusel is a PhD student at the University of Mannheim in the group of Heiner Stuckenschmidt. He holds a Master degree from the University of Mannheim in business informatics. His research is focused on semantic data structures for social networks and Web 2.0 platforms, as well as on maintenance of underlying concept hierarchies for data integration and homogenisation.

Andreas Papasalouros is a Lecturer at the Mathematics Department, University of the Aegean, Greece. He holds a PhD in Electrical and Computer Engineering from the National Technical University of Athens. His research interests include e-learning, hypermedia design, and Web engineering. He has a degree in Physics from the University of Athens and a degree in Electrical and Computer Engineering from the National Technical University of Athens. He has participated in several research and development European and national projects and is a co-author of a number of articles published in scientific journals and conference proceedings.

Xiaojun Qi received her MS and PhD degree in Computer Science from Louisiana State University in 1999 and 2001, respectively. Since 2002, she has been with the faculty of the Department of Computer Science at Utah State University, where she is currently an associate professor. Her research interests include content-based image/video retrieval, image processing and pattern recognition, computer vision, and bioinformatics. She has published over 50 peer-reviewed journal and conference publications. She has been served as the reviewers for 23 international scientific journals, 21 international conferences, two textbooks, and one book chapter. She also served as the NSF panelist, the NSF ad hoc reviewer, and the reviewer for other funding agencies. She has been served as technical program committees for 14 international conferences. She is a senior member of IEEE.

Marian-Andrei Rizoiu received the BE degree in Computer Science from Bucharest Polytechnic University, Romania in 2009. In parallel, he followed the courses of the Master KDD (Knowledge Discovery in Databases) and received his MS degree from Lumière University, Lyon France in 2009. He is currently pursuing the PhD degree in the ERIC laboratory at the University Lumière of Lyon, France. The subject of his thesis is the semi-supervised clustering of complex documents, with application to historical data. His research interest also includes textual mining, topic extraction, natural language processing, automatic image description, and classification.

Arno Scharl is the Vice President of MODUL University Vienna, where he also heads the Department of New Media Technology (www.modul.ac.at/nmt). Prior to his current appointment, he held professorships at the University of Western Australia and Graz University of Technology, was a Key Researcher at the Austrian Competence Center for Knowledge Management, and a Visiting Fellow at Curtin University of Technology and the University of California at Berkeley. Arno Scharl completed his doctoral research and habilitation at the Vienna University of Economics and Business Administration. Additionally, he holds a PhD and MSc from the University of Vienna, Department of Sports Physiology. His current research interests focus on the integration of semantic and geospatial Web technology (www.geospatialweb.com), Web mining and media monitoring (www.weblyzard.com), virtual communities, and environmental online communication (www.ecoresearch.net).

Heiner Stuckenschmidt is full Professor for Computer Science (non tenured) at the University of Mannheim where he is heading the Artificial Intelligence group. The group is performing foundational and applied research on applying AI methods to data and information management. Before being appointed as a full professor in 2009, Heiner Stuckenschmidt graduated in Computer Science from the University of Bremen (Germany) in 1999. He finished his PhD on Ontology-Based Information Sharing at the Vrije Universiteit Amsterdam in 2003. From 2003 to 2005, he worked in the Knowledge Representation and Reasoning group headed by Frank van Harmelen as Postdoctoral researcher. In 2005, he moved to the University of Mannheim as a Junior Professor to set up a research group funded by an Emmy-Noether Elite Scholarship from the German Science Foundation (DFG) on the topic of distributed knowledge representation and processing on the World Wide Web. In the course of his scientific career, Heiner Stuckenschmidt has created more than 120 peer-reviewed publications, including five books, 18 International Journal publications, and more than 40 papers at international peer-reviewed conferences, including papers at AAAI, IJCAI, and the WWW conference.

Benjamin Tsou received an MA from Harvard and PhD in Linguistics from U.C. Berkeley. He is now the Chair Professor of Language Sciences in Hong Kong Institute of Education, and Emeritus Professor of City University of Hong Kong. He is also a corresponding member of the Royal Academy of Overseas Sciences of Belgium, the founding president of Asian Federation of Natural Language Processing (AF-NLP). He is serving as the editorial board member or editorial advisory committee member of numerous reputable monograph series and journals. His research interests have focused on the quantitative and qualitative studies of language, and in recent years have been extended to developing search engines and algorithms to enable meaningful parallel linguistic comparison and mediation between Classical Chinese and Modern Standard Chinese, bilingual, technical, and legal texts in special domains, such as patents and judicial judgments. He has published widely in these areas.

Victoria Uren is currently a Senior Research Fellow at Sheffield University working in the OAK (Organisations, Information and Knowledge) Group at the University of Sheffield, where she leads the work on the SmartProducts project as well as participating in other research activities such as the GrassPortal project. Her research field concerns the use of structured information, particularly ontologies, in knowledge management. She worked for about eight years at the Knowledge Media Institute on research projects such as X-Media, DotKom, AKT, and ScholOnto. She holds a PhD from the University of Portsmouth, England, on the topic of text categorization. Prior to that, she worked on the production of scientific and engineering databases.

Julien Velcin received his PhD degree in Computer Science, specializing in Artificial Intelligence, from the University of Paris 6 in 2005. Until 2007, he worked on unsupervised learning models for extracting stereotypes from partially described data such as in newspapers. He is now an Associate Professor with the University of Lyon 2, doing his research in the ERIC laboratory. Dr. Velcin is currently working on data mining and machine learning research. His other interests include text mining, Web mining, topic models, and text clustering. Since 2007, he is the head of a Master programme in Knowledge Discovery in Databases.

Martin Volk is Professor of Computational Linguistics at the University of Zurich and at Stockholm University. His research focuses on language technology in multilingual text analysis. He has worked on machine translation, cross-language information retrieval, multilingual terminology, and ontology extraction. He is currently heading a project on compiling and annotating a large multilingual corpus of alpine heritage texts which includes the construction of a corresponding ontology. He is also involved in developing domain-specific machine translation systems; for example, for mountaineering reports and for film subtitles. Martin Volk has presented papers at numerous international conferences throughout Europe. He has been invited to give talks in Europe, USA, and Australia.

Wei Wang is a lecturer at the School of Computer Science, Faculty of Science, the University of Nottingham Malaysia Campus. He obtained his BSc and PhD in computer science at the University of Nottingham in 2006 and 2009, respectively. His research focuses on knowledge acquisition and semantic search. His general research interests include information retrieval, Semantic Web, ranking, ontology learning, social Web modeling, and machine learning.

Albert Weichselbraun is an Assistant Professor at the Department of Information Systems and Operations of the Vienna University of Economics and Business (www.wu.ac.at). He leads the technical development of the RAVEN project with a focus on the analytical methods involved. Prior to his current appointment, he held the position of a visiting Research Fellow at the University of Western Australia, where he joined webLyzard, a platform to gather, aggregate, and analyze unstructured textual data. His current research interests focus on ontology evolution and learning, text mining, and the application of semantic technologies to information retrieval.

Gerhard Wohlgenannt is a postdoctoral researcher at the Department of Information Systems and Operations of the Vienna University of Economics and Business. He recently completed his PhD thesis in the field of ontology learning on a method for learning ontology relations by combining corpus-based techniques and reasoning on data from Semantic Web sources. Gerhard Wohlgenannt participated in a number of research projects at the Vienna University of Economics and Business such as RAVEN, IDIOM, and AVALON, where he extended the webLyzard architecture and semantic services and used his expertise in technologies such as the Python programming language and the PostgreSQL DBMS.

Changhui Yan is an Assistant Professor at the Department of Computer Science of North Dakota State University. He received his PhD from Iowa State University in 2005. In his research, Dr. Yan applies data-mining techniques to explore the sequence-structure-function relationships in biological molecules.

Ziqi Zhang is a Research Associate at the University of Sheffield. He is a member of the Organisations, Information, and Knowledge (OAK) Group. His research field concerns human language related technologies with focus on information extraction, text mining, and natural language processing. He has worked on a number of information extraction and knowledge management related projects and produced a number of relevant publications in some major conference venues such as Knowledge Engineering and Knowledge Management by the Masses (EKAW) and Language Resources Evaluation Conference (LREC). He currently holds a Master degree from the University of Birmingham, and is pursuing his PhD in the field of Information Extraction.

Jingbo Zhu received a PhD in computer science from Northeastern University, P.R. China in 1999, and has been with the Institute of Computer Software of the same university since then. Now he is a full professor in the Department of Computer Science, and is in charge of research activities within the Natural Language Processing Laboratory. He has published more than 100 papers, and holds four United States and two China patents. Dr. Zhu was supported by Program for New Century Excellent Talents in

University (NCET) of China in 2005. His current research interests include natural language parsing, statistical machine translation, knowledge engineering, machine learning, and intelligent systems.

Amal Zouaq is a Postdoctoral Researcher at Simon Fraser University and Athabasca University. She obtained her PhD in 2008 from the University of Montreal. Her expertise and interest lie in the field of artificial intelligence in the areas of knowledge acquisition and information retrieval, using techniques from natural language processing and data mining. The overall goal is to contribute to the field of the Semantic Web and knowledge-based systems in general, and to the semi-automatic generation of ontologies from texts, in particular.

Index